Principles of Physiology
A Scientific Foundation of Physiotherapy

Principles of Physiology
A Scientific Foundation of Physiotherapy

DOUGLAS L. BOVELL BSc, PhD
Lecturer in Physiology,
Department of Biological Sciences,
Glasgow Caledonian University,
Glasgow, UK

MYRA A. NIMMO BSc, PhD
Professor of Exercise Physiology
Department of Physical Education, Sport and Outdoor Education,
Strathclyde University,
Glasgow, UK

LESLIE WOOD BSc, PhD
Senior Lecturer in Physiology,
Department of Biological Sciences,
Glasgow Caledonian University,
Glasgow, UK

Contributions by

MORAG THOW MCSP, BSc
Lecturer in Physiotherapy,
Department of Physiotherapy, Podiatry and Radiography,
Glasgow Caledonian University,
Glasgow, UK

LORNA SHAW MCSP, BSc
Lecturer in Physiotherapy,
Department of Physiotherapy, Podiatry and Radiography,
Glasgow Caledonian University,
Glasgow, UK

Edited by
DOUGLAS L. BOVELL

WB Saunders Company Ltd
London • Philadelphia • Toronto • Sydney • Tokyo

WB Saunders Company Ltd 24–28 Oval Road
London NW1 7DX, UK

The Curtis Center
Independence Square West
Philadelphia, PA 19106–3399, USA

Harcourt Brace & Company
55 Horner Avenue
Toronto, Ontario M8Z 4X6, Canada

Harcourt Brace & Company, Australia
30–52 Smidmore Street
Marrickville, NSW 2204, Australia

Harcourt Brace & Company, Japan
Ichibancho Central Building, 22–1 Ichibancho
Chiyoda-ku, Tokyo 102, Japan

A catalogue record for this book is available from the British Library

ISBN 0-7020-1936-4

Design by Landmark Design Associates

Typeset by J&LComposition Ltd, Filey, North Yorkshire

Printed and bound in Great Britain by Butler & Tanner Ltd, Frome, Somerset, UK

Contents

Preface

For many years, physiotherapists and physiotherapy undergraduates have had to rely on general physiology textbooks to obtain the background physiological knowledge which underpins their professional practice. While teaching physiology to our undergraduate physiotherapy students and also to their qualified counterparts, it became apparent to us that the available textbooks, irrespective of title, encompassed a broad canvas of physiology and, in so doing, addressed areas of physiology that were only indirectly applicable to the study of physiotherapy. Perhaps more importantly, they did not cover in sufficient depth the areas of physiology which physiotherapists encounter on a regular basis in their undergraduate and working life.

In developing *Principles of Physiology*, we set out to produce a physiology title that was specifically targeted at physiotherapists and physiotherapy students, and also to create a text which emphasized the applied nature of physiology as it relates to physiotherapy practice. This book, therefore, presents to the reader the underlying principles of physiology which serve as a scientific basis for physiotherapy. It has been prepared in close collaboration with our physiotherapy colleagues in order to provide a text which specifically deals with those areas of particular relevance to physiotherapy, and to do so at a level which reflects the importance of these areas. Most of the topics, therefore, take the reader beyond the fundamental aspects of the subject area towards a more detailed approach. It has been designed to present the important features of human physiology in a clear and concise way, such that it can be read by both undergraduates and qualified physiotherapists, and in a format that we hope proves suitable regardless of academic background. However, the importance of those physiological topics we have omitted from the text should not be underestimated, but they impinge only indirectly on the day-to-day application of physiotherapeutic practice, and readers who wish to obtain more information on these areas are referred to other physiology books.

For many people physiology seems a daunting subject on first encounter. The task for us as teachers of physiology, is to balance the depth and breadth of the topics covered while including new findings but without going to a level of detail that would leave the non-physiologist uninterested. We have borne these principles in mind with regards to the applicability of the subject matter for undergraduate study, but we have also tried to introduce detailed information that the final-year student and the qualified practitioner would find both interesting to read and useful as an information source. To achieve these goals, the book progresses from the broad aspects of cells and tissues through to body systems and, finally, to a chapter on exercise. The information given in the exercise chapter draws together material from the previous chapters and is designed to provide information for the steadily increasing number of physiotherapists who have roles, not only in the rehabilitation of injured sportspersons, but also in the development of their training regimes.

We would like to acknowledge the contributions of colleagues who assisted by reading and commenting on early drafts of the book and to express our thanks to Marie Wood and Heather Watt for their support and help during the preparation of the manuscript.

DOUGLAS L. BOVELL
MYRA A. NIMMO
LESLIE WOOD

1

Cells and Tissues

Cells
•
Tissues

Cells

Several levels of structural organization exist within the human body, progressing from the level of atoms to cells, tissues, organs and finally to body systems. The atom/chemical level consists of non-living chemical matter, such as the elements carbon, hydrogen, oxygen and nitrogen, combining to create what are called **molecules**. Millions of molecules make up a cell by forming small or large accumulations known as **macromolecules** and on which the living unit is built. These macromolecules combine to form the basic substances **lipids, nucleotides, carbohydrates** and **proteins,** which in conjunction with **water,** form the basic components of a cell.

The cell is the key structural and functional component of all living organisms and is the basic unit of organization in the human body (see Figure 1.1)

The body's tissues, organs and systems are all derived from cells. Cells have evolved to perform specific tasks such as **contraction, reproduction, communication, metabolism, excitation, growth** and **differentiation**. Because of the specialization of cells into organs or systems, isolated cells survive by relying on the functions of other cells and systems to support their existence.

The size, shape and structure of individual cells varies considerably depending on their function.

Sizes can range from approximately 1–100 μm (1 μm = 0.000001 m). Much of the internal structure of cells was invisible to early microscopists and those structures which could be seen appeared unrelated and unconnected. The advent of electron microscopy demonstrated that there exists a series of complex structures which have connections and interrelated functions.

Figure 1.1   Structural relationships. The different levels of organization in the body. (Redrawn from Tortora GJ and Anagnostakos NP (1990) *Principles of Anatomy and Physiology,* 6th edn. Harper Collins, New York.)

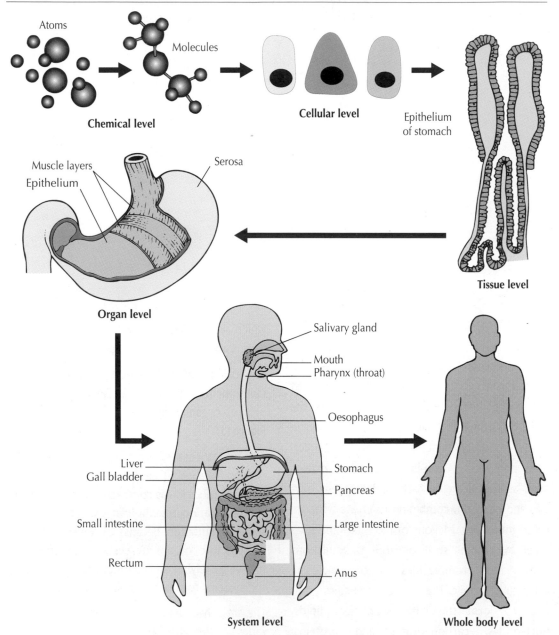

A cell, therefore, is not merely a container of chemicals, fluid and macromolecules, but can be regarded as having an outer covering called the **plasma (cell) membrane**, a **cytoplasm** which refers to the material inside the cell, specific identifiable functional structures (**organelles**) within the cytoplasm and **deposits**, molecules that are temporarily stored inside the cell.

Plasma Membrane

The plasma membrane is the structure which encloses and supports structures inside the cell as well as regulating what leaves or enters the cell (see Figure 1.2).

The membrane is a very thin elastic structure, ~ 4–10 nm (1 μm = 1000 nm) thick which is

Figure 1.2   Plasma membrane structure. Diagrammatic representation of the plasma membrane illustrating the bilayered lipid structure and the insertion of both integral (i) and peripheral (p) proteins.

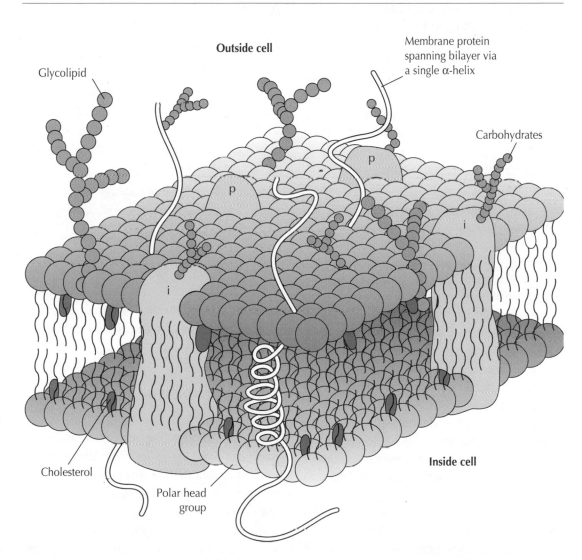

Outside cell

Glycolipid

Membrane protein spanning bilayer via a single α-helix

Carbohydrates

p

p

i

i

Cholesterol

Polar head group

Inside cell

composed almost entirely of proteins and lipids bound together. The majority of the lipids are phospholipids and glycolipids (lipids with phosphate and carbohydrate molecules attached, respectively), with some cholesterol.

A single phospholipid molecule has a polar head group, which makes it **hydrophilic,** with two non-polar **hydrophobic** acyl fatty acid chains attached (see Figure 1.2). Hydrophilic molecules can have electrostatic interactions with water, while hydrophobic molecules cannot. Therefore, when there are a lot of these molecules in an aqueous environment they spontaneously form a structure with all the hydrophilic 'heads' facing outwards towards the water molecules and all the hydrophobic 'tails' facing inwards towards each other. This arrangement of the lipid molecules makes the membrane a barrier to permeability for substances entering or leaving the cell. These substances must, therefore, pass through either the membrane or protein channels within the membrane.

Two kinds of proteins are associated with the membrane: **integral** and **peripheral** (see Figure 1.2).

1. Integral proteins span the width of the membrane with portions of the protein exposed to both the outside and the inside of the cell. Integral proteins may form water-filled channels which link the outside of the cell to the inside. These channels allow the movements of water-soluble substances, such as ions, in and out of the cell.
2. Peripheral proteins do not span the entire width of the membrane but are located either in the outer or inner membrane surfaces. Many of the peripheral proteins are actually bound to integral proteins.

Membrane proteins can act as cell receptors for hormone or neurotransmitter stimulation, where the binding of such substances to the protein causes an alteration in the cell's internal activity (e.g. increases in intracellular enzyme activity). Some proteins act to bind cells together, while others can act as carriers contributing to the movement of materials across the membrane, either by active or passive processes. Also, peripheral proteins linked together inside the cell act as a scaffold (cytoskeleton) contributing to cell shape and size.

Both integral and peripheral proteins on the outside of the cell may have molecules attached to them which may facilitate the recognition of cells from the same organism (self) or the identification of foreign cells (non-self).

The membrane is not a rigid structure; the lipid molecules of each layer are freely mobile in that layer but are not free to move from layer to layer. This is described as the 'fluid mosaic' theory of membrane structure.

More details of the biochemistry of the plasma membrane can be found in the bibliography.

Adaptations of the plasma membrane occur which are related to the different functions of the cells. A highly folded membrane increases the surface area of a cell, which is useful for absorption or for chemical reactions, e.g. microvilli on the epithelial membrane of cells in the small intestine (Figure 1.3).

PASSAGE OF MATERIALS THROUGH THE MEMBRANE

Movement through the membrane allows the passage of materials to and from the cell, which will help sustain the cell. The permeability of the membrane is influenced by several factors: (1) the size of the molecule (smaller molecules will pass more easily than larger molecules); (2) the solubility of the substance in lipid (the greater the lipid

Figure 1.3 Surface adaptations. Microvilli on the plasma membrane of a cell.

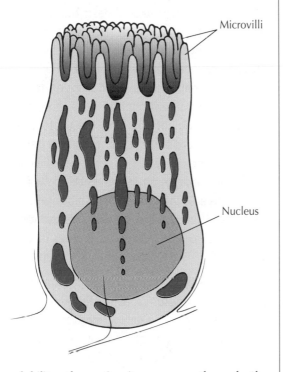

Figure 1.4 Diffusion. A soluble substance when placed in water slowly dissolves with the molecules becoming evenly dispersed throughout the solution.

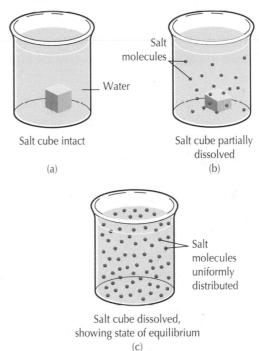

solubility, the easier it can pass through the membrane) and (3) the electrical charge of the substance (substances with similar electrical charges to the charged particles in the membrane will be repelled and therefore more difficult to transport across the membrane).

Movement through the membrane can be divided into mechanisms that require the presence and action of a protein carrier molecule, or mechanisms that do not require a carrier molecule. Carrier-dependent transport mechanisms include facilitated diffusion and active transport, while carrier-independent transport includes simple diffusion.

Carrier–independent Transport

Diffusion Diffusion is a passive process whereby movement of a substance occurs as a result of its concentration (Figure 1.4). Sub-

stances diffuse from regions where their concentration is higher to areas where their concentration is lower. Those substances that are lipid-soluble, i.e. non-polar, can pass easily across the membrane by simple diffusion while those substances which are water-soluble, i.e. polar, will have great difficulty crossing the membrane. The rate at which diffusion occurs is affected by how great the concentration difference between the two areas is, the substance's environmental temperature (i.e. the higher the temperature, the faster the rate of diffusion), size of the diffusing molecules and viscosity of the solution.

The integral proteins of the plasma membrane form channels that allow ions to diffuse across the membrane which would otherwise not be able to diffuse or diffuse only with difficulty. Ions such as sodium, potassium, chloride and calcium can pass through channels across the membrane. Different cells have differing capabilities in allowing these ions to pass through. This means that not all membranes have the same types of channels present or the same number of the same type.

The channels are not permanently open for diffusion of these ions and so have to be opened in some way. Different channels respond to different stimuli to facilitate opening. These stimuli consist of factors which can alter the protein structure to open the channel, either by chemicals binding to receptors on the channel (**receptor-mediated opening**), or a change in the membrane potential (**voltage-mediated opening**, see later) or mechanical change (**stretch-mediated opening**).

Osmosis Osmosis is the diffusion of water across a membrane. The movement of the water is also based on its concentration gradient, i.e. in an area with water molecules at a high concentration and solutes in a low concentration, water will move across a membrane to an area with a low water concentration and a high solute concentration.

The term 'osmotic pressure' describes the force required to prevent the net movement of water across a permeable membrane selective for water. This process is extremely important to cells as a large movement of water can disrupt or destroy the cells internal environment. Thus the greater the concentration of a solution, the greater is the osmotic pressure of the solution, and the greater is the tendency for water to move into the solution. Normally, the osmotic pressure of the fluid inside the cell is the same as the osmotic pressure of the fluid surrounding the cell. This balance of pressures across the membrane ensures that the volume of the cell remains the same (Figure 1.5).

A solution which has a higher concentration of solutes has a greater tendency for water molecules to move across a semipermeable membrane into it from a solution of lower solute concentration and is therefore termed 'hyperosmotic'. A solution with a lesser concentration of solutes has a greater tendency for water molecules to move from it across a semipermeable membrane

Figure 1.5 Osmosis. Water will move across a membrane separating pure water from a solution containing dissolved substances that cannot cross the membrane.

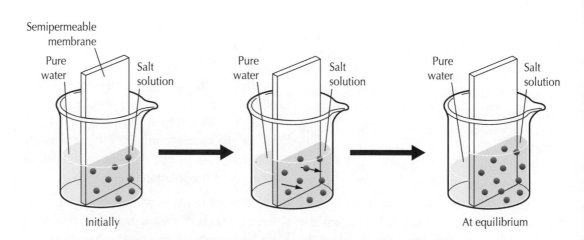

to a solution with a higher solute concentration and is termed 'hypoosmotic'.

Filtration Filtration is also a passive process which results in the movement of molecules in and out of cells. Molecular movement is the result of gravity or a hydrostatic pressure forcing water and dissolved molecules across a membrane via pores or channels, from an area of high pressure to an area of low pressure.

Carrier–dependent Transport Many of the essential molecules that the body requires for its continued functioning are too big to pass through the membrane, either through pores or channels. To accommodate the movement of these molecules across the membrane, there are transport mechanisms which will facilitate their passage.

Facilitated Diffusion A substance can move across the membrane, down its concentration gradient, by integral proteins present in the cell membrane acting as transporters. The substance will bind to a site present on the integral protein, which results in the protein transporter altering its configuration. The change in configuration facilitates the movement of the substance across the membrane to its other side. This can be a much faster process than simple diffusion, but is dependent on several factors such as the concentration of the substance, the number of transporters present on the membrane and how quickly the substance and carrier can bind and alter shape. Membrane carriers in general are specific for in-transporting substances.

Active Transport Mechanisms Active transport mechanisms are carrier-mediated processes where carrier function requires energy provided by adenosine triphosphate (ATP) molecules. The energy for the movement of the substance across the membrane and its release

Figure 1.6 Transport mechanisms across a membrane. The illustration shows a protein carrier molecule across a membrane exhibiting varying states of change during which a molecule is moved from one side of the membrane to the other.

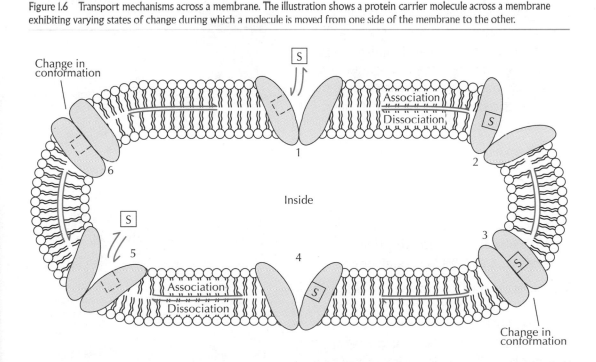

from the carrier protein is supplied by the breakdown of ATP. Active transport mechanisms are important in moving substances across the membrane against their concentration gradient.

There are **primary** and **secondary active transport processes** which are distinguished by their use of ATP in moving the substance across the membrane. Primary active transport relies on the energy released from the breakdown of the ATP molecule altering carrier function and moving the substance across the membrane. In secondary active transport processes, ionic gradients can move substances across the membrane. These ionic gradients are maintained by primary active transport mechanisms pumping the ions back against their concentration gradients. An example of a secondary active mechanism is the co-transport of glucose and sodium across the epithelial lining of the small intestine. A primary active transport mechanism pumps the sodium out of the cell, thereby maintaining the ionic gradient for sodium to move into the cell. The sodium and the glucose must both bind to the carrier to get the appropriate change to bring about their transport; the sodium enters the cell down its concentration gradient via the carrier, taking glucose with it.

Carriers can move more than one substance at a time in the same direction; this type of carrier is regarded as a **symporter**. Some carriers can also move two substances simultaneously in opposite directions, e.g. one molecule into the cell while another molecule is being removed from the cell; these carriers are referred to as **antiporters**.

Substances which are too large even for carriers to move them across the membrane can be moved into and out of cells by a further set of processes. **Endocytosis** refers to the bulk transport of materials into the cell, of which there are two pro-

cesses, **phagocytosis** and **pinocytosis**. The basis of these two processes is that the membrane envelops the substance forming a complete membrane pouch (vesicle) around the substance to be moved inside the cell. This pouch of membrane then fuses with the existing cell membrane resulting in the contents of the vesicle being released to the inside of the cell. Phagocytosis ('cell eating') is where large substances are moved into the cell, while pinocytosis ('cell drinking') results in a minute droplet of extracellular fluid being taken into the cell (Figure 1.7).

Figure 1.7   Phagocytosis and pinocytosis. Phagocytosis and pinocytosis are forms of endocytosis, where particles of differing size can be taken into the cell's cytoplasm. Large particles are taken in by phagocytosis (cell-eating) while small particles dissolved in fluid are taken in by pinocytosis (cell-drinking). Membrane folds develop, engulfing the particles before finally fusing to form membrane-bound vesicles inside the cell.

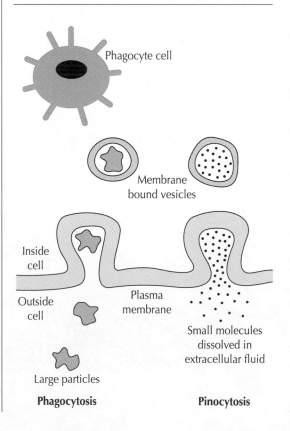

Exocytosis is the reverse of endocytosis where cell products are exported from the cell by packaging them in vesicles inside the cell. These vesicles then fuse with the plasma membrane releasing their contents to the outside of the cell. This is a common and important process within the body. Many important substances are released in this manner such as digestive enzymes or the chemicals that allow nerve-to-nerve, nerve-to-muscle and nerve-to-gland communication (Figure 1.8).

Defects of the plasma membrane and its associated structures are related to such diseases as cystic fibrosis (defects in the regulation of a chloride channel controlling the movement of

Figure 1.8   Exocytosis. Membrane-bound vesicles filled with material to be exported are formed in the Golgi apparatus. The vesicles migrate to the cell's surface where they fuse with the plasma membrane releasing their contents to the outside of the cell.

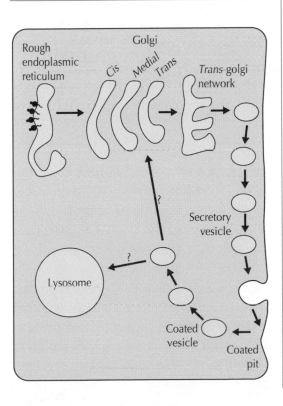

chloride ions across the membrane). Reversible interference of ion-channel function is involved in such things as anaesthesia, pain control and reduced output from cells (Figure 1.9).

Cytoplasm

The cytoplasm (see Figure 1.4) is regarded as the fluid-like environment which occupies the inner space of the cell. As the cell is approximately 75% water, the water contributes to the cytoplasm by creating a fluid matrix which is called the **intracellular fluid**. The cell organelles (cellular organs) along with the cytoskeleton (cellular framework; see later in this chapter) and dissolved or suspended molecules are located in the cytoplasm. The cytoplasm provides a matrix in which many of the cell's vital chemical reactions can occur.

Cell Organelles

Cell organelles are distinctive structures with specific functions which account for such processes as growth and development, maintenance, repair, control and defence of the cell. The numbers and types of organelles present in each cell vary according to the function of that particular cell. The various organelles are discussed below.

NUCLEUS

The nucleus is the largest structure, which is usually centrally placed and spherical, ovoid or lobed in shape. It can vary in size from 3 to 10 μm depending on the type of cell and its function.

The nucleus is bound by a double membrane where each membrane is a phospholipid bilayer. The nuclear membrane has many water-filled gaps or **pores** in it, which allow access between the

Figure 1.9   Generalized animal cell. The diagram is composite, encompassing all the organelles that can be found in animal cells. Not all cells have all these organelles; the type and amount of organelles present will differ between cells of different tissues.

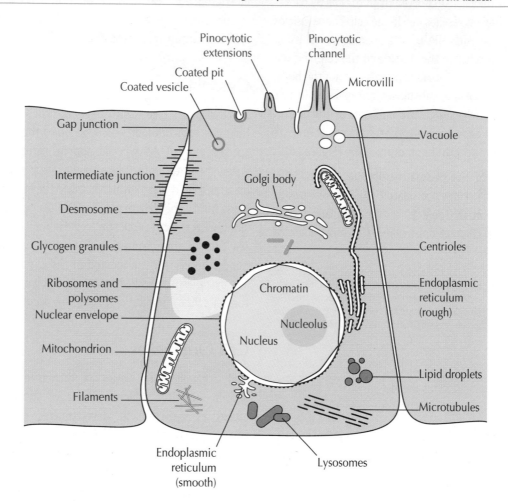

inside of the nucleus and the cytoplasm. These pores allow most water-soluble molecules or ions to move into or out of the nuclear compartment. The pores are much larger than the protein channels of the plasma membrane and so much larger molecules can pass through the nuclear membrane. The nuclear membrane is continuous in places with the membrane of the endoplasmic reticulum (see later).

The nucleus contains **deoxyribonucleic acid (DNA)**, the molecule of hereditary information, also called **genes**. The genes direct and control many of the actions of the cell. DNA is therefore involved in cell differentiation, cell growth and cell division. All mature cells in the human body have a nucleus except the red blood cells, while some cells have more than one nucleus per cell, e.g. skeletal muscle cells. In non-dividing cells or cells that are in a phase between the division process, DNA and associated proteins are loosely packed and diffuse within the nucleus and are referred to as **chromatin**. When the cell starts the process of cell division, the DNA condenses into structures called **chromosomes**.

Also present in the nucleus is an internal structure referred to as the **nucleolus**. The cell may have more than one nucleolus, which contains DNA, **ribonucleic acid** (RNA) and proteins which are involved in the production of **ribosomes** (see next section). This structure will disperse during the process of cell division and reappear afterwards.

RIBOSOMES

Ribosomes are the sites of protein synthesis and are found either free in the cytoplasm or bound to the **endoplasmic reticulum** (ER; see below). Unlike most other organelles, ribosomes are not bound by membrane but are composed of a large and a small subunit of RNA, called **ribosomal RNA**, attached to one another. The subunits are assembled in the nucleus and can then be either free ribosomes or bound ribosomes. Free ribosomes are found singly or in small groups in the cytoplasm, and are concerned with the synthesis of proteins for use inside the cell. Bound ribosomes are attached to the ER and are involved in the synthesizing of proteins for use inside the cell or for export from the cell.

ENDOPLASMIC RETICULUM (ER)

The ER is a system of interconnected membrane-bound channels called **cisternae** which branch and extend throughout the cell. The membrane of the ER is continuous in places with the nuclear membrane (Figure 1.10a,b). The system acts as an intracellular transport mechanism allowing materials to pass from one part of the cell to another as well as providing a route for materials to reach the plasma membrane and leave the cell. Additionally, the highly folded nature of the ER provides a greater surface area for chemical reactions to take place.

There are two types of ER:

1. **Rough** or **granular** ER has ribosomes attached to its outer surface. Rough ER serves as a temporary storage site for the proteins synthesized by the attached ribosomes. During storage, the proteins can be adapted by enzyme-catalysed reactions which may add other molecules, e.g. carbohydrates to the existing protein structures.
2. **Smooth** or **agranular** ER has no ribosomes attached. The smooth ER is the site of fatty acid, phospholipid and steroid synthesis. In some cells the smooth ER can function to inactivate or detoxify chemicals, such as alcohol (e.g. in liver cells), while in others (e.g. in muscle cells), modified smooth ER act as a calcium storage site for the contractile mechanism (see Chapter 6).

GOLGI APPARATUS (OR COMPLEX)

The Golgi apparatus is a series of four to eight flattened membranous sacs called **cisternae** stacked one on top of the other (Figure 1.10c). The cisternae are close to the endoplasmic reticulum as well as near to the nucleus. In cells with a high secretory output there is an extensive apparatus throughout the cytoplasm.

The Golgi apparatus modifies, sorts, packages and distributes throughout the cell, molecules which have been manufactured in the endoplasmic reticulum, either for internal cell use or for export from the cell. Irrespective of whether the molecules are for internal or external use they tend to follow the same pathway through the Golgi complex. Proteins assembled in the endoplasmic reticulum are transferred to the first of the Golgi apparatus cisternae, in small membrane-bound vesicles. As the protein passes through the cisternae it is modified according to its final function. The protein is

Figure 1.10   Cell organelles. The structure of (a) the nuclear envelope; (b) endoplasmic reticulum with ribosomes attached, (c) Golgi apparatus and (d) mitochondrion.

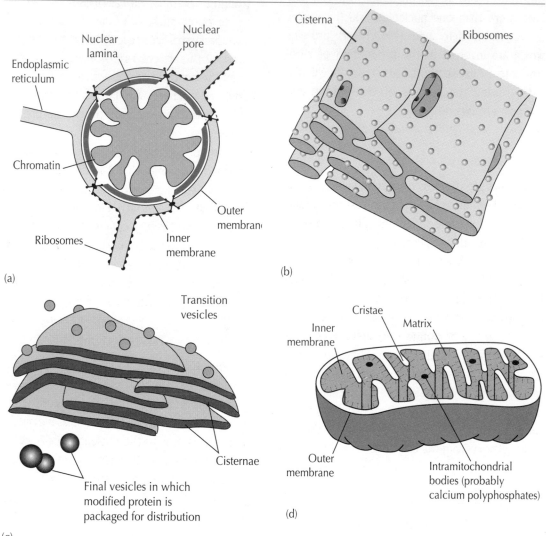

(a)

(b)

(c)

(d)

passed from one cisterna to the next by vesicles. Finally, when the modified protein has passed through all the cisternae it is packaged into a final vesicle for distribution within or to the outside of the cell. The contents of the vesicle can be exported by exocytosis or the vesicle itself can be released from the cell.

MITOCHONDRIA

Mitochondria are rod or oval-shaped organelles that are involved in the formation of the high-energy molecule adenosine triphosphate (ATP), from the energy stored in nutrient molecules. ATP is the body's major energy source for its endergonic chemical reactions and for this reason mitochondria are often referred to as the cell's 'powerhouses'.

The mitochondrion has two distinctive membranes, an inner and an outer membrane, separated by an intramembranous space (Figure 1.10d). The outer membrane is smooth in appearance while the inner membrane is highly infolded, creating partitions called **cristae**. The infolding increases the membrane surface area available for the chemical reactions involved in the generation of ATP. The inner membrane surrounds the mitochondrial cytoplasm (or **matrix**) which contains the many enzymes involved in the chemical reactions that create ATP during the **Krebs** or **tricarboxylic acid** (TCA) cycle. The enzymes involved in energy-releasing reactions (**electron-transport chain**) that form greater amounts of ATP are located on the cristae. (More detailed information on ATP production can be found in the biochemistry texts quoted in the bibliography).

The mitochondria contain strands of DNA which allow them to be self-replicating, i.e. they can divide and generate new mitochondria from existing ones. The stimulus for this to happen is the cell's increased demand for ATP. Cells which are very active such as kidney, liver and muscle cells, usually have a high number of mitochondria present because of their energy needs.

LYSOSOMES

Lysosomes are membrane-bound vesicles, released by the Golgi complex, which are filled with digestive enzymes. The lysosomes function by phagocytosis so that the enzymes can digest bacteria and other substances which may enter the cell. They can also be used to break down old organelles to recycle their component parts for the manufacture of new organelles. The membrane around the vesicle protects the cell's contents from being damaged by these powerful enzymes. Disorders of lysosome function can have a variety of effects from increased self-destruction of cells to defective development.

PEROXISOMES

Peroxisomes are very similar to lysosomes in that they are membrane bound and contain powerful enzymes. However, these enzymes are involved with the break down of hydrogen peroxide and the detoxification of potentially harmful substances like alcohol. The peroxisomes are found in cells of organs that are involved in detoxification, e.g. liver and kidney cells.

CYTOSKELETON

The cytoskeleton is the framework inside the cell which acts as a support for the various cell organelles, maintains shape and allows cellular movement. It is composed of **microfilaments, microtubules** and **intermediate filaments**.

Microtubules are hollow cylindrical structures composed of the protein **tubulin,** which offer support to internal structures and help maintain cell shape. This can be seen particularly in nerve cells where microtubules are found in the long processes of the nerve, maintaining their shape. The microtubules also provide a means for cellular movement and are found in the cellular structures known as **cilia** and **flagella** (Figure 1.11b).

Cilia are small, membrane-bound hair-like projections extending from the cell surface. They have a central core of microtubules arranged in a precise pattern which gives the cilia the ability to move back and forwards. This movement can best be described as a 'beating' action where, on the forward stroke, the cilia is rigid, while on the return stroke it is soft and flexible. Due to this 'beating' action, the cilia can achieve a one-way movement of materials across the cell surface.

Cilia are found on the cells lining the airways of the respiratory system and the female oviduct.

In contrast, the flagella are larger structures which have a more 'whip-like' action that can move the entire cell from one point to another. Movement of sperm is an example of flagellar action.

Functional defects of cilia and flagella can result in a variety of different conditions. Sperm which have defective flagella are unable to move properly and may not be able to reach the ovum and achieve fertilization. Defective cilia would hinder the passage of both the released ovum in the fallopian tube and mucus in the respiratory passages.

When a cell divides, the separation and movement of chromosomes appears to be related to the assembly and disassembly of tubular proteins. The **centrosome** is a region of material near the nucleus which serves as a microtubule organizing centre and contains a pair of microtubular structures, at right angles to one another called **centrioles** (Figure 1.11c). These structures organize the microtubules that facilitate chromosomal movements during cell division.

Microfilaments are rod-like structures composed of the protein **actin** which was first described in muscle tissue for its role in contraction; however, it has been demonstrated in nearly all cells. In muscle cells, actin, in conjunction with another microfilament **myosin,** are both involved in the mechanism facilitating contraction (see Chapter 6).

The role of intermediate filaments is as yet still unclear but appears to be concerned with structural support as they are extensive in cells subjected to mechanical stresses.

Clinically, conditions of the cytoskeletal filaments can affect the structural integrity of the membrane and the cell. For example, a lack of **dystro-phin,** a cytoskeletal protein, is thought to be one factor in the genetically inherited disease muscular dystrophy.

Disorders of cell organelles will obviously have detrimental affects on cell functions. If the disorder is widespread, then tissue and organ dysfunction may result.

Cell Deposits

A deposit is a substance in the cell cytoplasm and which is generally organic, and may appear or disappear many times during the life span of the cell. These inclusions comprise materials such as melanin deposits (which give us skin, hair and eye colour), glycogen granules (a highly branched polysaccharide molecule) stored in liver and skeletal muscle cells as a rapidly available energy store, and lipids stored in fat cells, also an energy store.

Tissues

Cells are grouped into tissues where each cell is specialized to perform a particular function and the tissues are then specialized to perform specific tasks. The structure of cells and the contents of the matrix surrounding the cells (extracellular matrix) is used to classify cellular groups into tissues. The tissues of the body can be classified into four basic categories: (1) **epithelial tissues;** (2) **connective tissues;** (3) **muscular tissues;** and (4) **nervous tissues.**

Epithelial Tissues

A characteristic of epithelial tissues is that they have very little extracellular matrix, with the cells closely packed together either in sheets of single

Figure 1.11   (a) Cell organelles. Cytoskeletal proteins provide a scaffolding that supports other intracellular structures. (b) Diagrammatic representation of the structure of a cilia/flagellum. The structure is surrounded by plasma membrane enclosing a specific pattern of nine microtubular pairs around two central microtubules at the top. At the bottom of the structure, the microtubules form nine sets of three. The protein dynein connects pairs of microtubules together. The dynein arms can move past one another; this facilitates movement of the whole structure. (c) The structure of a centrosome containing centrioles.

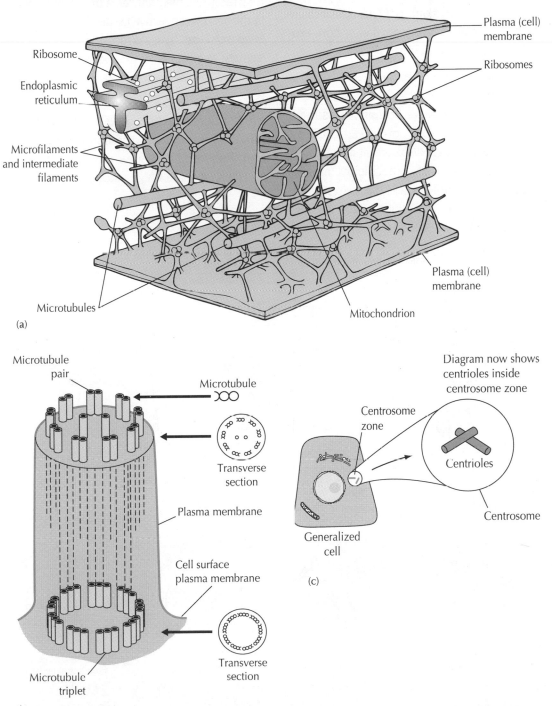

Plasma (cell) membrane

Ribosome

Ribosomes

Endoplasmic reticulum

Microfilaments and intermediate filaments

Plasma (cell) membrane

Microtubules

Mitochondrion

(a)

Microtubule pair

Microtubule

Transverse section

Plasma membrane

Cell surface plasma membrane

Transverse section

Microtubule triplet

(b)

Diagram now shows centrioles inside centrosome zone

Centrosome zone

Centrioles

Generalized cell

Centrosome

(c)

cells or as multilayers. Epithelial tissues can be classified into either (1) **covering** and **lining tissues** which line all the internal and external surfaces of the body (e.g. blood vessels, respiratory and digestive tracts, skin) and (2) **glandular tissue** which forms the secretory portion of both **exocrine** and **endocrine** glands (see later).

The exposed surface of epithelial cells is not in direct contact with other cells, and is called the **apical** or **free** surface. The bottom-most surface of a single or multilayer is normally attached to a basement membrane. The basement membrane is a specialized type of extracellular material, secreted by the epithelial cells themselves, which anchors the cells in position. Cells are also attached to one another at their lateral surfaces by means of strong cell junctions.

The epithelial cells have no direct blood supply; they receive all their nutrients from blood vessels in the nearby connective tissues. Groups of cells, in contrast, can have a direct nerve supply. Some sensory receptors in the body are modified epithelial and nerve cells.

Epithelia also have a diverse range of functions which include **secretion, absorption, protection, filtration, lubrication, digestion** and **reproduction.** They also have a great capacity for renewal and therefore have a high mitotic activity.

Figure 1.12   Examples of the different types of epithelial tissues and some of their locations.

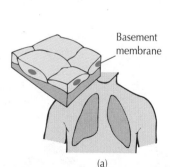
(a)
Simple squamous

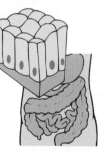
(b)
Simple columnar

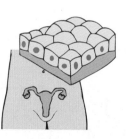
(c)
Simple cuboidal

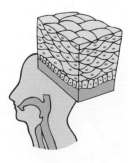
(d)
Stratified squamous

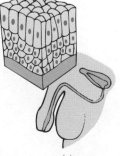
(e)
Stratified columnar

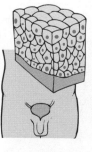
(f)
Transitional

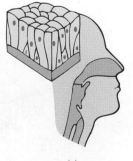
(g)
Pseudostratified
columnar ciliated

COVERING AND LINING TISSUES

Cells are arranged according to their location and function (Figure 1.12). An area of filtration or absorption would have only a single layer of cells to facilitate the passage of materials through the cell layer. Too thick a layer would hinder the passage of materials. A single-layer arrangement is regarded as being a **simple epithelium,** while an area that undergoes wear and tear would have multiple layers and would be regarded as a **stratified** or **compound epithelium**. One further type of cell arrangement exists where all the cells present in the epithelial lining are attached to the basement membrane but not all of the cells reach the free surface. This arrangement of cells, when viewed under the microscope, gives the appearance of having many layers, when in fact it is only a single layer of cells. It is therefore referred to as a **pseudostratified epithelium** and is much less common in the body than the other types.

Epithelial cells can be further classified according to their shape (Table 1.1). If the cell is flattened and scale-like it is regarded as being a **squamous** cell type. Cells which have a cubed shape are called **cuboidal** cells, while those that are tall and cylindrical are called **columnar** cells. Cells which exhibit a variety of shapes and which change their shape due to stretching are called **transitional** cells.

Table 1.1
Categories of Epithelial Tissue

Simple	Stratified	Pseudostratified
Squamous	Squamous	Columnar
Cuboidal	Cuboidal	
Columnar	Columnar	
	Transitional	

Examples of Cell Types and Locations

- Simple squamous cells line blood and lymph vessels, air sacs of the lungs and the glomerular capsule of the kidney.
- Simple cuboidal cells are found on the surface of the ovaries, the front of the eye lens and the kidney tubules.
- Simple columnar cells line the gastrointestinal tract from the stomach to the rectum as well as the ducts of some glands. There may also be present **goblet cells** (unicellular glands – see later) which secrete **mucus,** and **microvilli** in some places. Simple columnar cells with cilia present are found in the upper respiratory tract, oviduct and the uterus.
- The Stratified squamous type is a multiple layer of cells forming the lining of the oesophagus, mouth, vagina and tongue. Stratified squamous cells are also found on the skin; however, the layers are more numerous and the cells produce a tough waterproof protein called **keratin**.
- Stratified cuboidal cells line parts of the sweat gland duct and ovarian follicle.
- Stratified columnar cells are found in parts of the mammary and salivary glands.
- Transitional cells line the urinary bladder and parts of the urethra and ureter.
- Pseudostratified columnar cells line the large ducts of many glands, while the ciliated type with goblet cells present, line most of the major airways.

GLANDULAR EPITHELIUM

These are cells or tissues which secrete material. Glands can either consist of a single cell or be multicellular with the secretory products being released into ducts or directly into the blood. If the secretory products from the cells are released into a duct then the gland is classified as an **exocrine gland**. Glands that are ductless and

Figure 1.13   Glandular development. Both types of gland are derived from epithelial cells. As development continues, endocrine glands lose their connection with the epithelial layer, whereas exocrine glands are still part of the epithelial layer. Endocrine secretion passes into blood vessels that have permeated between the cells, while exocrine secretions pass onto the epithelial surface via a duct.

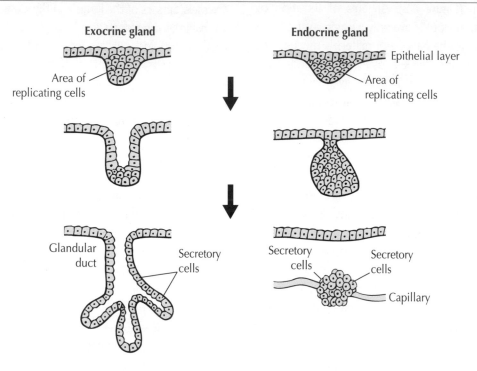

release their products directly into the blood are classed as **endocrine glands**. Glands are formed by downgrowths from the epithelial layer in the developing embryo. As the downgrowths develop, those secretory cells which retain cellular links (ducts) to the surface layer become exocrine glands. Those secretory cells which lose any links with the epithelial layer, eventually become endocrine glands (Figure 1.13).

Exocrine glands are further classified on the basis of their shape and the mode of their secretion. Examples of exocrine glands are shown in Table 1.2. If the duct of the gland does not branch then it is a **simple** type of gland; however, if the duct branches then it is a **compound** gland. If the gland forms a tube it is a **tubular** gland, while

those glands that form sacs are called **acinar** glands (Figure 1.14).

Secretion by exocrine glands is thought to be achieved by three different mechanisms (Figure 1.15):

Table 1.2
Examples of Exocrine Glands

Gland	Secretion
Salivary glands	Saliva
Sweat glands	Sweat
Goblet cells	Mucus
Part of the pancreas	Enzymes
Mammary glands	Milk
Sebaceous glands	Sebum

Figure 1.14　An illustration of variations found in the gross structure of exocrine glands.

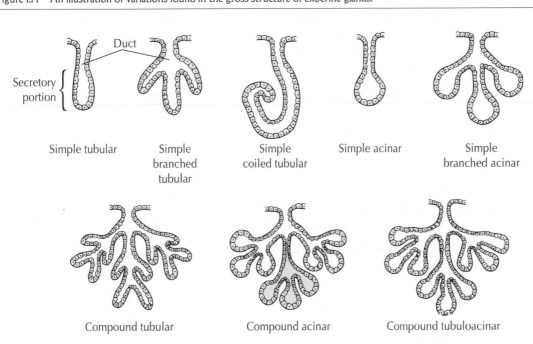

Simple tubular

Simple branched tubular

Simple coiled tubular

Simple acinar

Simple branched acinar

Compound tubular

Compound acinar

Compound tubuloacinar

1. **Apocrine** secretion. The cells accumulate their secretory products at their apical surface; the cell membrane of that portion then pinches off from the rest of the cell, containing the secretion.

2. **Holocrine** secretion. The secretory products accumulate throughout the whole of the cell; the cell then dies and the secretory products are released.

3. **Eccrine** secretion. The secretion passes from the cell through the membrane out into the duct without any loss of membrane or cell death.

Endocrine glands are ductless, so secretory products diffuse from the glandular tissue into the

Figure 1.15　Glandular secretion. Glands export their secretions by three apparent methods. (a) Holocrine, (b) eccrine and (c) apocrine.

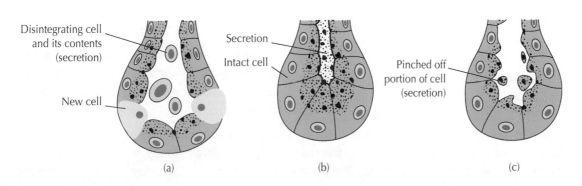

Disintegrating cell and its contents (secretion)

New cell

Secretion

Intact cell

Pinched off portion of cell (secretion)

(a)

(b)

(c)

extracellular fluid and from there directly into the bloodstream. The secretions of endocrine glands are always **hormones,** the body's chemical means of controlling physiological functions. Examples of endocrine glands include the pituitary, thyroid and adrenal glands. We will not discuss the endocrine system here; those readers wishing more information are referred to physiology texts in the bibliography.

The genetically inherited disease cystic fibrosis affects the body's secretory epithelia. As mentioned earlier, the defect causes types of chloride channels present in the membrane of the cells to be missing or not to function properly. One result is that the glands of the respiratory tract produce a viscous mucus which the cilia cannot easily remove from the airways. This thick mucus builds up in the lungs, blocks the airways and leads to infection, inflammation and subsequent cell damage, where the epithelial cells are replaced by connective tissue. Sufferers require physiotherapy to help remove the mucus and maintain unobstructed airways.

Connective Tissues

Connective tissues **support, bind, separate, strengthen, protect** and **insulate** the tissues of the body. Because of these functions it is found throughout the body in large amounts.

The connective tissue is made up of three basic components: **cells, ground substance** and **fibres**. The essential characteristic that makes it different from the other three types of tissue is that the cells are separated from each other by a non-living **extracellular matrix** which is composed of ground substance and fibres. The cells of the different connective tissues are specialized to produce the extracellular matrix, which give the tissues their functional characteristics. Blood is a connecting tissue between the external and internal environments. It is therefore an exception in that the extracellular matrix does not contain fibres.

CONNECTIVE-TISSUE CELLS

All the cells of the connective tissues are derived from one type of tissue called **mesenchyme**. Mesenchyme is the embryonic precursor of all the adult connective tissues. Cells are named according to their function in the connective tissue. Cells associated with the extracellular matrix may be either 'blasts' which produce the matrix, 'cytes' which maintain the matrix, or 'clasts' which disassemble the matrix. For example, osteoblasts form bone, while osteocytes maintain the bone and osteoclasts break the bone matrix down.

There are other cells present in connective tissues. **Plasma cells** develop from a type of white blood cell called a **B lymphocyte**. Plasma cells produce **antibodies,** a defence mechanism against infections. **Mast cells** are abundant cells which produce the chemical **histamine** which causes blood vessels to dilate (increase in diameter) during inflammation. **Macrophages** develop from certain white blood cells and have a role in engulfing and destroying bacteria and other foreign bodies. The different types of connective-tissue cells are shown in Figure 1.16.

CONNECTIVE-TISSUE FIBRES

Collagen, reticular and **elastic** fibres help to provide strength and support to tissues and form the basis of connective tissues. The fibres are all comprised of types of protein.

Collagen fibres are composed of the protein collagen and are tough and resilient, enabling them to be flexible while resisting stretching

Figure 1.16 Connective tissue origins. Diagram illustrating the origins and development of the main types of connective tissues from the embryonic mesenchyme cell.

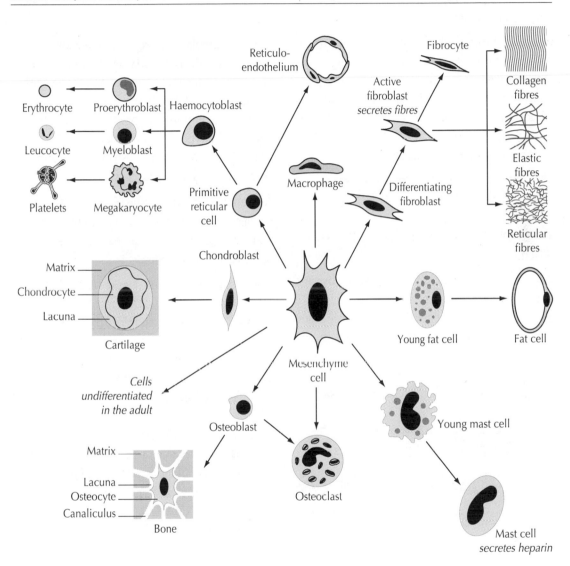

forces. The fibres are usually bound together in bundles giving them greater strength in the same way that a single thread is weak, but many threads bound together are much stronger. These fibres are abundant in connective tissues such as bone, tendons and ligaments.

Elastic fibres are composed of the protein **elastin** and as the name suggests they can stretch. Elastic fibres are smaller than collagen fibres and freely branch and rejoin to one another while still retaining strength. Once stretched or compressed, the fibres can return to their original size and shape, providing the tissue with a stretchable quality. Elastic fibres can be found in blood-vessel walls, lung tissue and skin.

Reticular fibres are also composed of the protein collagen, but are much smaller and thinner in size than collagen fibres. They too branch and form meshworks for support in areas such as the sites of accumulated blood cells (e.g. lymph nodes, spleen). They also contribute to the basement membrane in epithelial tissues.

The different fibres in connective tissues are shown in Figure 1.17.

TYPES OF CONNECTIVE TISSUES IN THE ADULT BODY

Adipose tissue (Figure 1.18a) is a fat depository. There are two types of adipose tissue: white adipose tissue (WAT) and brown adipose tissue (BAT). White adipose tissue is involved in the storage of energy while brown tissue is involved in temperature control. The fat does not lie free but is enclosed inside fat cells or **adipocytes**.

Figure 1.17   Connective tissue fibres. Different connective tissue fibres shown diagrammatically.

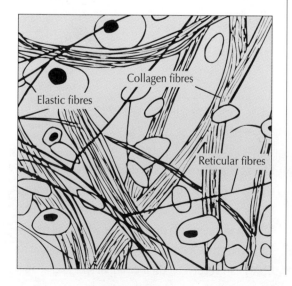

Adipose tissue, as well as acting as an energy store, also helps to insulate, cushion and protect internal organs.

Loose or **areolar** connective tissue is one of the most widely distributed types of connective tissue. It forms the foundation on which the epithelial cell basement membrane rests. In this tissue all three types of fibres are present, loosely woven, with several types of cells dispersed between the fibres. Cells found in the mesh include fibroblasts, macrophages and plasma cells.

Reticular connective tissue (Figure 1.18b) is made up of entwined reticular fibres forming a network to bind together tissues as the blood cells in the spleen and lymph nodes.

Dense connective tissue (Figure 1.18c,d) has fibres in greater numbers in either regular or irregular arrays. The greater the number of fibres bundled together, the greater the density of the tissue. In the regular array, collagen fibres are bundled together in a parallel arrangement, in tissues such as tendons and ligaments. The parallel arrangement offers great strength while maintaining some flexibility. The irregularly arranged fibres are enmeshed to cope with tensile forces occurring in a variety of directions. This offers strength to tissues such as the dermis of the skin, the bone coverings, joint capsules and the outer capsules of many organs.

Elastic connective tissue (Figure 1.18e) consists of branching elastic fibres which can stretch and return to their original shape and size allowing the structures that they are present in to do likewise. Elastic tissue forms components of elastic arteries (e.g. the aorta), lung tissue, trachea and vocal chords.

Cartilage is a fairly flexible and resilient tissue with the cells and collagen fibres surrounded by a relatively dense matrix of a chemical substance

Figure 1.18   Connective tissues. Diagrams portraying the different types of connective tissue found in the human body. (a) Adipose; (b) reticular; (c) dense irregular; (d) dense regular. (*continued over*)

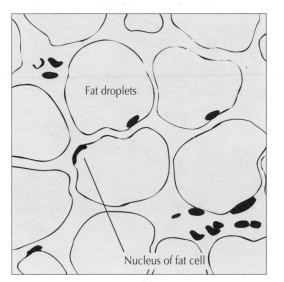

(a)

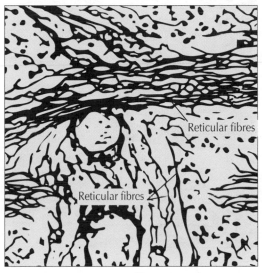

(b)

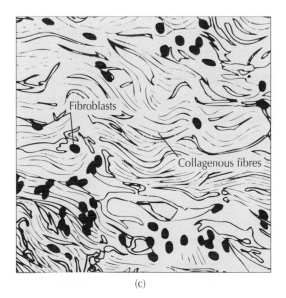

(c)

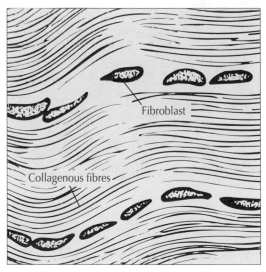

(d)

Figure 1.18 *Continued.* (e) elastic; (f) fibrocartilage; (g) elastic cartilage.

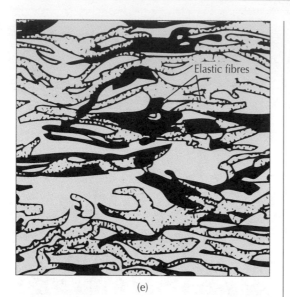

(e)

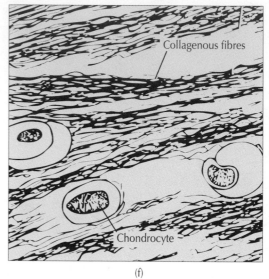

(f)

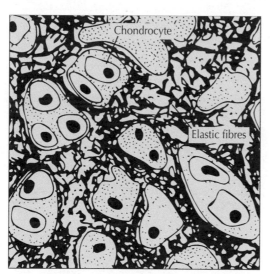

(g)

three distinguishable types of cartilage: (1) **hyaline**, (2) **fibrocartilage** and (3) **elastic**.

Hyaline cartilage is the commonest type found in the body. It serves to reduce friction and absorb shock on the ends of bones at joints, ribs, parts of the larynx, trachea, bronchii and the nose.

Fibrocartilage (Figure 1.18f) comprises chondrocytes dispersed amongst arrays of collagen fibre bundles. It is found at the joining point of the two hip bones, in the invertebral discs and the knee joint.

Elastic cartilage (Figure 1.18g) is found in the ear and epiglottal tissue of the throat. It is composed of cells surrounded by many elastic fibres and helps support and maintain shape in these tissues.

Unlike other connective-tissues cartilage is **avascular,** that is blood vessels do not permeate the tissue. Therefore when cartilage is damaged the repair process is slow because the nutrients and cells required for repair reach the damaged area only with great difficulty.

called **chondroitin sulphate**. The collagen fibres give the tissue strength while the chondroitin sulphate gives it resilience. The cells of the cartilage are called **chondrocytes** and occupy spaces in the matrix called **lacunae**. The chondrocytes are responsible for the production of the resilient extracellular matrix of the cartilage. There are

BONE

Bone (Figure 1.19) is a highly specialized form of connective tissue which not only forms about 22% of the body mass but is the hardest tissue containing living cells. Bone forms most of the skeleton providing **movement, support, protection, mineral homeostasis** and **blood cell production**. It consists of cells surrounded by a matrix which is both **organic** and **inorganic** in composition. The matrix consists of approximately 25% water, 25% protein and 50% minerals. The protein forms fibres which makes up the organic component and are surrounded by mineral deposits of calcium, carbonate and phosphate, known as **hydroxyapatite,** as well as magnesium, sodium and potassium which are also present in varying amounts forming the inorganic portion.

The tensile and compressional strength of bone is due to the layout of the hydroxyapatite and the collagen fibres.

Bone has four associated cell types: (1) **osteoprogenitor** cells which are the precursor cells for the other cells; (2) **osteoblasts** which secrete collagen and other organic components of the intercellular matrix; (3) **osteocytes** which are the principal cells involved in the day-to-day maintenance of cellular activities, e.g. exchange of nutrients and waste products; and (4) **osteoclasts** whose primary function is to resorb bone either allowing remodelling of the bone or the release of calcium into the blood supply. The osteocytes are located in lacunae in the matrix, similar to the lacunae in cartilage.

Figure 1.19   Bone. Stylized diagram showing the structure of compact and spongy bone.

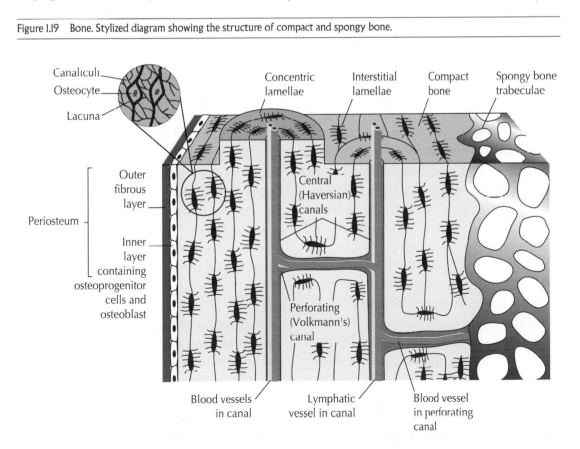

Bone tissue is described as either **compact** or **spongy** (see Figure 1.19), depending on how the cells and the matrix are deposited. Compact bone is extremely hard and is found largely in the shafts of long bones and has few spaces within the matrix. Spongy bone has interlacing bone partitions called **trabeculae** enclosing cavities and is found in the vertebrae, flat bones and ends of long bones.

Long bones consist of: (1) the **epiphyses** or ends of the bone; (2) the **diaphysis** or shaft; (3) the **metaphysis**, a region in mature bone where the diaphysis joins with epiphyses; (4) the **periosteum**, the outermost connective tissue covering of the bone, which contains blood vessels and nerve fibres; (5) the **articular cartilage**; (6) the **endosteum**, the membranous layer containing osteoprogenitor cells which lines the cavity; and (7) the **marrow cavity**.

Compact bone is arranged in concentric circles (**Haversian system**) of matrix with calcium and phosphate deposits. The minerals give the bone its hardness, while the protein fibres gives it its strength. Because the matrix of the compact bone is so dense it is difficult for nutrients and gases to diffuse to and from the osteocytes. Blood vessels, lymphatic vessels and nerves enter from the periosteum via perforating canals called Volkmann canals. The blood vessels of these canals connect with blood vessels and nerves of the cavity and those of the central canals called Haversian canals. These canals run longitudinally through the length of the bone. Around the canals are the concentric rings of hard calcified matrix while between layers are spaces called lacunae. Emanating from the lacunae in all directions are minute canals called **canaliculi** which are filled with extracellular fluid. The canaliculi extend through the matrix linking individual osteocytes to one another providing a network for the passage of nutrients to, and waste products away from, the cells.

Spongy or cancellous bone does not have the Haversian arrangement of compact bone, but has instead plates of bone (trabeculae) which contain the osteocytes and their spaces, along with canaliculi. It is called spongy bone because its appearance resembles that of a naturally occurring sponge with many holes throughout the tissue. These holes in the bone are normally filled with red bone marrow.

Both compact and spongy bone are normally found together. For example, a long bone of the body consists of thick compact bone surrounding a cavity. The cavity is normally filled with bone marrow. The epiphyses consist of a thin layer of compact bone overlying the spongy bone. At the epiphyses there is no clearly defined cavity. However, the spaces in the spongy bone link to the main cavity and are normally filled with bone marrow. In adult years, the marrow of the long cavity in the shaft contains numerous adipose cells and takes on a yellowish appearance while the marrow of the spongy bone remains red bone marrow.

Bones are important reserves of calcium and other minerals. In times of need the calcium can be resorbed from the bone and distributed around the body. Parathyroid hormone secreted by the parathyroid glands, regulates the exchange of calcium between the bones and the interstitial fluids.

Bone Growth or Ossification Ossification is the process of bone formation and begins around the 6th week of embryonic development. Bone grows in two ways: (1) **intramembranous**, where the bone is formed inside the fibrous connective layers; and (2) **endochondrial**, where the bone develops in the hyaline cartilage.

Early in embryonic life, a cartilage model or **template** of the future bone is laid down, which is covered by a membrane called the **perichondrium**. Midway along this shaft, a blood vessel penetrates the perichondrium supplying blood to the osteoprogenitor cells stimulating them to enlarge and become osteoblasts. The cells then begin to lay down matrix and form a periosteal collar of bone around the middle of the shaft of the cartilage model. Once the bone starts to form, the perichondrium becomes the periosteum.

When cartilage becomes calcified, nutritive materials cannot diffuse through the intercellular space and so the cells die, leaving large cavities. Blood vessels grow into these spaces and enlarge the cavities even further. Eventually these spaces link up to form the marrow cavity.

As the developmental changes occur, the osteoblasts of the periosteum are laying down successive layers of bone on the outer surface so that the periosteal collar gets thicker. The cartilage model continues to grow at its ends, increasing in length. Bone grows in length and diameter.

Blood Supply to the Bone Bone has three basic blood supplies: (1) **nutrient artery** which arises from the main circulation; (2) **metaphyseal** and **epiphyseal** arteries: and (3) **periosteal** arteries. The main vessels vary in number according to the bone, with the femur having many while the tibia has only one.

Skeletal Homeostasis Bone undergoing ossification is continuously remodelled from the time of initial calcification. The process of remodelling is the replacement of old bone with new bone tissue. Bone is perpetually deposited and reabsorbed throughout our lives. The normal rate of deposition and resorption of bone is usually equal; however, remodelling occurs at different rates in different areas of the body (e.g. the distal portion of the femur is replaced approximately every four months). Remodelling allows worn or injured bone to be replaced.

The continual deposition and absorption of bone has a number of physiologically important functions.

1. Bone ordinarily adjusts its strength in proportion to the degree of bone stress. Consequently, bone thickens in response to increased loading.
2. Shape can be rearranged for the proper support of mechanical forces in response to stress patterns.
3. Old bone becomes relatively weak and brittle and so new organic matrix is required. In this way the toughness of bone is maintained.

Bone is deposited in proportion to the compressional load that the bone must carry. Bones of athletes become considerably more heavy than those of a non-athlete and a limb that is in plaster will become thinner and may become as much as 30% decalcified.

The deposition of bone at points of compression is thought to be caused by a **piezoelectric** effect. This occurs as follows: compression of the bone causes a negative potential at the compressed site and a positive potential elsewhere in the bone. Minute quantities of current flowing in the bone cause osteoblastic activity to increase at the negative end, which is thought to be the reason for the increase in bone deposition.

Normal Bone Growth Normal bone growth in the young and bone replacement in adults depends on several factors. These include sufficient quantities of minerals such as calcium, phosphate, boron, manganese and magnesium in the diet. A good supply of vitamins is also required, particularly vitamin D which has roles in the absorption of calcium from the gastro-intestinal tract, calcium removal from bone and kidney reabsorption of calcium that might otherwise be lost. Hormones such as growth hormone and the sex hormones aid osteoblast activity and promote new bone development. Hence the typical growth spurt at the onset and throughout puberty.

Repair of damaged tissues is dealt with in a later section of this chapter.

Muscle Tissues

Movement of the body and within the body is achieved by muscle tissue which is composed of cells which create a force by contracting. This specialized tissue utilizes the interaction of protein filaments (contractile proteins) and chemical energy within the muscle cells to produce the contraction. Contraction is an active process while relaxation in general is a passive process.

Contraction of muscle will lead to such diverse things as bodily movement and posture, the

Figure 1.20   Muscle types. The structure of the three different types of muscle highlighting cell structure and organization.

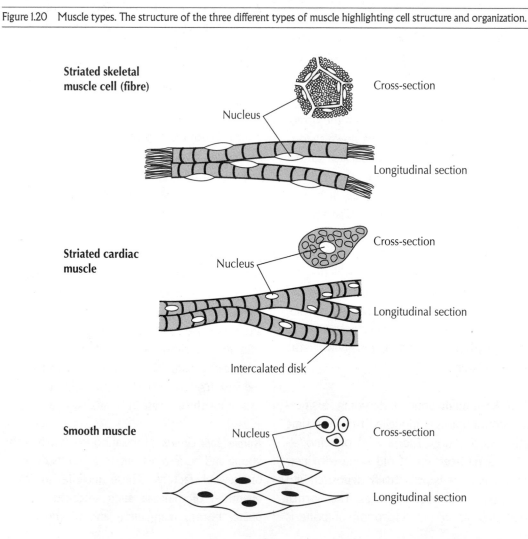

movement of ingested food through the gastro-intestinal tract, the pumping of blood around the cardiovascular system, the generation of heat and the regulation of blood pressure.

There are three types of muscle tissue in the human body (Figure 1.20): (1) **skeletal** — attached primarily to bone and so supports and moves the skeleton; (2) **cardiac** — which forms most of the wall of the heart and is responsible for pumping blood around the body; and (3) **smooth** — located in the walls of the hollow internal organs such as blood vessels and the gastrointestinal tract and can regulate the diameter of the hollow organs or propel the contents, respectively.

The muscles are classified according to their location, structure and functional characteristics. Skeletal muscle (Figure 1.21) is regarded as a voluntary type of muscle because in general we have conscious control over it and can decide when and how it will be moved. Cardiac and smooth muscle are regarded as involuntary muscle tissues because we have no conscious control over their contraction. Structurally, skeletal and cardiac muscle share a similar regular contractile protein architecture, which demonstrates alternating light and dark bands or stripes when examined under the light microscope, and are thus referred to as **striated**. Smooth muscle has an irregular array of the contractile proteins and does not exhibit a striated pattern, and is thus called **non-striated**.

Irrespective of the type, muscle tissue has four functional characteristics: **contractility, excitability, elasticity** and **extensibility**. The term 'contractility' refers to the muscle's capacity to contract or shorten producing a force. Its excitability comes from the fact that it can respond to stimulation by nerves and, in some muscle types, hormones. Muscle tissue is extensible because it can be stretched and elastic because it will return to its original length.

SKELETAL MUSCLE

Skeletal muscle is composed of bundles of muscle fibres lying parallel to one another. A muscle fibre is a single cylindrical structure which can range in diameter from 10 to 100 μm and up to 25 cm in length. Each fibre is a cylindrical accumulation of cells fused end to end, making it a multinucleated structure which lies parallel to other fibres in a bundle called a **fasiculus**. This is surrounded by a connective-tissue sheath called the **perimysium**. Numerous fasiculi bound together by connective tissue (the **epimysium**) make up the bulk of a skeletal muscle.

Each skeletal fibre or cell has a membrane which is referred to as the **sarcolemma** which encloses the fibre's cytoplasm or **sarcoplasm**.

Examination of a single skeletal muscle fibre under the electron microsope shows that the fibre is composed of small parallel subunits called **myofibrils** which run the whole length of the fibre. The myofibrils are the contractile elements of both skeletal and cardiac muscle fibres and are about 1–2.5 μm in diameter. They are composed of two types of protein filaments (myofilaments) called **actin** and **myosin**. The actin, or **thin filaments**, are composed of two strands of protein molecules twisted together, with an additional series of proteins attached — **troponin** and **tropomyosin**. Troponin has three components, one which binds the troponin to the actin filament, one which binds to the tropomyosin and one which binds calcium ions. During the relaxed state the troponin anchors the tropomyosin over a site on the actin filament where attachment between the myosin and actin filaments can occur, thereby blocking any attachment of the two filaments.

Figure 1.21 Skeletal muscle structure. (a) Organization of a skeletal muscle down to the level of a sarcomere. (b) The layout of the sarcomere and the two contractile proteins actin and myosin. (c) The alignment and location of the regulatory proteins troponin and tropomyosin on the actin filament.

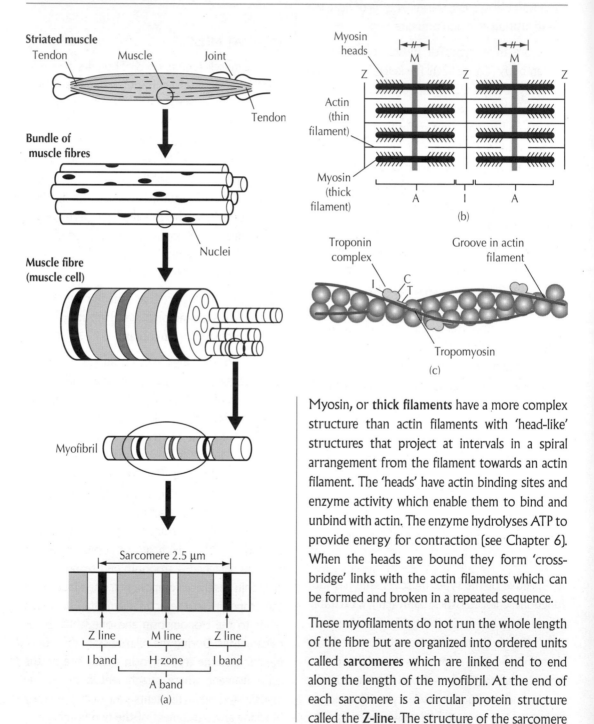

Striated muscle
Tendon   Muscle   Joint
Tendon

Bundle of muscle fibres
Nuclei

Muscle fibre (muscle cell)

Myofibril

Sarcomere 2.5 µm

Z line   M line   Z line
I band   H zone   I band
A band
(a)

Myosin heads
M   M
Z   Z   Z
Actin (thin filament)
Myosin (thick filament)
A   I   A
(b)

Troponin complex   Groove in actin filament
I   C   T
Tropomyosin
(c)

Myosin, or **thick filaments** have a more complex structure than actin filaments with 'head-like' structures that project at intervals in a spiral arrangement from the filament towards an actin filament. The 'heads' have actin binding sites and enzyme activity which enable them to bind and unbind with actin. The enzyme hydrolyses ATP to provide energy for contraction (see Chapter 6). When the heads are bound they form 'cross-bridge' links with the actin filaments which can be formed and broken in a repeated sequence.

These myofilaments do not run the whole length of the fibre but are organized into ordered units called **sarcomeres** which are linked end to end along the length of the myofibril. At the end of each sarcomere is a circular protein structure called the **Z-line**. The structure of the sarcomere is such that the actin and myosin filaments overlap one another to a greater or lesser degree depending on whether the muscle is contracted or relaxed. The pattern of the filaments overlap is what gives the muscle a striated appearance, when viewed under the light microscope. The thin filaments are anchored to the Z-line, while the myosin filaments are linked to one another by proteins in their central region (the **M-line**). An end-on view of the actin/myosin overlap shows that each thick filament is surrounded by a hexagonal array of thin filaments.

The sarcolemma has along its surface numerous tube-like invaginations called **transverse tubules** or **T-tubules** which are filled with extracellular fluid linking the sarcolemma with the inside of the muscle fibre. In the sarcoplasm between adjacent T-tubules is a highly specialized membrane-bound structure similar to smooth endoplasmic reticulum called the **sarcoplasmic reticulum (SR)**. The SR actively stores calcium ions from the sarcoplasm, thereby reducing calcium levels present in the vicinity of the myofibrils when the muscle is relaxed. Present on the SR membrane are calcium 'pumps' which utilize the hydrolysis of ATP to pump calcium back into the SR. This calcium can be released in response to the depolarization of the T-tubule membrane following stimulation of the muscle by an action potential.

More detailed information regarding skeletal muscle is given in Chapter 6.

CARDIAC MUSCLE

Cardiac muscle, while similar to skeletal muscle in its striated appearance due to the presence of actin and myosin filaments, has a number of differences, not least of all its location. Cardiac muscle is the principal tissue of the heart wall and unlike skeletal muscle is an involuntary muscle that can remain contracted 10–15 times longer.

The fibres are quadrangular in shape and much shorter in length ($\sim 100\,\mu m$) than those of a skeletal muscle. They are approximately $14\,\mu m$ in diameter with a single centrally placed nucleus, a much more abundant sarcoplasm and numerous mitochondria. Another difference is that the fibres may branch and interconnect to adjacent cells with irregular thickenings of the plasma membrane called **intercalated discs**. The discs act as sites for cell-to-cell adhesion and contain **gap junctions** which are, as their name implies, holes in the adjoining cell's membrane. Intercalated discs allow mechanical and electrical connections between adjacent cells.

Cardiac muscle has less SR than skeletal muscle and a loose association between that and the T-tubules. Because of this, action potentials are not carried from the surface to the SR as efficiently as in skeletal muscle and the released calcium has further to diffuse. Calcium also enters from the extracellular fluid, which is a much slower process and this partly accounts for the slower onset of a cardiac muscle cell contraction and the prolonged phase of contraction.

Cardiac muscle has many more mitochondria than skeletal muscle indicating that cardiac muscle is dependent on aerobic production of ATP. Cardiac muscle derives its energy principally by generating ATP aerobically. However, lactic acid, a by-product of skeletal muscle metabolism, can be utilized as an energy source by cardiac muscle cells.

SMOOTH MUSCLE

Smooth muscle is an involuntary muscle whose activity is influenced by nerves of the autonomic nervous system. Smooth muscle is distributed widely throughout the body and has a greater range of functions than the other types of muscle. Two major types of smooth muscle exist:

visceral (single unit) and **multi-unit**. Visceral is the more common type and is found in sheets that form parts of the walls of hollow organs such as blood vessels and the gastrointestinal tract.

Each smooth-muscle cell is generally spindle shaped with a single centrally located nucleus, sparse SR and no transverse tubules.

Smooth muscle lacks the striated pattern of the other two types. However, this does not mean that smooth muscle has no actin or myosin filaments. The thick and thin filaments are present but are arranged somewhat differently. Smooth muscle cells also contain intermediate filaments. Present in smooth muscle cells are structures called **dense bodies** which serve as anchor points for the actin filaments.

Due to the lack of a well-developed SR, the calcium required to initiate contraction is derived mainly from the extracellular fluid. This process takes time; therefore, smooth muscle cells are slower to contract than skeletal muscle cells. The calcium ions that enter bind to a protein called **calmodulin**; this binding initiates cross-bridge formation between the actin and myosin filaments.

The single unit smooth muscle cells are electrically coupled by gap junctions in a manner similar to cardiac muscle cells. Contractions within these cells are initiated by pacemaker cells within the tissue itself. Neurones of the autonomic nervous system regulate rather than instigate contractions in single unit smooth muscle cells. Contraction of multi-unit smooth muscle cells is initiated by neural connections as these cells have very few gap junctions.

Hormones, may also stimulate smooth muscle contraction; for example, oxytocin will increase smooth muscle contractions in the uterus during child birth. Local factors such as oxygen levels can also influence smooth muscle contraction.

Nervous Tissue

The nervous system detects (sensory function), integrates (associative function) and generates (motor function) responses to a vast array of inputs from within the body and from the outside environment.

The nervous system can be divided into two main parts: the **central nervous system** (which includes the brain and the spinal cord) and the **peripheral nervous system** (which includes the nervous structures located outwith the CNS). This latter can be further subdivided into the **somatic** nervous system and the **autonomic** nervous system. The autonomic system innervates tissues other than skeletal muscle. It has two branches with opposing physiological effects – the **sympathetic** and the **parasympathetic** branches.

Despite the complexity of the system that has evolved to cope with all the different inputs, the nervous system consists of only two principal kinds of cells: **neurones** and **neuroglia**. The neurones, or nerve cells, are highly specialized cells that are sensitive to various stimuli, capable of converting stimuli into nervous signals and transmitting these signals, or impulses (see Chapter 2), to other nerve cells, muscles and glands. The structure of the neurone is adapted for its function, but consists of three basic components: a **cell body** (which contains the nucleus and other organelles) and two cytoplasmic processes called **axons** and **dendrites**. Because of the arrangement of the nervous system, certain processes transmit impulses to the cell body (dendrites) while others carry impulses away from the cell body (axons). The dendrites function primarily to receive information from other nerves or sensory receptors. Axons, on the other hand, function to conduct and pass on information to other cells.

Most axons of the peripheral nervous system are

covered by a fatty substance called **myelin** and are called myelinated fibres. Those that have no covering of myelin are classed as **unmyelinated** fibres. Because of the lipid content of myelinated fibres they have a white appearance. The myelin sheath is composed of folds of membrane from **Schwann cells** (see Figure 1.24), which are located at intervals along the length of the axon and which wrap around the nerve axon, insulating it from the extracellular fluid. The myelin sheath is not continuous the entire length of the nerve axon but is separated at intervals called **nodes of Ranvier**. The myelin sheath and the nodes of Ranvier are instrumental in increasing the speed of conduction of nerve impulses. (Loss of myelin results in the clinical condition known as multiple sclerosis.)

NEURONES

There are considerable differences in neuronal structure which makes it difficult to describe an arrangement that relates to all nerves. Structural classification is based on the number of processes that extend from the cell body and three types are identifiable (Figure 1.22).

Unipolar neurones have one single process which emerges from the cell body of the nerve; however, this separates into two branches, one functioning as the axon and the other as the dendrite. Examples of this type of neurone can be found in the sensory neurones that enter the spinal cord.

Bipolar neurones have two processes which arise from different poles of the cell body. One process is the dendrite and the other the axon. Bipolar neurones are those associated with the senses of sight, smell and sound.

Multipolar neurones are the most common type of neurone where numerous processes emerge from the cell body. One of these processes acts as the axon while the rest form dendrites.

Figure 1.22   Nerve cells. Nerves are classified according to their general structure. (a) Bipolar neurone. (b) Unipolar neurone. (c) Multipolar neurone.

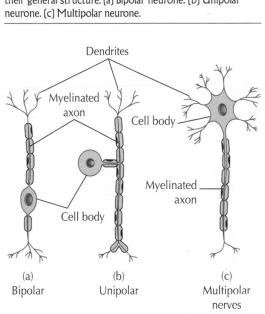

(a) Bipolar   (b) Unipolar   (c) Multipolar nerves

Functionally, there are three types of neurones: **sensory neurones** which conduct signals to the CNS; **motor neurones** which conduct the impulses away from the brain to muscles or glands; **interneurones** (association neurones) which relay information within the CNS. A neurone can be excitatory where it increases the activity of the cells it transmits its impulses to, or it can be inhibitory, where it decreases the activity of the cells.

Neurones are not distributed in a random nature throughout the body but in a highly organized architecture. Neuronal cell bodies and axons tend to be amalgamated into groups. The term 'nucleus' is used to describe a collection of cell bodies of neurones within the CNS. This should not be confused with a cell nucleus which is a completely different structure. A 'ganglion' is a collection of cell bodies of neurones within the peripheral nervous system. A 'tract' describes a bundle of axons in the CNS and the term 'nerve' describes a collection of axons in the peripheral nervous system.

The structure of a typical nerve is shown in Figure 1.23.

NEUROGLIAL CELLS

Neuroglial cells (Figure 1.24) do not transmit impulses but perform supportive and protective functions. Neuroglial cells are plentiful and are widely distributed amongst the neurones. They insulate and hold in place the neurones as well as attaching nearby blood vessels.

There are four major types of neuroglial cells:

Schwann cells (or neurolemmocyte) provide electrical insulation for axonal processes in the peripheral nervous system. Schwann cell function was described in an earlier section discussing myelinated nerves. The CNS does not contain Schwann cells but other cells called **astrocytes, oligodendrocytes, ependymal** and **microglial** cells.

The astrocytes form a supporting network within the CNS attaching blood vessels to the neurones. Oligodendrocytes support the neurones as well as producing a phospholipid myelin sheath around the axons. Microglia acts as macrophages phagocytosing microbes and cellular debris.

Ependymal cells form a continuous lining of the ventricles of the brain and the central canal of the spinal cord and seem to assist the flow of CSF.

Clinical conditions which affect the functioning of nerves will be mentioned throughout Chapter 4.

Skin

The skin as such is not just a single tissue but an organ in its own right and in conjunction with its ancillary structures such as hair, nails, glands and sensory receptors, is regarded as the integumentary system. The skin comprises epithelial cells, exocrine glands, connective tissues and small amounts of muscle and nerves, which are joined to perform specific functions (Figure 1.25).

As well as providing a tough waterproof covering for the body, the skin also regulates body tem-

---

Figure 1.23   Peripheral nerve structure. Connective-tissue sheaths bind neurones together to form a nerve.

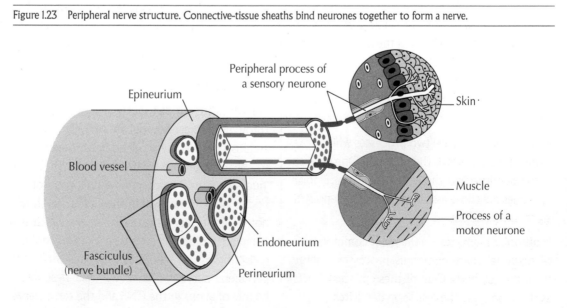

Figure 1.24   Schwann cells and the myelin sheath. The membrane from Schwann cells wrap around the axon several times, forming the myelin sheath. The myelin sheath is not continuous, but breaks are present between the different Schwann cells. These interruptions in the myelin sheath are known as the nodes of Ranvier.

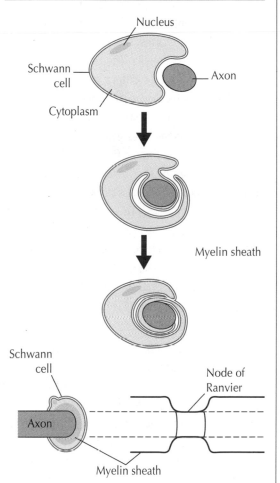

Figure 1.25   Epidermis, dermis and ancillary structures of the skin.

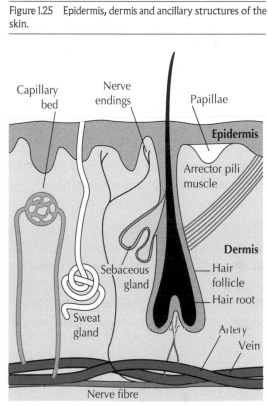

perature, provides protection, is involved in vitamin D synthesis and provides a means of excretion (salt and water). Being the outermost layer, the skin also has to endure a great deal of wear and tear. The skin has an abundance of sensory nerve endings and receptors that provide us with the ability to detect touch, pressure, pain and temperature. The sensory receptors of the skin are dealt with in more detail in Chapter 3.

The skin consists of two main layers, an epithelial surface layer called the **epidermis** and an underlying layer of connective tissues called the **dermis.**

The epidermis is composed of tightly packed keratinized stratified squamous epithelia several cells thick. The close nature of the packed cells restricts blood vessels from passing in between the cells; therefore the epidermis is avascular, with no direct blood supply. Blood vessels in the dermis supply nutrients and remove waste products for the cells. The cells of the basal layers are mitotically active and new cells move towards the surface, replacing those that have been damaged or lost through natural wastage. As the cells near the uppermost portion of the epidermis, they die and in conjunction with the keratin produced by the cells, form this tough waterproof coating that prevents loss of too much water and invasion by microorganisms. Also present in the epidermis are melanocytes, pigment cells, which give our skin a coloration.

The dermis consists of areolar connective tissue with a rich supply of blood vessels and sensory nerve endings permeating through the layer. Fat cells are located in the lower portion of the dermis. The subsidiary structures of the skin are located in this layer or pass through the layer (e.g. sweat glands and hair follicles).

The epidermis does not lie flat on top of the dermis, but has a wavy appearance (Figure 1.25). Ridges of the dermal connective tissue (known as **papillae**) push up into the epidermal layer displacing some of the cell causing epidermal ridges. These epidermal ridges are what appear as fingerprints.

Ancillary Structures

Sweat glands are exocrine organs that are found over most of the body surface and which empty their secretions onto the skin surface. There are thought to be two main types of sweat glands, the **eccrine gland** which is found on the general body surface and the **apocrine gland**, which is localized in specific areas such as the axillae, pubic and anal regions. Modified sweat glands are also found in the eyelids. Eccrine secretion produces, in response to thermal stimulation, the watery fluid termed 'sweat'. The apocrine secretion tends to be more viscous and is secreted at times of emotional stress and sexual arousement. Sweat is composed of a mixture of water, salts, urea and ammonia.

Sebaceous glands are mostly connected to hair follicles and produce the oily substance known as **sebum** that helps maintain the skin surface as a flexible waterproof covering. Oversecretion of sebum after puberty is the common cause of blocked pores (blackheads or comedons) and the common skin disease acne.

Hair develops from undifferentiated epithelial cells in the region of the papillae. Hair occurs in most areas of the body though it is not always apparent. Exceptions are the red part of the lips, the palms of the hands, the soles of the feet and portions of the genitalia. The texture of the hair throughout the body differs substantially from very fine hairs to very coarse hairs. Each hair is surrounded by a hair follicle which is a continuation of the epidermal layer. The follicle has a plexus of blood vessels and nerve fibres which penetrate into the bottom of the follicle. Attached to the hair follicle are very small smooth muscles called **arrector pili** muscles. These muscles contract, raising the hair into a vertical position, in response to cold temperature, fright and other emotional stresses. The contraction of the arrector pili muscles is what is responsible for 'goose bumps', the elevations of the skin at the follicle sites.

The skin plays a major role in thermoregulation. As mentioned earlier, all the blood vessels of the skin lie in the dermis either just under the epidermis or deep in the dermis. The deep plexus supplies the sweat glands and the hair follicles. The blood vessels have a rich sympathetic nerve supply from the autonomic nervous system. These nerves release noradrenaline from the nerve endings; this agent has a vasoconstrictor effect on the blood vessels. There is no parasympathetic stimulation of the blood vessels in the skin, so vasodilation is passive and the result of reduced sympathetic output.

The internal temperature of the body (around 37°C) is controlled very carefully to avoid extremes of temperature that would otherwise affect the body's metabolic functions. The skin's role is in controlling heat loss from the body. The large surface area, ancillary structures and blood supply lend themselves to this task.

The body can lose heat by four different physical processes:

1. **Conduction:** For example, placing the hand on a cold piece of metal will result in heat leaving the hand by conduction to the cold metal.
2. **Radiation:** A central heating radiator radiates heat. Similarly, our bodies radiate heat when the surrounding environment is cooler than ourselves.
3. **Convection:** The air surrounding the body is warmed by both conduction and radiation. As this warm air rises, cooler air will replace it. Winds and breezes will enhance this process increasing heat loss.
4. **Evaporation:** Water or sweat evaporated from the body cools the body down. The heat of the body is transferred to the water, or the sweat, by conduction and is lost as the fluid is evaporated.

How does the heat get to the skin to be lost? Temperature like many other processes in the human body is controlled by homeostatic mechanisms. Thermoreceptors in the skin, for both heat and cold, detect the temperature of the skin's surface while central receptors in the hypothalamus respond to changes of internal temperature. The temperature input from the receptors is coordinated by the hypothalamus so that an appropriate response can be effected. The effector organs are the blood vessels and sweat glands of the skin.

When body temperature is too high, the hypothalamus reduces the autonomic nervous system's output to the skin's blood vessels causing vasodilation, thereby allowing more blood to enter these vessels. Also, capillary beds that had minimal blood flow due to arteriovenous shunts are opened up to accept an increased blood flow. This means that more blood is now in closer proximity to the skin's surface and more heat can be lost by the methods already discussed.

The sympathetic stimulation also results in sweat glands producing sweat to facilitate heat loss by evaporation.

When the temperature is too cold then it is essential to conserve heat. The body does this by limiting the amount of blood passing through the dermal blood vessels and hence near the skin's surface. The rate at which heat is produced is also raised by increasing voluntary and involuntary muscular activity. Involuntary muscle contractions are known as 'shivers'. Also, the hormones which affect body metabolism (thyroxine and adrenaline) are secreted in greater amounts, raising cellular metabolism and the amount of heat produced. This should raise body temperature back to its homeostatic level.

The skin also functions in vitamin production. Vitamin D is a group of chemicals found in the body and involved in calcium homeostasis. One such substance is vitamin D_3 which is a steroid found in a limited number of foods. Vitamin D_3 can also be formed in the skin by the action of ultraviolet light on a compound present there, called 7-dehydrocholesterol. The 7-dehydrocholesterol is converted to vitamin D_3, which is biologically inactive, just like the ingested form of vitamin D. This molecule is modified by reactions that then occur in the liver and the kidneys, to produce the activated form of vitamin D_3, the compound 1,25-dihydroxycholecalciferol.

The skin's secretions facilitate the skin's ability to protect us. For a long time, the skin's secretory glands were thought to have unrelated functions, i.e. sweat glands produced sweat in response to thermal stimulation, while sebaceous glands secreted oils for maintaining hair follicles and shafts. Not only does sebum maintain hair, it also helps maintain the skin and in conjunction with keratin helps to keep the skin waterproof. When sebum and sweat mix an emulsion is formed, which creates both a physical and chemical barrier against microorganisms. Components of both the sweat and the sebum have antibacterial properties which provide the chemical barrier.

Tissue Repair

The different categories of tissues that we have discussed so far in this chapter do not all respond to damage and injury in exactly the same way. Tissues that are exposed to greater wear and tear (e.g. the skin), have a greater ability to replace cells that have been lost or damaged. Others can less readily replace cells while in some cases damage results in the permanent loss of that type of cell.

A tissue response to damage can be divided into three basic types:

1. Cells which under normal conditions continually undergo the process of dividing to form new cells have the capacity to repair easily. Tissues such as epidermis, intestine, uterine and urinary tract epithelium fall into this group. Cells at the base of the epithelial lining continually divide to produce new cells.

2. Some cells can retain their ability to mitotically divide even after normal cell division associated with growth has ceased. Cells in this group can therefore be stimulated to divide to regenerate the tissue upon damage. This group includes tissues such as the liver and the pancreas.

3. Some cells lose their ability to divide from an early stage of development and therefore cannot regenerate to repair damage that has occurred. The best example of this is the neurone.

When tissue repair occurs, cells of that tissue reproduce to replace worn or damaged cells with exact replicas of the original cells thereby allowing the tissue to retain its functional capabilities. However, repair can occur where damaged cells are replaced by cells produced in the underlying connective tissue layer supporting the damaged tissue. In this case new collagen is deposited by fibroblasts, resulting in the formation of **scar** tissue. The scar tissue, being different from the original tissue, can not perform in the same way and so function is impaired. An illustration of this is wound healing in the skin.

Healing and repair can be influenced by a number of factors:

1. Blood supply. A disruption of the local blood supply slows down the repair process. Avascular tissues or those with a minor blood supply will heal at a much slower rate than those with a profuse blood supply. Cartilage which is avascular and relies on nutrients diffusing from other nearby tissues takes a very long time to heal in comparison to the skin which is highly vascular and can repair very quickly.

2. Nutrition. The blood being delivered to the tissues must have an adequate supply of nutrients to facilitate repair. Lack of protein and vitamins in the diet will adversely affect repair mechanisms.

3. Hormones may speed up the repair process in the early stages of growth and development (e.g. growth hormone). However, excess glucocorticoids from the adrenal cortex have an adverse effect on repair processes by reducing the numbers of new fibroblasts and the formation of collagen.

REPAIR AND REGENERATION OF NERVOUS TISSUE

Mature cells in the central nervous system, once damaged, cannot be replaced. Nerve cells lose the mitotic capabilities early in development and so upon damage, both the cell body and the axon degenerate. In contrast, the peripheral nerves can be repaired and retain their functional capabilities. This of course depends on the type and severity of the damage. Transection of a peripheral nerve results in the myelin degenerating at the exposed ends of the axon with increased Schwann cell activity within the connective tissue sheath (endoneurium) surrounding the nerve. The proliferation of the Schwann cells forms pathways for the axons to regrow along. Axonal appendages then grow from the exposed ends towards one another.

The process is very slow and re-innervation of the nerve endings may take quite some considerable time to repair depending on the severity of the damage. If the nerve fibres only are damaged, while the rest of the nerve components remain intact, then the regenerating axons can grow along their original endoneurial tubes. However, if there is considerable derangement of internal structures so that the continuity of the endoneurial tubes is lost, fibrosis occurs which acts as a barrier to regeneration of the axon. Some of the regenerating axons cannot cross this barrier while those that do may not re-attach to its original counterpart. This then results in complete loss of appropriate innervation or the development of inappropriate innervation.

BONE REPAIR

A previous section discussed bone on the basis of growth and maintenance. Utilizing this information, this section deals with the way bone can recover from an injury such as a fracture.

The basic process of healing in bones is similar to that of general repair but with obvious tissue-specific differences. After the initial haemorrhage, a clot or haematoma forms and acute inflammation develops, possibly with some death of the bone and the periosteum, depending on the severity of the initial injury. This is due to the reduction in blood supply after the tearing of blood vessels in the periosteum and the medullary cavity. The amount of cell death will depend on the site of the injury and the blood vessels that are damaged and how much bone is without a proper blood supply.

It usually requires a great deal of force to fracture a bone and this normally results in fragments of the bone being displaced. There is immense proliferation of fibroblasts and osteogenic cells of the inner periosteal layer around a wide area over the break. These cells then deposit a collar of bone and collagen around the broken ends of the bone, referred to as a callus. Underneath this callus, bone is deposited with blood vessels permeating through the bone. This deposition of new bone is dependent on blood supply.

As the two sets of new bone develop over the broken ends, they grow towards one another until finally they unite forming a callus. This attachment of the fractured ends of the bone does not bring the bones into alignment; it merely anchors the ends to one another. Remodelling of the bone will take place in response to the mechanical stresses placed upon the bone as it is rehabilitated. Surgeons utilize the phenomenon of bone stress to accelerate the rate of fracture healing. A fixing device holds the bones together allowing use of the bone; this increases stress, thereby increasing recovery.

REPAIR OF ARTICULAR CARTILAGE

Articular cartilage is a dense avascular connective tissue. Yet despite this, it remains metabolically active throughout our lives, relying on diffusion of nutrients from other nearby tissues for its survival. This means that upon injury repair occurs from two main sources: (1) the chondrocytes themselves and (2) from surrounding connective tissues.

After damage, the chondrocytes will proliferate, generating new matrix to replace the damaged matrix. As the manufacture of the new matrix relies on the diffusion of nutrients from surrounding tissues, it is therefore a slow process. Despite the formation of new matrix it is not enough to completely repair any damage. Further repair will occur from the outermost layer of the fibrous connective tissue resulting in the deposition of collagen fibres and the generation of fibrocartilage. The overall result is that the amount and quality of the replacement tissue may not be adequate enough to cope with normal functional demands.

REPAIR OF TENDONS

To be functionally active after damage, a tendon must have a strong re-attachment and have a full range of movement of the dense connective tissue fibres that make up its structure.

Repair occurs by the development of blood vessels permeating from surrounding tissues and increased fibroblast activity. The new fibres are arranged randomly at first, but become properly oriented along the line of the tendon as repair progresses. This proliferation of fibroblasts and the synthesis of new fibres and collagen, may continue for some weeks after the injury. The downside of this is the increased chance of adhesions developing. These are abnormal tissue bindings which can affect the functional capabilities of any tissue under repair. In the case of tendons, if the adhesions are long then functional capabilities remain good. However, if the adhesions are small with large numbers of fibres, then the tendon has a limited range of movement.

REPAIR AND REGENERATION OF MUSCLE

In general, the different types of muscle have little capacity to regenerate. Normal development of muscle after birth is due to the enlargement of existing cells rather than any increase in their numbers.

The ends of skeletal muscle fibres that have been damaged can develop 'finger-like' appendages that reach out from the ends of the damaged fibres to reconnect them to other fibres. Skeletal muscle also contains satellite cells which are stem cells that lie between the muscle fibres. These cells have the ability to form with one another to produce new skeletal muscle fibres. However, there is a finite number of these cells and once utilized there is no further replacement available. This means that there is only a little capability to repair severe damage to skeletal muscle, and when damage is excessive, fibrous replacement occurs resulting in scar tissue formation in the muscle.

Similarly, cardiac muscle damage is repaired by the deposition of fibrous scar tissue rather than regeneration of muscle cells.

Some smooth muscle types appear to have the ability to regenerate by cellular division while some fibres are regenerated from stem cells of an unclear origin.

Bibliography

General Reading

CHEMISTRY

General Chemistry, Principles and Structure. Brady, JE, Humiston, GE (1982) 3rd Edition, Wiley, New York.

BIOCHEMISTRY

Biochemistry. Stryer, L (1988) 3rd Edition, Freeman, New York.

Textbook of Biochemistry. Devlin, TD (1992) Wiley–Liss, New York.

Molecular Biology of the Cell. Alberts, A *et al.* (1994) 3rd Edition. Garland Publishing, New York.

CELLS

Human Anatomy and Physiology. Spence, AD & Mason, EB (1992) 2nd Edition, West Publishers, St Paul, MN.

Molecular Biology of the Cell. Alberts A *et al.* (1994) 3rd Edition, Garland Publishing, New York and London.

Organelles. Carroll, M (1989) Macmillan Molecular Biology Series, London.

Principles of Anatomy and Physiology. Tortora, G, Grabowski, SR (1993) Harper Collins, New York.

The Cell. Fawcett, DW (1981) WB Saunders, Philadelphia.

TISSUES

Anatomy and Physiology. Seeley, RR, Stephens, TD, Tate, P (1991) Mosby Yearbook Inc., St Louis & London.

A Textbook of Histology. Fawcett, DW (1994) 12th Edition. Chapman Hall, New York & London.

Bone: Fundamentals of the Physiology of Skeletal Tissue, McLean, FC, Urist, MR (1973) 3rd Edition. University of Chicago Press, Chicago & London.

Exocrine Secretion. Wong, PYD, Young, JA (1988) Hong Kong University Press.

Histology: A Text and Atlas. Ross, W, Reith, EJ, Romrell, LJ (1989) 2nd Edition. Williams & Wilkins, Baltimore & London.

Human Anatomy and Physiology. Spence, AD, Mason, EB (1992) 2nd Edition. West Publishers, St. Paul, MN.

Human Physiology. Vander, AJ, Sherman, JH, Luciano, DS (1994) 6th Edition. McGraw-Hill Inc., New York.

Muir's Textbook of Pathology. Edited by RNM MacSween, K Whaley (1992), 13th Edition. Edward Arnold, London.

Physiology of Smooth Muscle. Bulbring, E (1981) Edward Arnold, London.

Principles of Anatomy and Physiology. Tortora, G, Grabowski, SR (1993) Harper Collins, New York.

Skeletal Muscle in Health and Disease. Jones, A, Round, J (1990) Manchester University Press.

The Physiology, Biochemistry and Molecular Biology of the Skin. Goldsmith, LA (1991) 2nd Edition. Oxford Medical Publications, Oxford & New York.

The Physiology of Bone. Vaughan, J (1981) 3rd Edition. Clarendon Press, Oxford.

The Structure and Function of the Skin. Montagna, W (1974) 3rd Edition. Academic Press, New York.

Visceral Muscle. Huddart, H, Hunt, S (1975) Blackie, Glasgow.

2

The Nervous System: Structure and Basics

The Membrane Potential

•

Action Potential

•

The Synapse

•

General Organization of the Nervous System

The Membrane Potential

The distribution of ions across the plasma membranes of nerve cells and the semipermeability of the membrane to specific ions means that an electrical potential difference exists across the membrane — the **membrane potential**. Nerve cells are excitable cells, in that they can respond to an appropriate stimulus, by altering the cell membrane permeability to certain ions, thereby altering the membrane potential. This change in membrane potential occurs rapidly and can serve as a mechanism for the nerve cell to transmit information within the nervous system.

Ionic Basis of the Resting Membrane Potential

At rest, the distribution of ions across the nerve cell membrane is such that there is a high concentration of sodium ions (Na^+) outside the cell — about 145 mmol l^{-1} (mM) — and a high concentration of potassium ions (K^+) inside the cell (about 150 mM). Conversely, the concentration of sodium ions inside the cell is low — about 10 mM, and potassium ion concentration outside the cell is low (about 5 mM). There therefore exists a concentration gradient for potassium ions between the inside and the outside of the cell, and for sodium ions between the outside and the inside of the cell (Figure 2.1).

Figure 2.1 Distribution of sodium ions (Na$^+$) and potassium ions (K$^+$) in intracellular and extracellular fluid. The shaded wedges show the direction of concentration gradients for each ion.

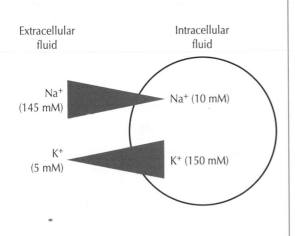

Figure 2.2 Distribution of positive and negative charges on either side of the resting cell membrane. The inner surface of the cell membrane displays an abundance of negatively charged particles, while the outer surface has an abundance of positive charge.

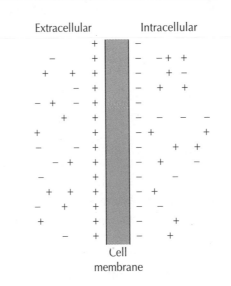

At rest the cell membrane is selectively permeable to potassium ions. This selectivity occurs through specific ionic channels in the cell membrane which allow potassium ions to move through, but not sodium ions. This therefore means that potassium ions will move out of the cell down their concentration gradient.

As these positively charged ions move out of the cell, they leave behind negatively charged ionic groups (mostly organic anions) within the cell and add to the overall positive charge outside the cell. The inside of the cell therefore has an overall greater negative charge than the outside of the cell, which has an overall positive charge. There is consequently a charge difference between the outside and inside of the cell, separated by the cell membrane. The cell membrane is therefore said to be **polarized** (Figure 2.2).

The charge difference — or voltage — between the inside and the outside of the cell can be measured by placing a microelectrode inside the cell, and measuring the voltage difference between that and another microelectrode placed in the extracellular fluid. If this is done, the voltage across the

cell membrane at rest is recorded as about 70 mV. This is written with respect to the overall charge inside the cell, which is negative. The resting membrane voltage — or **resting membrane potential** — is therefore −70 mV (Figure 2.3). This value is actually slightly less than what is expected for movement of potassium ions out of the cell — this

Figure 2.3 Measurement of resting membrane potential. A microelectrode of about 0.5 μm in diameter is inserted into the cell and another placed just outside the cell. The voltage between the inside and outside of the cell is recorded as −70 mV.

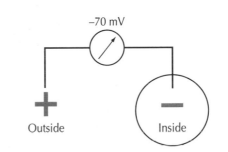

would be expected to be about −90 mV. This is because the resting membrane also has a slight permeability to sodium ions. There is therefore a small degree of leakage of sodium ions *into* the cell which reduces the overall intracellular negativity.

Action Potential

Ionic Basis

When nerve cells are stimulated, whether chemically, electrically or mechanically (see below), the ionic channels which are responsible for the selective permeability of the membrane alter their properties, reducing the movement of potassium ions out of the cell. The membrane potential therefore becomes less negative — the cell membrane becomes **depolarized**.

If the size of this depolarization is sufficient, i.e. if it reaches a **threshold potential**, a series of changes in membrane permeability occur which cause a rapid reversal of the membrane potential, followed by a rapid return to the resting potential. These rapid changes in membrane potential are termed the **action potential**.

When the threshold potential is reached, sodium channels in the cell membrane open, allowing a rapid flow of sodium ions down their concentration gradient into the cell. This rapid movement of positively charged ions into the cell therefore causes the inside of the cell to become positive and the outside of the cell to become negative — the opposite of the resting situation.

Gated ion channels are membrane proteins that can either be in the open state, allowing ions to pass from one side of the membrane to the other, or in the closed state, thus preventing movement of ions. The opening and closing of these channels depends on the value of the membrane potential, i.e. they are voltage dependent. Separate specific gated ion channels exist for different ions and differ from the (nongated) ion channels that determine a cell's resting permeability to different ions.

The movement of sodium ions inside the cell is such that the membrane potential rises from the resting −70 mV to +30 mV.

The sodium channels quickly begin to close, reducing the movement of sodium ions into the cell. This is followed by the opening of gated potassium channels. This, therefore, now allows potassium ions to flow out of the cell, restoring the membrane potential to its resting value — **repolarization**. In fact, these gated potassium channels (which are different to the nongated potassium channels responsible for generating the resting membrane potential) are relatively slow to close, and the membrane potential transiently undershoots the resting membrane potential. Since the cell membrane is even more polarized at this point, this phase is known as **hyperpolarization**.

The whole process of depolarization and repolarization (including hyperpolarization) takes about 1 millisecond (1 ms) to complete.

The amplitude (size) of the action potential is dependent on the relative concentrations of sodium and potassium ions outside and inside the cell. Since these relative concentrations are constant in normal situations, the size of the action potential is therefore constant. Subthreshold changes in membrane potential will not be sufficient to generate an action potential, whereas those which exceed threshold will always generate an action potential of the same amplitude. This is known as the **all-or-none law**. In simpler terms, this law states that an action potential of maximum amplitude is always generated when the membrane potential exceeds threshold *no matter how strong the stimulation,* but no action potential will be generated if threshold is not exceeded.

The changes in membrane potential and in ionic permeabilities during an action potential are summarized in Figure 2.4.

Figure 2.4   Upper panel: changes in membrane potential during an action potential, showing the phases of depolarization, repolarization and hyperpolarization. Small, subthreshold potentials, insufficient to generate an action potential are also shown. Lower panel: relative changes in membrane conductance to sodium and potassium ions during the action potential. The time scale for this panel is identical to that of the upper panel.

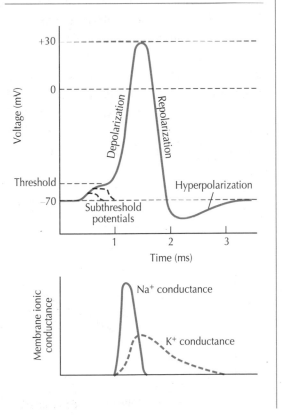

Refractory Periods

An action potential is followed by a period in which it is either impossible or more difficult to produce another action potential in the nerve cell. The **absolute refractory period** is the period of time immediately following an action potential in which it is impossible to elicit a further action potential in the nerve cell no matter how strong the stimulus. This refractory period lasts for about 1–1.5 ms. This is followed by the **relative refractory period**, lasting for a further 3–4 ms, during which an action potential may be elicited, but only by utilizing a stronger than normal stimulus, i.e. during the relative refractory period, the threshold for stimulation has been increased (Figure 2.5).

The existence of these refractory periods is due

Figure 2.5   Absolute and relative refractory periods. The lower panel shows changes in membrane threshold voltage relative to the time course of the action potential shown in the upper panel.

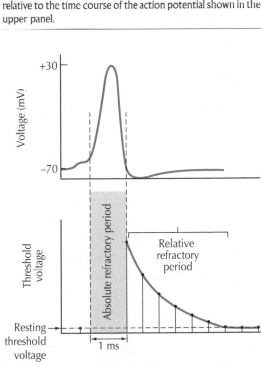

to the time taken for the gated ionic channels to close. During the absolute refractory period, the sodium channels are slowly closing and must complete this process before they can be re-opened to generate a further action potential. During the relative refractory period, the slow closure of the potassium channels means that the membrane potential is greater than at rest, and so a higher than normal stimulus strength is required to bring the membrane to threshold.

These refractory periods mean that maximum number of action potentials which can be generated in a nerve cell over a given period of time is limited. The frequency cannot exceed that which is governed by the duration of the absolute refractory period (about 750 per second). Frequencies of action potentials which exceed that governed by the relative refractory period (about 250 per second) can only be elicited if the stimulus strength is sufficient to raise the membrane potential above the increased threshold during this refractory period.

Frequency Coding

The frequency of action potentials in a nerve cell is related to the strength of the stimulus which activates the nerve. This is related to the changes in the membrane properties which accompany stimulation of the nerve cell. The **generator potential** is the change in membrane potential which is produced when the nerve cell is stimulated (in sensory receptors, the generator potential is referred to as the **receptor potential**). The stronger the stimulus, the greater the generator potential. If the generator potential exceeds the threshold for the nerve cell, action potentials will be generated. The frequency of these action potentials is related to the size of the generator potential. Since the size of the generator potential

is related to the size of the stimulus, it therefore follows that the frequency of action potentials is related to the strength of the stimulus (Figure 2.6).

In this way, the frequency of action potentials in a neurone codes for the strength of stimulation of the nerve.

Action Potential Propagation

The changes in ionic permeability of the nerve cell membrane which generate an action potential are restricted only to a small portion of the cell membrane of the nerve axon. However, the movement of the ions or **membrane currents** set up during an action potential can stimulate adjacent portions of the nerve cell membrane to reach threshold and therefore generate a 'new' action potential in this adjacent portion of the membrane. This, in turn, can stimulate the next portion of the membrane to threshold, generate a further action potential, and so on, along the length of the nerve axon. In this way, it appears that the action potential travels, or is **propagated**, along the length of the nerve axon (Figure 2.7). Non-myelinated nerves rely on this mechanism for the propagation of action potentials along

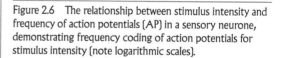

Figure 2.6   The relationship between stimulus intensity and frequency of action potentials (AP) in a sensory neurone, demonstrating frequency coding of action potentials for stimulus intensity (note logarithmic scales).

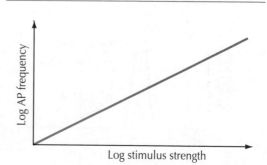

Figure 2.7 Generation of local currents in a nerve axon by an active portion of membrane (shaded area). Current flows from positive to negative regions through the nerve cell membrane, sufficient to depolarize adjacent regions of membrane to threshold and therefore generate an action potential in these regions. This process continues along the length of the axon.

Figure 2.8 Saltatory conduction in a myelinated axon. Current can only flow through the exposed regions of membrane at the nodes of Ranvier. This effectively increases the speed of conduction of action potentials along the axon. Conduction velocities in myelinated nerve axons can reach up to 100 m s^{-1}, compared to 0.5–2 m s^{-1} in unmyelinated nerves (see Tables 3.2 and 3.4).

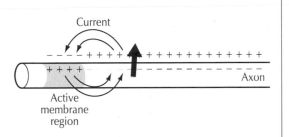

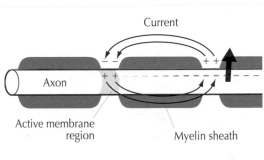

the nerve axon. The speed of action potential propagation, or **conduction velocity,** is relatively slow in these nerves. However, myelinated nerves are capable of faster conduction velocities by virtue of the myelin sheath which surrounds their axons.

The myelin sheath acts as an insulator around the axon, and prevents the leakage of electrical current into the surrounding extracellular fluid. This means that the membrane currents set up during an action potential cannot stimulate the adjacent area of membrane to reach threshold and therefore generate an action potential. Instead, the membrane currents can only leak out into the extracellular fluid at the points on the axon where there is no myelin present — the **nodes of Ranvier** (see p. 35). It is only at these exposed regions of the axon membrane that action potentials can be generated. Action potential propagation in myelinated nerves therefore occurs in such a way that the action potential appears to 'jump' from one node of Ranvier to the next. This is known as **saltatory conduction** (from the Latin *saltare* — 'to leap'), and significantly increases the speed of conduction of the action potential along the axon (Figure 2.8).

The Synapse

Action potentials are propagated along the length of the nerve axon until they arrive at the terminal portions of the nerve cell. In the nervous system, these terminals form a specialized area of contact between nerve cells — the **synapse.** The adjacent nerve cells do not make physical contact with each other, but are separated by a small gap (about 10–40 nm) — the synaptic cleft. Synapses between nerve cells allow communication from one nerve cell to another. This communication can be electrical or chemical. Electrical synapses are much less common than chemical synapses.

An axon can have several synaptic terminals making contact with one or several neurones at the same time. The synpase is usually between the axon terminal of the presynaptic nerve cell and the cell body or dendrites of the postsynaptic nerve cell (Figure 2.9).

At the synaptic terminal, the axon swells to form the synaptic bulb which has an accumulation of intracellular vesicles containing a chemical messenger — the **neurotransmitter.** A common

Figure 2.9   Synapses on the cell body and dendrites of a nerve cell. The location of the synapses is important in determining their effectiveness. The axon hillock of the nerve cell is the most sensitive portion and the synapses here are more likely to have a strong effect on the activity of the nerve.

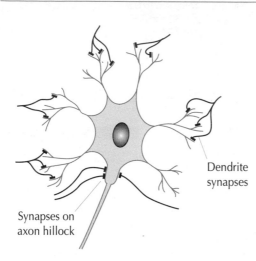

Dendrite synapses

Synapses on axon hillock

Figure 2.10   Transmitter release at a synapse.

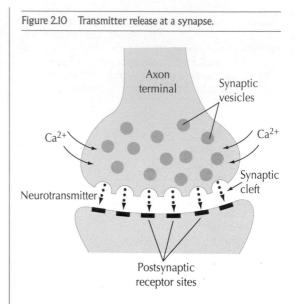

neurotransmitter which is found at several types of synapse in the nervous system, as well as at the nerve–muscle (neuromuscular) junction, is **acetylcholine.**

When the membrane of the synaptic bulb is depolarized, there is an influx of calcium ions from the surrounding extracellular fluid which causes these vesicles to fuse with the cell membrane of the neurone and release their contents into the synaptic cleft (Figure 2.10).

The neurotransmitter then diffuses across the synaptic cleft to bind to specific receptors on the cell membrane of the postsynaptic nerve cell. This subsequently affects the membrane properties of the postsynaptic cell, causing it to become depolarized or hyperpolarized according to the nature of the neurotransmitter released at the synapse.

Neurotransmitters which cause depolarization of the postsynaptic cell are said to be excitatory transmitters, since they bring the membrane potential of the postsynaptic cell closer to threshold for generation of an action potential, i.e. they produce an **excitatory postsynaptic potential (EPSP)**. Those which cause hyperpolarization are said to be inhibitory, since they move the postsynaptic membrane potential further away from threshold, i.e. they produce an **inhibitory postsynaptic potential (IPSP)**. Details of different excitatory and inhibitory neurotransmitters found throughout the nervous system are given in Table 3.3.

The amount of neurotransmitter released by the synaptic vesicles depends on the frequency of action potentials arriving at the synaptic terminal. The greater the action potential frequency, the greater the overall amount of neurotransmitter that is released. As the neurotransmitter is contained in distinct 'packets' (vesicles), an increase in the amount of transmitter released is achieved by having more vesicles release their contents into the synaptic cleft. The greater the amount of transmitter that is released results in a greater change in the postsynaptic membrane potential (postsynaptic potentials are graded in size according to stimulus strength, and therefore do not, like action potentials, obey the all-or-none law). In this way, information can be passed from one nerve cell to the next.

The synapse operates as a 'one-way valve' in that it only allows information to be passed from the presynaptic nerve cell to the postsynaptic nerve cell, but not the other way round. Information flow within the nervous system is therefore in one direction only.

When activity at the synaptic junction has ceased, the remaining neurotransmitter in the synaptic cleft is removed to prevent lingering effects on the postsynaptic cell. This removal occurs by diffusion of the transmitter out of the synaptic cleft, enzymic destruction of the transmitter (e.g. acetylcholinesterase splits acetylcholine into acetate and choline which is subsequently re-used by the presynaptic nerve) or by active transport of the transmitter back into the presynaptic cell.

Spatial and Temporal Summation

The amount of depolarization produced in the postsynaptic cell by the binding of neurotransmitter to the receptors in the cell membrane is not always enough to reach threshold and therefore generate an action potential in the postsynaptic neurone. However, the summation of postsynaptic potentials from the synaptic input of several neurones can be sufficient to bring the membrane to threshold and therefore produce an action potential.

Summation of excitatory postsynaptic potentials can occur in two ways. Firstly, consider a neurone which receives input from several presynaptic cells. Whilst the individual postsynaptic potentials generated by each of these inputs alone may not be enough to bring the postsynaptic membrane to threshold, if the input from several

cells is received simultaneously, the size of the accompanying postsynaptic potentials will be added together. This addition of postsynaptic potentials is known as **spatial summation** and may be sufficient to bring the membrane potential above threshold and so generate an action potential (Figure 2.11a).

Secondly, if inputs from several presynaptic neurones are received within a short period of time from each other (usually < 10 ms), the postsynaptic potentials which individually may not be sufficient to bring the membrane to threshold may overlap in time and so summate to produce a larger postsynaptic potential sufficient to reach threshold. This is known as **temporal summation** (Figure 2.11b).

Combinations of excitatory and inhibitory postsynaptic potentials produce changes in the membrane potential dependent on the relative sizes of the individual EPSPs and IPSPs (Figure 2.11c).

A single EPSP, which on its own would be sufficient to bring the membrane potential to threshold and generate an action potential, may be reduced in size below threshold by the influence of a simultaneous IPSP (Figure 2.11d).

Neurones within the central nervous system receive many inputs, both excitatory and inhibitory. The spatial and temporal combinations of these inputs ensure that a high level of integration of information occurs in these neurones. This is especially important for the modulation of nervous activity associated with motor output at the level of the spinal cord.

Presynaptic Inhibition

One further mechanism for modulation of synaptic activity exists. This is **presynaptic inhibition**. Here, synaptic input onto the axon terminal of

Figure 2.11 Spatial and temporal summation. The top of this figure shows a nerve cell which receives four separate synaptic inputs, A, B, C and D. Input C is shown in black to represent an inhibitory input. (a) Spatial summation – input from synapse A or synapse B alone produces only subthreshold potentials. Simultaneous inputs from A and B summate to elicit a greater postsynaptic potential which now exceeds threshold and generates an action potential. (b) Temporal summation – input from synapse A or synapse B alone produces only subthreshold potentials. Input from synapse A followed very shortly by input from synapse B is now sufficient to raise the membrane potential to threshold and generate an action potential. (c) Input from synapse A alone produces a subthreshold membrane depolarization, while input from synapse C (an inhibitory input) produces membrane hyperpolarization. Input from A and C simultaneously produces a small hyperpolarization. (d) Input from synapse D alone is sufficient to raise the membrane potential to threshold and generate an action potential. Simultaneous input from D and C produces only a subthreshold depolarization due to the hyperpolarizing influence of synapse C.

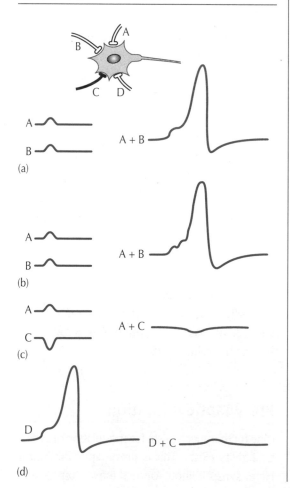

(a)

(b)

(c)

(d)

the presynaptic cell can depolarize the axon terminal, thereby reducing the amplitude of the presynaptic action potential. The outcome of this is less neurotransmitter will be released from the axon terminal, leading to a reduction in the postsynaptic potential generated (Figure 2.12). This will affect whether or not a postsynaptic action potential will be produced.

Pre- and postsynaptic modulation of nervous activity is essential in the normal functioning of the nervous system. Examples of the importance of this are illustrated in later sections.

General Organization of the Nervous System

The nerve cells which have been previously described here and in Chapter 1, together with cells adding structural support, make up the nervous system. The function of the nervous system is to process information from the external environment obtained through sensory

Figure 2.12 Effect of presynaptic inhibition on transmitter release at a synapse.

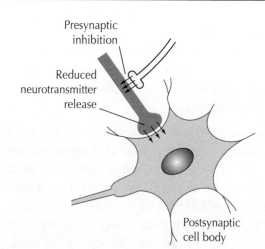

Presynaptic inhibition

Reduced neurotransmitter release

Postsynaptic cell body

receptors in the periphery, and to modulate motor function in response to this information. Higher cognitive functions also exist in the higher centres of the nervous system.

The general organization of the nervous system is summarized in Figure 2.13. The nervous system can be split into central and peripheral components. The central component comprises the brain and the spinal cord. The spinal cord receives sensory information from, and sends motor signals to, the periphery via the spinal nerves. The peripheral nervous system consists of the autonomic and somatic nervous systems. The autonomic nervous system coordinates involuntary and, to a large extent, unconscious motor responses in the smooth muscles of the body. This is achieved through the actions of sympathetic and parasympathetic nerves and hormones such as adrenaline. The somatic nervous system is concerned with sensory and motor nerve supply to different areas of the periphery.

The Brain

The brain is the main integrative centre of the nervous system, responsible for the complex processing of a huge variety of information and for such seemingly intangible concepts as thinking, feeling and imagination. Some of the principal structures of the brain are shown in Figure 2.14.

The most substantial of the brain structures are the cerebral hemispheres. The surface of these hemispheres is highly convoluted, throwing the surface into many folds which greatly increase the surface area of the hemispheres. This folding of the surface produces raised portions (the **gyri**) and hidden portions (the **sulci**).

The surface layer of the cerebral hemispheres is the **cortex**. The cortex is only about 0.5-cm thick, but it contains in total about 14 billion neurones. However, it is not the number of neurones alone which is important. Rather, it is the number of connections between the neurones that gives the cortex its vast integrating power. Each neurone can receive thousands of inputs from other neurones and, in turn, can send outputs to many thousands of other neurones. The total number of interneuronal connections within the cerebral cortex is therefore astronomical.

The cerebral hemispheres can be divided into several **lobes**. These are the **parietal, occipital temporal** and **frontal** lobes, each with some degree of functional specialization. In addition, the cortex can also be divided into different areas according to the types of cells found in each area.

Figure 2.13   General organization of the nervous system.

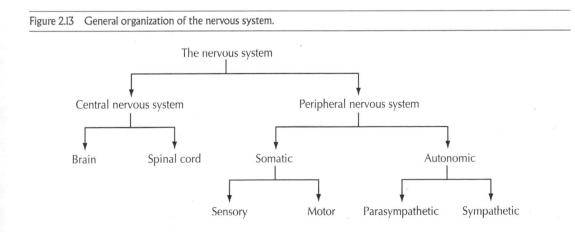

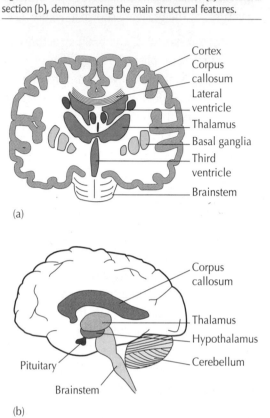

Figure 2.14 The brain shown in a frontal section (a) and lateral section (b), demonstrating the main structural features.

(a)

Cortex
Corpus callosum
Lateral ventricle
Thalamus
Basal ganglia
Third ventricle
Brainstem

(b)

Corpus callosum
Thalamus
Hypothalamus
Cerebellum
Pituitary
Brainstem

Details of the structure and function of some of these areas will be given below.

The two cerebral hemispheres are anatomically and functionally joined to each other by a bridge of nerve fibres known as the **corpus callosum**. This allows for interhemisphere communication, essential for normal functioning. Experiments in the 1960s, in which the corpus callosum was severed during surgery for the relief of severe epilepsy (so-called 'split-brain studies'), demonstrated the functional specialization of the right and left hemispheres. The left hemisphere is primarily concerned with language, speech and communication, abstract thinking and mathematical computation. In contrast, the right hemisphere is specialized for interpretation of spatial informa-

tion such as pattern recognition (e.g. face recognition), and sound perception and appreciation (e.g. music and voices).

There are several subcortical structures which play important roles in the normal functioning of the brain. The functioning of some of these, notably the thalamus, basal ganglia and the cerebellum, will be given later.

The Brainstem and Spinal Cord

The brain is in two-way communication with the peripheral nervous system via the brainstem and spinal cord.

The brainstem comprises several important structures – the **midbrain, pons** and **medulla oblongata**. Within these structures are nuclei of cells which have a significant role in motor control and which are influenced by descending and ascending inputs from the brain and spinal cord, respectively.

The spinal cord represents the lowest level of integrative power within the nervous system and is subject to a large amount of control from higher centres. Nevertheless, the neural organization within the spinal cord is still sufficient to enable a wide range of complex motor acts to be carried out without the need to involve higher centres. These can range from the generation of a pattern of nervous activity necessary to produce a rhythmical walking pattern, to the stereotyped nervous reaction to a particular stimulus – the spinal reflex.

In cross-section, the spinal cord shows a central portion of butterfly-shaped grey matter which contains the cell bodies of the spinal neurones. This is surrounded by the white matter which comprises the axons of nerve fibres passing up and down the cord (Figure 2.15a).

The spinal cord receives information from, and

Figure 2.15   (a) General structure of a spinal cord segment, showing the white and grey matter and dorsal and ventral spinal nerve roots. (b) Segmental organization of the spinal cord, showing cervical (C1–C8), thoracic (T1–T12), lumbar (L1–L5) and sacral (S1–S5) segments. The cauda equina (horse's tail) is the region in the spinal column where only the spinal nerves are present, the spinal cord itself actually being shorter than the spinal column. ((b) Adapted from Pansky and Allen (1980) *Review of Neuroscience*. New York, Macmillan.)

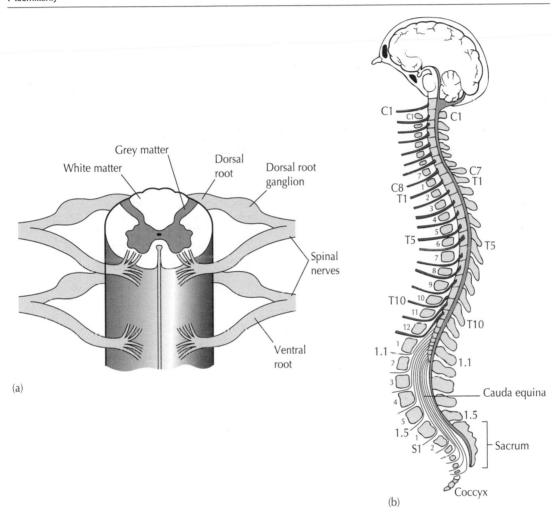

sends signals to, the periphery via the spinal nerves. Information passes into the cord along **afferent** nerve fibres via the dorsal root of the spinal nerve, and signals from the cord to the muscles in the periphery leave via the ventral root, travelling along **efferent** nerve fibres. The spinal nerves leave the spinal cord on both sides at particular levels throughout the length of the cord, effectively dividing the spinal cord into different segments. These are divided into cervical, thoracic, lumbar, and sacral segments depending on their point of exit from the vertebral column (Figure 2.15b).

The spinal nerves supply different areas of the body, providing a motor output to the muscles of that area and conveying sensory information from that area to the cord. There is therefore a **segmental innervation** of different body areas. This is perhaps best seen in the pattern of sensory innervation of different skin areas — the **dermatomes** (Figure 2.16).

A similar, but less distinct, pattern exists for the segmental innervation of the muscles.

The Autonomic Nervous System

The division of the peripheral nervous system which deals with the unconscious and involuntary control of many of the body's systems is the autonomic nervous system. This control serves to regulate the functions of the internal organs and blood vessels and adapt their activity to the immediate needs of the body.

The organs supplied by the autonomic nervous system include the heart, blood vessels, glands, alimentary canal and lungs.

The autonomic nervous system can be split into two anatomically and functionally separate divisions — the **sympathetic** and **parasympathetic** divisions. These two divisions leave the spinal cord at different segmental levels; the sympa-

Figure 2.16   Segmental innervation of different skin areas — the dermatomes. The spinal nerves which supply each area of the skin are indicated on the diagram. (Adapted from Pansky and Allen (1980) *Review of Neuroscience*. New York, Macmillan.)

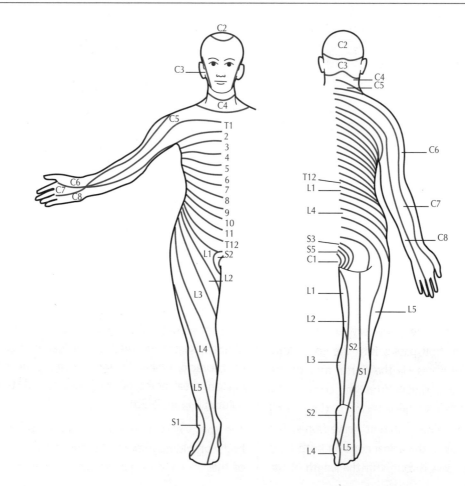

thetic fibres leave the cord at the thoracic and lumbar levels, while the parasympathetic fibres leave the cord from the lower portion of the brainstem – the cranial segments – and from the sacral segments. Organs still receive innervation from both divisions of the autonomic nervous system – dual innervation.

Both divisions of the autonomic nervous system are arranged in a two-neurone pathway. The synapses between these neurones occurs outside the central nervous system in groups of cell bodies, known as **ganglia**. The sympathetic ganglia lie close to the spinal cord in the **sympathetic chain** – a series of ganglia lying vertically alongside the vertebral column. There are also a number of other sympathetic ganglia which lie nearer to the target organ. The parasympathetic ganglia lie close to, or within, the target organ itself.

The two divisions of the autonomic nervous system also differ in the neurotransmitters that are used at the two synapses in the pathway. In both cases, the synapse at the ganglion, between pre- and postganglionic neurones, utilizes **acetylcholine**. However, in the sympathetic division, the transmitter used at the junction between the postganglionic fibre and the target tissue is **noradrenaline**. The parasympathetic division utilizes acetylcholine at the junction between the postganglionic fibre and the target tissue.

Figure 2.17 summarizes these details in diagrammatic form.

The actions of the autonomic nervous system on different target organs depend on a number of factors, including the transmitter released and the types of receptor for that transmitter which are present on the cell membranes of the target tissue.

The binding of a transmitter to postjunctional receptor sites alters the intracellular properties

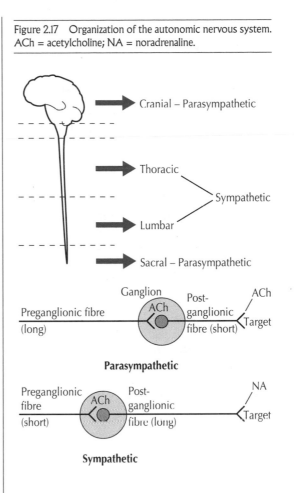

Figure 2.17 Organization of the autonomic nervous system. ACh = acetylcholine; NA = noradrenaline.

of the cell causing a modification of cellular function. Examples of this include smooth muscle contraction or relaxation, or an increase or decrease in the force of contraction of cardiac muscle.

There can be several types of receptor for the same transmitter, producing different responses to that transmitter in different target tissues. There are two types of receptor for acetylcholine – **nicotinic** and **muscarinic receptors**.

- Nicotinic receptors, as well as being stimulated by acetylcholine, are also stimulated by the drug nicotine. These types of receptors are found on the postsynaptic neurones of the

Table 2.1

Effects of the Sympathetic and Parasympathetic Systems on Various Organs

Organ	Sympathetic action	Parasympathetic action
Eyes	Dilates pupil (smooth muscle relaxation)	Constricts pupil (smooth muscle contraction)
Airways	Dilation (smooth muscle relaxation; beta-receptors)	Constriction (smooth muscle contraction)
Heart	Increased heart rate; increased contractility (beta-receptors)	Decreased heart rate; decreased contractility
Blood vessels (arterioles)	Constriction (smooth muscle contraction; alpha-receptors)	No major effect
Gut	Decreased motility, decreased secretion, contraction of sphincters	Increased motility, increased secretion, relaxation of sphincters
Adrenal medulla	Activation	No effect
Bladder	No major effect	Contraction
Genitalia	Ejaculation	Erection

autonomic ganglia and also on motor endplates at the neuromuscular junction.

- Muscarinic receptors are sensitive to the drug muscarine, as well as to acetylcholine. These receptors are found on parasympathetic target organs.

Similarly, different subtypes of receptors exist for noradrenaline. There are basically two types of these — alpha- and beta-receptors — although these can also be divided into further subgroups. Noradrenaline can therefore produce differing effects on target organs depending on which type of receptor is present. This is perhaps more obvious when the effects of both the parasympathetic and sympathetic systems on different organs are considered. In the majority of cases, the two systems work antagonistically to each other, but in some situations they can operate in parallel. Table 2.1 summarizes the effects of both systems on different organs.

In general terms, the parasympathetic system is regarded as energy-conserving, while the sympathetic system is concerned with energy expenditure.

Bibliography

Cohen, H (1993) *Neuroscience for Rehabilitation*. Lippincott, Philadelphia.

Kandel, ER, Schwartz, JH, Jessel, TM (1991) *Principles of Neural Science*. 3rd Edition. Appleton and Lange, Connecticut.

Kiernan, JA (1987) *Introduction to Human Neuroscience*. Lippincott, Philadelphia.

Nicholls, JG, Martin, AR, Wallace, BG (1992) *From Neuron to Brain*. 3rd Edition. Sinauer, Sunderland, MA.

Readings from *Scientific American* (1993) Mind and Brain. Freeman, San Francisco.

Rothwell, J (1994) *Control of Human Voluntary Movement*. 2nd Edition. Chapman and Hall, London.

3

The Nervous System: The Neurophysiology of Movement

Spinal Reflexes
•
The Spinal Cord
•
Cortical Control of Movement
•
Spasticity
•
The Basal Ganglia and the Extrapyramidal Motor System
•
The Cerebellum
•
Nervous System and Motor Control: Summary

Spinal Reflexes

Basic Principles

In studying the neurophysiology of movement, it is often a convenient starting point to deal with the simplest type of coordinated motor function, which also has the simplest type of neuronal circuits: the spinal reflexes. These can also serve as a basis for the description and interpretation of the more complicated motor acts which are brought about by the action of higher centres in the nervous system. The spinal reflexes, and their modulation, are also the basis for several therapeutic techniques such as proprioceptive

neuromuscular facilitation (PNF) and cutaneous stimulation techniques.

The basic organization of a reflex can be summarized as follows:

- Input to the spinal cord
- Relay circuitry
- Output from the spinal cord

The basic anatomical organization of these elements is shown in Figure 3.1.

INPUT TO THE SPINAL CORD

Input to the spinal cord initially arises from peripheral sensory receptors which have been activated by some form of external stimulus. This information from the sensory receptors is con-

Figure 3.1 Basic organization of spinal reflexes. (1) Afferent input to the spinal cord via sensory nerves. (2) Central relay within the spinal cord via interneurones. (3) Efferent output from the spinal cord via motoneurones. The cell bodies of the sensory afferents are located in the dorsal root ganglion. Neurones in this, and subsequent, diagrams are illustrated by a circle representing the cell body, a line representing the nerve axon and a V representing the synaptic terminal of the axon.

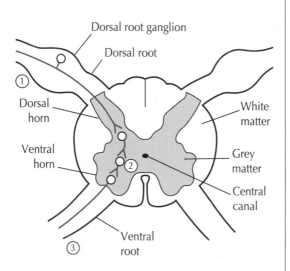

veyed to the spinal cord via **afferent nerves** (afferent: conveying information *towards* the central nervous system). These afferent nerve fibres arrive at the spinal cord via the spinal nerves and enter the cord via the dorsal roots. Some of these sensory receptors and the stimuli to which they are sensitive are summarized in Table 3.1.

The afferent nerves which connect these various receptors to the spinal cord vary in their diameter and in their speed of conduction of action potentials (or impulses) to the cord. The larger the diameter of the nerve fibre, the faster the impulse conduction velocity. These diferences in diameter and conduction velocity form the basis of classification of afferent nerve fibres. The characteristics of these afferent types are summarized in Table 3.2.

RELAY CIRCUITRY

The elements responsible for relaying incoming information to the output stage of the reflex are the **interneurones**. The number of interneurones in the spinal cord outnumber the motoneurones by about 30:1.

The number of interneurones participating in a reflex can vary. There may be none. A reflex which involves no interneurones therefore has only one synapse between the input stage and the output stage of the reflex and is therefore termed a **monosynaptic reflex**. Reflexes involving one, two or more interneurones are termed **disynaptic**, **trisynaptic** and **polysynaptic** reflexes, respectively, depending on the number of synaptic connections in the reflex circuit.

The actions of interneurones in the spinal cord can be either excitatory or inhibitory, depending on the transmitter substance released at the synapse with the next neurone in the pathway. Table 3.3 illustrates some excitatory and inhibitory neurotransmitters found in spinal cord interneurones and elsewhere in the central nervous system.

The large number of interneurones in the spinal cord and the subsequent convergence of input from various sources onto different components of the output stage of the reflex illustrate that there is a vast opportunity for a high degree of neuronal integration to occur within the spinal cord. The importance of this possibility for integration will be dealt with later (p. 68–70).

OUTPUT FROM THE SPINAL CORD

The function of the reflex output from the spinal cord is to somehow modify motor behaviour or muscle activity. The final output stage of the reflex is therefore the motoneurones. These nerve fibres leave the spinal cord to travel to the muscles and are termed **efferent nerve fibres** (efferent: conveying information *away from* the central nervous system). These nerve fibres leave the spinal cord

Table 3.1
Examples of Some Sensory Receptors Found in The Body and The Stimuli to Which They Respond

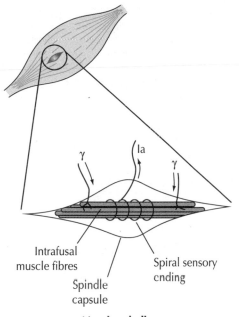

Muscle spindle

Muscle spindles are encapsulated receptors (up to 10 mm in length) located within skeletal muscles and which are sensitive to changes in muscle length. Stretch of the muscle elongates the spindle and so distends the spiral sensory ending. This increases the discharge of the Ia afferent fibre, thereby signalling the length change to the central nervous system. The muscle spindle also contains specialized skeletal muscle fibres – the Intrafusal fibres – which are supplied by gamma (γ) fusimotor motoneurones. When the intrafusal muscle fibres contract, they can increase the sensitivity of the spiral ending to stretch. Gamma motoneurone activity also maintains spindle discharge during skeletal muscle contraction. In addition to the spiral sensory ending, the muscle spindle also possesses secondary sensory endings (not shown) which are located nearer the poles of the spindle. These give rise to slower group II afferent fibres. The primary spiral endings signal the rate of change of muscle length as well as the final length change, i.e. they are velocity-sensitive as well as length-sensitive. The secondary endings are more sensitive to the final length change and have little velocity-sensitivity. The number of muscle spindles present in different in different muscles is variable – a large muscle such as quadriceps can have over two hundred spindles

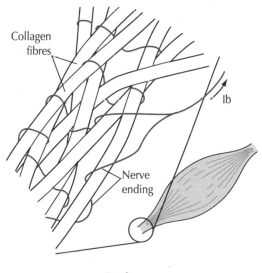

Tendon organ

Golgi tendon organs (GTOs) are sensitive to changes in muscle tension and are located within the collagen fibres of the muscle tendon. The nerve endings interweave throughout the network of collagen fibres. When the muscle contracts the collagen fibres straighten out, thereby compressing the nerve endings running between them. This compression increases the discharge of the nerve endings, thereby signalling the increase in tension. This information is transmitted to the central nervous system via the Ib afferent fibres

Table 3.1 (*Continued*)

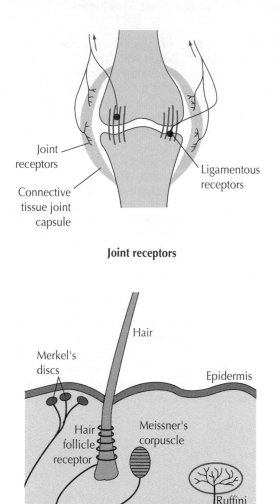

Joint receptors are mechanoreceptors located within the connective tissue capsule of the joint and within the joint ligaments. Movement of the joint causes deformation of the capsule or ligaments, thereby altering the discharge of the joint receptors. The joint receptor discharge is position sensitive, and so signals changes in joint position to the central nervous system via group II afferent fibres. Different classes of joint receptor are rapidly- and slowly-adapting and therefore contribute to the sensitivity to rate of change of joint angle and static joint position

Joint receptors

The skin contains many different types of sensory receptor, some of which are shown in this diagram. Merkel's discs and Ruffini endings are pressure receptors located in the upper portions of the skin which signal the intensity of the pressure being applied. Hair follicle receptors respond to movement of the hairs on the skin surface and are velocity-sensitive. Meissner's corpuscles and Pacinian corpuscles are rapidly-adapting receptors which respond to vibratory stimuli applied to the skin. The free nerve endings are nociceptors which respond to noxious mechanical and chemical stimuli. In each of these cases, the nature of the receptor's accessory structure associated with the nerve ending is important in determining the receptor's function

Cutaneous receptors

Table 3.1 (*Continued*)

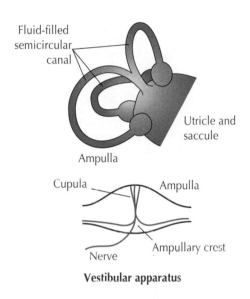

Fluid-filled semicircular canal

Utricle and saccule

Ampulla

Cupula

Ampulla

Nerve

Ampullary crest

Vestibular apparatus

The vestibular apparatus is located in the inner ear and consists of the semicircular canals and the utricle and saccule. The vestibular system is sensitive to changes in the position of the head and body in space. The three semicircular canals are oriented at roughly right angles to each other, parallel to each of the three x, y and z axes. They are fluid-filled and have a widening — the ampulla — which contains the sensory portion of the canal. Within the ampulla, there is a crest (or crista) which projects up into the ampulla. The upper surface of the crest contains numerous specialized hair cells which project into the jelly-like cupula. Since the semicircular canals are fluid-filled, any movement of the head will induce movement of the fluid inside the canals. This fluid movement pushes on the cupula causing it to bend. As it does so, it also bends the hairs which are embedded in it. This alters the discharge of the nerve fibres associated with the hair cells, thereby signalling the change in head position to the central nervous system. These receptors are most sensitive to acceleration and deceleration of the canal. Since the canals are oriented in each of the three planes, movement of the head in any direction can be detected by the summation and integration of the nervous activity from all three canals, together with the activity in the canals on the opposite side of the head. The utricle and saccule are collectively known as the otolith organ which signals the direction of the force of gravity. The sensory portions of the otolith organ are known as the maculae — one macula in the saccule oriented vertically and the other in the utricle oriented horizontally. Each macula consists of numerous hair cells projecting into a sheet of gelatinous material which contains calcium carbonate crystals. As the head moves relative to the force of gravity, the gelatinous sheet shifts over the hair cells, bending them. As with the semicircular canals, this alters the discharge of the nerve fibres associated with the hair cells, and so signals the change in head position to the central nervous system

via the ventral roots and travel to the periphery in the spinal nerve fibres.

Like the afferent nerve fibres, the motoneurones are also classified according to their diameter, conduction velocity and the type of muscle fibre which they supply. This classification is summarized in Table 3.4. The organization of this motor output is important in terms of the final alteration in muscle activity. To explain this, it is first useful to define the functional element of motor output — the **motor unit**. The motor unit is defined as a

Table 3.2

Classification of Afferent Nerve Fibres, Based on Axon Diameter and Conduction Velocity

Afferent type	Diameter (μm)	Conduction velocity (m s^{-1})	Examples
Group I	12–20	70–12	Ia from muscle spindle, Ib from tendon organ
Group II	5–12	30–70	Spindle secondary ending, joint receptors, touch, pressure receptors in skin
Group III	2–5	12–30	Some pressure receptors, thermoreceptors, nociceptors
Group IV	0.5–2	0.5–1	Nociceptors, some thermoreceptors

Table 3.3

Neurotransmitters Found Throughout the Central Nervous System and their Synaptic Actions.

Acetylcholine	Excitatory and inhibitory
Amino acids	
Glutamate	Excitatory
Aspartate	Excitatory
Gamma-aminobutyric acid	Inhibitory
Glycine	Inhibitory
Amines	
Dopamine	Excitatory and inhibitory
Noradrenaline	Excitatory and inhibitory
Adrenaline	Excitatory and inhibitory
Histamine	Excitatory and inhibitory
5-Hydroxytryptamine (serotonin)	Excitatory and inhibitory
Peptides	
Substance P	Excitatory
Enkephalins	Inhibitory
Endorphins	Inhibitory

For those neurotransmitters which can display both excitatory and inhibitory actions, the nature of the action is determined by the type of receptor for the transmitter found on the postsynaptic cell membrane

Table 3.4

Classification of Motoneurones According to Axon Diameter and Conduction Velocity

Motoneurone	Diameter (μm)	Conduction velocity (m s^{-1})	Examples
Alpha	9–17	50–100	Extrafusal muscle fibres
Beta	10–15	60–90	Extra- and intrafusal muscle fibres
Gamma	1–8	10–35	Intrafusal muscle fibres

Figure 3.2 Organization of a motor unit. In this case, the motor unit comprises a single motoneurone which branches to supply four separate muscle fibres.

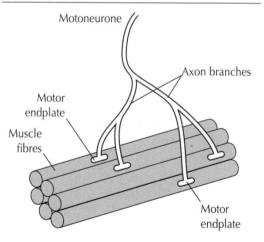

single motoneurone plus the muscle fibres which it supplies (Figure 3.2). The size of individual motor units is very variable: a small motor unit would be defined as a single motoneurone supplying only a very few muscle fibres; a large motor unit would be defined as a single motoneurone supplying up to several hundreds or, in some cases, thousands of muscle fibres.

It will be clear that the smaller the motor unit, the more finely controlled will be the movement produced by activation of that motor unit, since it involves the activation of only a few muscle fibres. In contrast, activation of larger motor units will produce much coarser movements, since many more muscle fibres will be activated. Muscles which are used for fine delicate movements (e.g. finger muscles, extra-ocular muscles of the eye) have a higher proportion of small motor units whereas muscles involved in more gross movements of the limbs or trunk (e.g. gastrocnemius, soleus) consist mainly of large motor units.

This type of organization of motoneurones and muscle fibres allows for two methods for the regulation of motor output:

- **Recruitment:** an increase in muscle tension is produced by bringing gradually more and more motor units into action.
- **Rate coding:** an increase in muscle tension is produced by increasing the rate of motoneurone firing (increased motoneurone action potential frequency).

Recruitment of motor units occurs in an orderly fashion such that small motoneurones and small motor units are recruited first (smaller-diameter motoneurones have the lowest threshold to activation). Increasing the afferent input to the spinal cord, or increasing descending activation of motoneurones will recruit gradually larger and larger motoneurones and motor units. This pattern of motor unit activation is known as the **Henneman size principle**. The size principle means that the recruitment of motor activity allows for finer degrees of motor control to be implemented first before the coarser movements occur.

Rate coding of motoneurone firing ensures that the active motor units and muscle fibres can participate in the summation of muscle twitches to provide a greater force of contraction (see Chapter 6, p. 107).

Reflexes Involving Ia Afferents

MONOSYNAPTIC EXCITATION

Monosynaptic excitation is the basis of the stretch reflex (or tendon jerk) and involves the excitation of alpha motoneurones by Ia afferents arising from muscle spindles (Figure 3.3). The purpose of this reflex is to cause muscle contraction which resists an original length change in the same muscle. Since this reflex involves excitation of motoneurones supplying the same muscle from which the stimulus arises, this is known as **homonymous excitation**. It must be borne in mind here that Figure 3.3 shows an oversimplified version of the spinal reflex circuit, and that each Ia afferent from a single muscle spindle makes monosynaptic connections with up to 90% of the alpha motoneurones supplying that muscle, i.e. it is not simply a one-to-one connection as illustrated or implied in the diagram.

Ia afferents can also elicit **heteronymous** excitation, i.e. excitation of alpha motoneurones sup-

Figure 3.3 The monosynaptic stretch reflex.

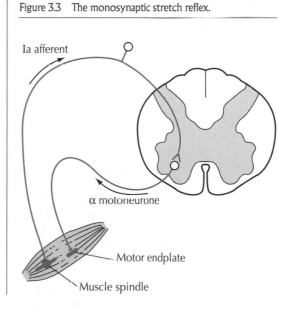

plying muscles different to that in which the original length change occurred. These connections are also monosynaptic and are with alpha motoneurones supplying **synergist** muscles (i.e. muscles which have the same action at the same joint). This group of muscles is known as the Ia synergists.

DISYNAPTIC INHIBITION

Ia afferents also make excitatory connections with interneurones which have an inhibitory input to alpha motoneurones of muscles which are antagonistic in their actions to the homonymous muscle (Figure 3.4). That is, impulses in the Ia afferents can switch on the inhibition of antagonist muscles via an interneurone. This interneurone is known as the **Ia inhibitory interneurone**.

This inhibition of antagonist muscles makes functional sense since it allows a particular movement to occur (stimulated by activation of the agonist muscle and its synergists) without producing

activity in those muscles which have an opposite action. This reflex action is known as **reciprocal inhibition**. Figure 3.4 summarizes the reflex actions of Ia afferents on homonymous, synergist and antagonist muscle groups.

Reflexes Involving Ib Afferents

Ib afferents, arising from Golgi tendon organs are activated by increasing levels of muscle tension. The reflex effect of activating these Ib afferents is to produce an inhibition in the homonymous and synergist motoneurones. This inhibition is achieved by activation of an inhibitory interneurone – the **Ib inhibitory interneurone**. The Ib afferents also disynaptically excite the motoneurones supplying the antagonist muscle groups, thereby causing these muscles to contract. These connections are summarized in Figure 3.5.

The function of the Ib reflex is therefore to act as a tension feedback system. Negative feedback is produced when the tension in the muscle exceeds a certain level and reflexly prevents the

Figure 3.4 Monosynaptic excitation of homonymous and synergist motoneurones and disynaptic reciprocal inhibition of antagonist motoneurones via the Ia inhibitory interneurone. Inhibitory interneurones are indicated by a black cell body and a small dot to represent the synapse. Excitation is indicated by ⊕ and inhibition is indicated by ⊖

Figure 3.5 Disynaptic inhibition of homonymous and synergist motoneurones via the Ib inhibitory interneurone and disynaptic excitation of antagonist motoneurones. Excitation is indicated by ⊕ and inhibition is indicated by ⊖

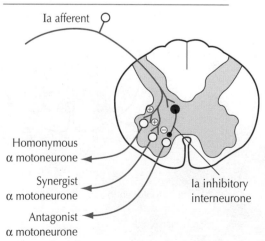

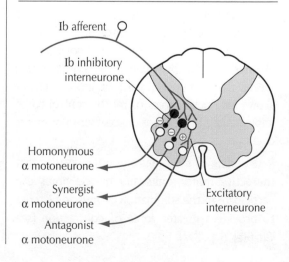

muscle from producing any further tension. This can have a protective function in the prevention of muscle damage caused by excessive muscle tension.

Reflexes involving Ib afferents are not always seen in normal situations as the reflex effects can often be overridden by voluntary input to the spinal cord from higher centres. However, when this voluntary override facility is not present, for example in some instances of spasticity (see p. 82), the true effects of Ib inhibition can sometimes be observed. One such situation involves the **clasp-knife reflex**. This reflex is observed in spastic subjects when an attempt is made to lengthen an extensor muscle. Initially, a resistance to lengthening is observed as the muscle contracts due to the presence of an abnormal stretch reflex. If the attempt to lengthen the muscle is continued, the tension in the muscle suddenly gives way, allowing the muscle to be lengthened freely. This sudden melting of resistance to lengthening is similar to that experienced when attempting to close a penknife — hence the name 'clasp-knife reflex'. The clasp-knife reflex therefore avoids excessive tensions (which may damage the muscle fibres) building up in the muscle due to abnormal stretch reflexes when the muscle is lengthened.

Recent work in this area has indicated that this reflex may also involve afferent contributions from muscle group II (non-spindle), III and IV afferents arising in the stretched muscle.

A further possibility is that changes in Ib afferent input to the spinal cord may have a role in the maintenance of muscle tension during fatigue in sustained contractions. Any sudden decrease in muscle tension due to fatigue would result in a decrease in activation of the Golgi tendon organs and therefore a decrease in the Ib afferent discharge. This decreased Ib afferent input to the

cord will result in a decrease in the inhibitory input to the homonymous and synergist muscle groups (via the Ib inhibitory interneurone) and therefore allow the muscle to develop extra tension.

The Ib inhibitory interneurone also acts as an important relay interneurone for several other types of input to the spinal cord as will be seen later (p. 69).

Reflexes Involving Group II Afferents

The group II classification of afferents covers a wide range of nerve fibres including muscle afferents, cutaneous afferents and joint afferents.

REFLEX CONTRIBUTIONS FROM MUSCLE GROUP II AFFERENTS

Muscle group II afferents arise from muscle spindle secondary sensory endings. Activation of these fibres produces, in general, an excitation of flexor muscle groups and an inhibition of extensor muscle groups. This pattern persists independent of whether the muscle group II afferents arise in flexor or extensor muscles. The excitatory effects from muscle group II afferents on to flexors are mediated by a disynaptic pathway, while the inhibitory effects on to extensors are mediated by a trisynaptic pathway (Figure 3.6). Muscle spindle group II afferents also contribute monosynaptically to activation of the stretch reflex.

Group II afferents from muscle spindles are also thought to play a role in the lengthening reaction observed in the clasp-knife reflex. The reflex inhibition of the extensor mediated by activation of the Ib inhibitory interneurone produces a sudden decrease in the tension which originally

Figure 3.6 Effects of group II afferents on flexor and extensor motoneurones.

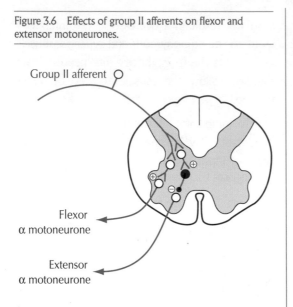

Group II afferent

Flexor
α motoneurone

Extensor
α motoneurone

activated the Golgi tendon organs. It might therefore be thought that this sudden decrease in tendon organ activation would reduce the input to the Ib inhibitory interneurone, thereby allowing muscle tension to redevelop. This does not happen, however, and the muscle remains relaxed and lengthened. It is thought that the sudden lengthening of the extensor muscle will activate

the spindle secondary endings, causing activation of muscle group II afferents which maintain the inhibitory input to the extensor muscle. In this respect, the clasp-knife reflex probably consists of two components — an initial inhibition of the extensor due to tendon organ activation followed by a maintenance of inhibition from activation of spindle secondaries.

REFLEX CONTRIBUTIONS FROM CUTANEOUS GROUP II AFFERENTS

Input from group II afferents arising in the skin also produces excitation of flexor motoneurone pools and inhibition of extensor motoneurone pools. Again, this pattern is consistent and independent of the location of the cutaneous afferents.

The general response of flexor muscles when these group II afferents are activated has led to the term **flexor reflex afferents** (FRAs).

Group III and group IV afferents from skin and muscle also come under the umbrella of flexor reflex afferents since, again, they produce similar

Figure 3.7 Ipsilateral and contralateral reflex effects from flexor reflex afferents — flexor withdrawal and crossed extension. Ipsilateral flexor motoneurones and contralateral extensor motoneurones are excited. Ipsilateral extensors and contralateral flexors are inhibited.

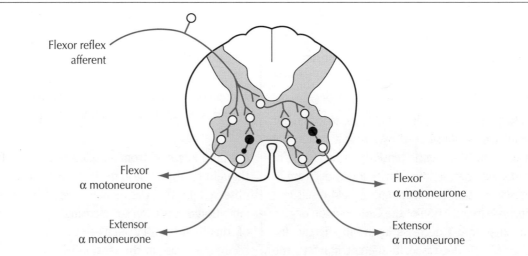

Flexor reflex
afferent

Flexor
α motoneurone

Extensor
α motoneurone

Flexor
α motoneurone

Extensor
α motoneurone

responses. These can range from a slight twitch of the flexors caused by light stimulation of the skin to complete **flexor withdrawal** of the whole limb if the stimulus is noxious.

Accompanying these flexor responses is excitation of extensor motoneurone pools on the contralateral side of the spinal cord, causing **crossed extension** (Figure 3.7). This pattern of activity makes sense since it allows the weight of the body to be supported by contralateral limb extension while the ipsilateral limb is withdrawn from the noxious stimulus.

Electrical stimulation of flexor reflex afferents can be produced in a coordinated pattern in order to elicit motor responses in some subjects with spinal cord injury who have no normal motor control in the lower limbs. This **functional electrical stimulation (FES)** produces motor responses that are coordinated in a functional pattern so that stance and some semblance of gait may be restored in these subjects. Electrically elicited flexor withdrawal responses may be able to produce hip flexion in both limbs in an alternating pattern which can be used to propel the patient.

REFLEX CONTRIBUTIONS FROM SLOWLY-ADAPTING JOINT AFFERENTS

There are several types of slowly-adapting group II joint afferents, with the discharge pattern of each type being dependent on the range of joint angles in which it is active. Some joint receptors display increased activity when the joint is moved towards flexion (**flexion receptors**) whilst others increase their activity as the joint is moved into extension (**extension receptors**). Between these two extremes are other populations of slowly-adapting receptors whose discharge is modulated by mid-range joint angles (Figure 3.8). These joint

Figure 3.8   Action potential firing frequencies in several knee joint afferents at different joint angles in the cat. (From Skoglund (1956) Anatomical and physiological studies of knee joint innervation in the cat. *Acta Physiologica Scandinavica* **36** (suppl. 124) 1–101.) More recent research has demonstrated that the majority of joint receptors discharge at the extremes of joint position, with mid-range joint receptors being rarer.

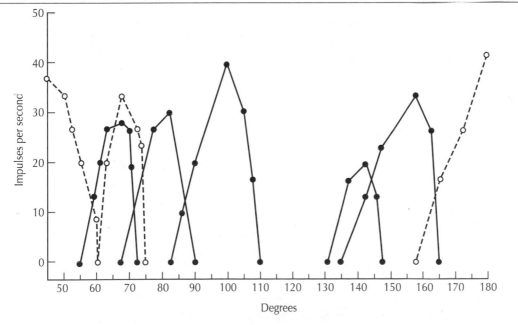

receptors can modulate the activity of spinal reflexes affecting muscles acting at or around that joint. Flexion receptors are capable of inhibiting the excitability of flexion reflexes, whilst extension receptors can inhibit the excitability of extension reflexes. That is, these receptors can modulate reflexes in such a way that the joint will not be moved too far in a particular direction by other reflex activity. For example, if a joint is held in an almost fully flexed position, the strength of any reflex which produces further flexion will be reduced by the modulating influence of flexion receptors. This has an obvious protective role in preventing reflexes from moving the joint into potentially damaging positions. Recent work has demonstrated that the activation of nociceptive group IV joint afferents by inflammation may reduce this influence of group II joint afferents on these flexion and extension reflexes. Subjects with joint inflammation or other joint diseases may, therefore, be more at risk of reflexly moving their joints into potentially damaging positions, which may further exacerbate their condition.

Activation of joint afferents by pathological conditions can also have reflex effects on muscle activity. Increased fluid volume within the joint will stretch the joint capsule and activate joint mechanoreceptors. This is known to be able to inhibit the strength of contraction of the muscles acting at that joint. Such increase in fluid volume within a joint accompanies disease conditions such as rheumatoid arthritis, and may account for muscle weakness and postural changes associated with this disease.

The Spinal Cord

Integration and Convergence

Many interneurones in spinal reflex pathways can receive inputs from more than one source, i.e. these interneurones are not linked exclusively to a particular reflex. These other inputs can include different afferent sources or descending inputs from higher centres. The effect of these other inputs is to modulate the excitability of particular reflex pathways through spatial and temporal summation.

CONVERGENCE ONTO IA INHIBITORY INTERNEURONE

The Ia inhibitory interneurone receives input not only from Ia afferents, but also from higher centres and from antagonistic Ia inhibitory interneurones (Figure 3.9).

Descending inputs onto Ia inhibitory interneurones also make connections with alpha and

Figure 3.9 Convergence of inputs on to Ia inhibitory interneurones (Ia IN) of agonist and antagonist muscles. See text for details.

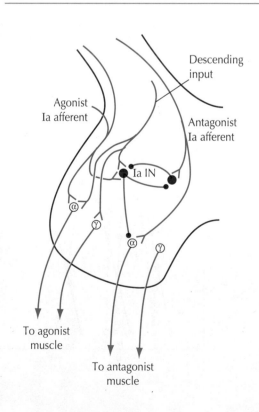

gamma motoneurones supplying the same muscle. These three spinal neurones together form a functional unit. Activation of the functional unit will produce co-activation of alpha and gamma motoneurones as well as reciprocal inhibition of antagonistic muscles. This type of activity is important in voluntary muscle activity since, when the agonist muscle contracts, Ia input from the muscle spindles will be maintained by the gamma input and antagonist stretch reflexes will be inhibited. Additionally, since the agonist Ia inhibitory interneurone converges onto the antagonist Ia inhibitory interneurone, no reciprocal inhibition of the agonist can arise as a consequence of stretch of the antagonist during agonist shortening.

CONVERGENCE ONTO IB INHIBITORY INTERNEURONE

As well as receiving Ib input from tendon organs, the Ib inhibitory interneurone also receives input from a variety of sources: low-threshold cutaneous and joint afferents, excitatory descending inputs (corticospinal, rubrospinal) and inhibitory descending inputs (reticulospinal) (Figure 3.10).

Activation of skin and joint afferents can therefore alter the excitability of reflexes and motoneurone pools via the Ib inhibitory interneurone. The functional importance of these inputs concerns the ability to reflexly inhibit muscle contraction when joints are moved to the limits of their range of movement or when obstacles are encountered during a particular movement.

The presence of these varied inputs to spinal interneurones and their capability of modulating the excitability of reflex pathways has important implications for physiotherapy practice. Techniques such as proprioceptive neuromuscular facilitation, the Rood techniques and passive and active stretching techniques will all in some way

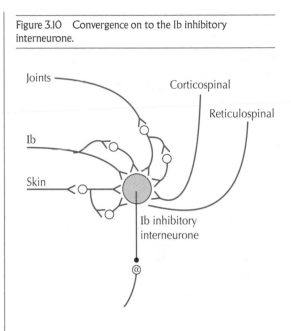

Figure 3.10   Convergence on to the Ib inhibitory interneurone.

alter afferent input to the spinal motoneurones and, in doing so, will alter motor output.

Recurrent Inhibition

One further way in which motoneurone activity can be influenced by interneurones is by **recurrent inhibition**. Axonal branches of the alpha motoneurones can excite a special population of interneurone — the **Renshaw cell**. These are inhibitory interneurones which feed back to the pool of homonymous alpha motoneurones which originally excited them (Figure 3.11). The Renshaw cells release the neurotransmitter glycine to produce inhibition of the alpha motoneurones. The Renshaw cells also project to the motoneurones of synergist muscles.

The function of this recurrent inhibition is to limit the output of motoneurones so that only strongly activated motor units will remain active, with activity in weakly activated motor units being suppressed. Rapid alterations in the firing rate of motoneurones is also controlled by recurrent

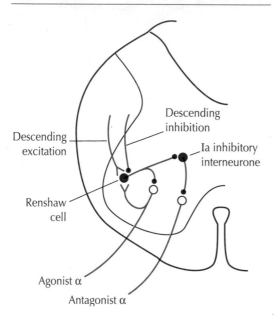

Figure 3.11 Recurrent inhibition. The Renshaw cell and connections with agonist and antagonist neurones. The Renshaw cell also receives descending excitatory and inhibitory inputs.

inhibition; as the firing rate of a motoneurone increases, so too will the amount of recurrent inhibition increase, thereby limiting the change in firing rate.

Renshaw cells also send branches to the Ia inhibitory interneurones acting on the motoneurones of antagonist muscles (Figure 3.11). This therefore means that they also reduce the Ia inhibition acting on the antagonists.

The excitability of Renshaw cells can also be influenced by descending inputs, thereby altering the overall excitability of the motoneurone pool.

Descending Inputs to the Spinal Cord

As well as convergence from afferent fibres arising from peripheral sensory receptors, spinal moto-

neurones also receive descending input from higher centres in the central nervous system. These descending inputs can directly control the activity of the spinal motoneurones, or can modulate the excitability of spinal reflexes affecting these motoneurones. Figure 3.12(a) shows the main descending inputs to the spinal cord. Figure

Figure 3.12 (a) Descending inputs to the spinal cord. (b) Cross-section of spinal cord showing location of descending spinal tracts in the white matter.

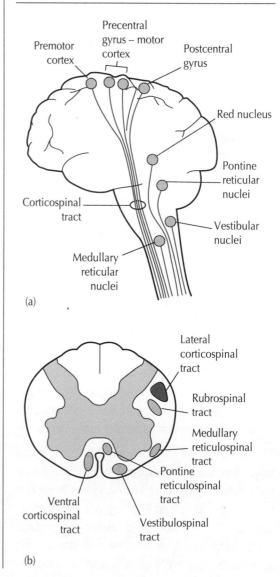

3.12(b) shows the location of the nerve tracts from these higher centres in the spinal cord white matter. The tracts are always named with the source of the nerve fibres given first followed by their destination (e.g. corticospinal tract fibres originate in the cortex and terminate in the spinal cord; rubrospinal tract fibres originate in the red nucleus and terminate in the spinal cord). The location of these tracts within the spinal cord white matter is important when considering spinal cord lesions and which tracts might be affected by these.

The descending tracts terminate and make synaptic connections within the spinal cord grey matter. The grey matter can be divided into several layers, based on the types of cells found in each layer. These are known as Rexed's laminae, after the Swedish neuroanatomist who proposed these divisions. These laminae will be dealt with in more detail later, but for now can be grouped into two main regions (Figure 3.13).

Region A represents the ventromedial portion of the grey matter and contains motoneurones which innervate proximal muscle groups. Region B represents the dorsolateral portion of the grey matter and contains motoneurones which supply the distal muscle groups of the extremities.

Figure 3.13   Grouping of spinal cord grey matter laminae. Region (A), ventromedial portion; region (B), dorsolateral portion.

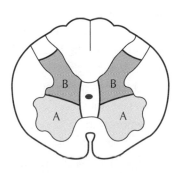

Medullary and pontine reticulospinal tract fibres and vestibulospinal tract fibres terminate in region A of the grey matter and therefore collectively form the ventromedial pathways in the spinal cord. The rubrospinal tract terminates in region B and therefore forms a dorsolateral pathway.

The ventromedial pathways are important in the control of balance and posture, which relies on the activity of proximal muscles, and are also important in the integration of body and limb movements, orientation movements for the body and head and are important in maintaining the direction of locomotion. The ventromedial pathways have a wide distribution of terminals throughout the grey matter, with some terminating on both sides of the spinal cord, and sending branches to different spinal segments via long propriospinal interneurones.

The dorsolateral pathways are important in the coordination of movement in guiding the extremities and for providing fine control of movement, which relies on distal muscle groups. There is some degree of intersegmental diffusion via short propriospinal interneurones.

CORTICOSPINAL TRACT

The main descending pathway involved in motor control is that which leaves the motor cortex and travels to the lower motoneurones in the spinal cord. This is the **corticospinal tract** (or pyramidal tract). The axons which run in the corticospinal tract are also known as the upper motoneurones and originate in several cortical areas which lie close to the central sulcus of the cerebral hemispheres. Thirty per cent of the axons originate in area 4 (the precentral gyrus), which is the primary motor cortex. Thirty per cent of the axons originate in area 6 (the premotor cortex) while 40% of the axons originate in areas 1, 2, 3 (the sensorimotor cortex) and area 8, which is concerned with coordination of eye movements (Figure 3.14).

The corticospinal axons travel down to the medulla, where the majority of fibres cross the midline at the pyramidal decussation. These crossed fibres travel in the dorsolateral fasciculus of the spinal cord to form the **lateral corticospinal tract**. Uncrossed corticospinal fibres originate mainly in area 6 (with some originating in area 4 which are concerned with neck and trunk movements). These fibres run in the ventral columns of the spinal cord, forming the **ventral corticospinal tract**. Of the crossed fibres, a few terminate on both sides of the spinal cord, while more of the uncrossed fibres will do this (Figure 3.15).

The terminations of these corticospinal fibres are slightly different for the two corticospinal tracts. Lateral corticospinal tract fibres terminate on interneurones in the intermediate zone and motor nuclei of the spinal cord grey matter – specifically the motoneurone pools supplying distal limb muscles. The lateral corticospinal fibres also project to sensory neurone terminals in the dorsal horn (laminae IV and V). Ventral corticospinal fibres project to motoneurone

Figure 3.14 Brodmann's classification of motor areas in the cerebral cortex. The numbers of the different cortical areas are derived from Brodmann's original classification based on cortical cell architecture.

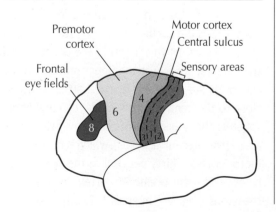

Figure 3.15 Organization of the lateral and ventral corticospinal tracts. The lateral corticospinal tract carries crossed motor fibres from the motor areas of the cerebral cortex and terminates in the intermediate zone and motor nuclei of the spinal cord grey matter. The ventral corticospinal tract carries uncrossed motor fibres from the motor cortex and terminates in the motoneurone pools of the proximal and axial muscle groups.

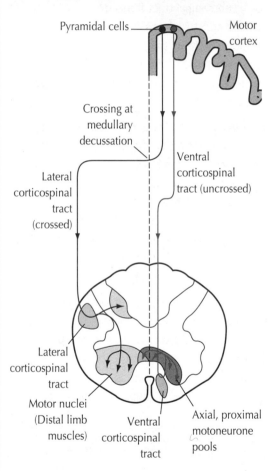

pools on both sides of the spinal cord which supply axial and proximal muscle groups, and also to interneurones in the intermediate zone. Recent evidence suggests that this corticospinal innervation of bilateral motoneurone pools is especially important for those muscle groups which must demonstrate a coordinated bilateral activity, such as the respiratory muscles and jaw muscles. Ventral corticospinal tract fibres also send branches to the brainstem nuclei.

Since corticospinal tract fibres can terminate directly on spinal cord motoneurones, the motor cortex therefore has the ability to control individual muscles and muscle groups independently of each other. This is known as **fractionation of movement**.

EFFECTS OF SPINAL CORD LESIONS ON DESCENDING PATHWAYS

Lesions of the corticospinal tracts may be due to vascular disease, tumours, trauma or as a result of demyelinating diseases. The consequences of corticospinal tract lesions are displayed as negative signs (where there is some loss of normal motor function) or positive signs (where there is an abnormal motor response as a result of removal of normal descending inhibitory influences on the spinal cord; these positive signs are sometimes referred to as 'release phenomena').

One example of a negative sign is the loss of fractionation observed in lesions of the lateral corticospinal tract. Here, there is a loss of direct descending control of the spinal motoneurones. Experiments on sectioning the lateral corticospinal tracts of monkeys have shown that subjects, as well as demonstrating weakness and generally slow voluntary contractions, are no longer able to perform precision movements of the distal muscle groups, and are therefore unable to grasp small objects between two fingers, most noticeably the thumb and forefinger. When grasping is attempted, the hand acts as a crude shovel, or all fingers contract simultaneously. There is, however, no impairment to posture or balance, as these involve the axial and proximal muscle groups controlled by the ventral corticospinal tracts. When lesions affect the ventral tracts, subjects have difficulty in sitting or standing and maintaining an upright posture.

An example of a positive sign accompanying lesions of the lateral corticospinal tract is the Babinski sign. Here, stroking of the outer sole of the foot results in fanning of the toes and extension of the big toe. The normal response is to produce flexion of all of the toes, including the big toe. This response is an enhanced withdrawal reflex which has been 'released' due to the corticospinal tract lesion removing the normal descending inhibition of this reaction. The Babinski sign is only seen in normal situations in infants, where there is incomplete myelination of the corticospinal tracts.

Complete transection of the spinal cord results in a complete and immediate loss of all motor activity below the level of the section. Both voluntary and reflex motor control are lost. This condition is known as 'spinal shock', and it can persist for several weeks or months. After this time, reflex activity returns in the spinal segments below the lesion. This reflex activity is considerably abnormal, however, with exaggerated flexion reflexes (hyperreflexia) and clonus (rhythmical and repetitive contraction and relaxation of muscle when stretched). Even slight cutaneous stimulation can trigger a mass reflex, involving a generalized contraction of all flexor muscles, sometimes accompanied by reflex emptying of the bladder and rectum. In later stages after spinal transection, spasticity may appear in muscles supplied by spinal segments below the level of the lesion.

The mechanism for hyperreflexia is not fully understood. There are several possible causes. One of these is that the complete transection of the spinal cord has removed descending inhibitory inputs to the lower motoneurones, causing them to be more readily excited by reflex inputs. Another is that there is an increased sensitivity of the motoneurones and interneurones to neurotransmitters. A further suggestion is that the synaptic terminals from descending inputs onto the interneurones degenerate, leaving synaptic 'vacancies' on the interneurones. These 'vacancies' are subsequently utilized by incoming afferent nerve terminals from the periphery, leading to an increased afferent input onto the interneurones. The recovery of reflex function following spinal shock is therefore not the restoration of normal reflexes, but the creation of new, abnormal reflexes.

Corticospinal tract lesions can therefore lead to the loss of some normal functions, or the release of other abnormal functions which are normally held in check by descending influences.

Lesions of the corticospinal tract will also lead to loss of voluntary motor control below the level of the lesion. It is therefore important to know at which level the lesion exists. Table 3.5 lists some of the muscle groups in the body, together with the level of their spinal segmental innervation.

Any lesion of the corticospinal tracts above the

Table 3.5
Muscle Groups in Relation to the Level of their Spinal Segmental Innervation

Muscle group	Segmental innervation
Diaphragm / trapezius	C4
Deltoid / biceps	C5
Wrist extensors	C6
Triceps	C7
Finger flexors	C8
Hand intrinsic muscles	T1
Chest and trunk muscles	T2–L1
Iliopsoas	L2
Quadriceps	L3
Tibialis anterior	L4
Extensor hallucis	L5
Gastrocnemius	S1
Bladder / bowel	S2–S4

level of innervation for a particular muscle will affect the voluntary control of that muscle group, with an attendant loss of function – paralysis. Complete spinal section at a high spinal level (for example, C5) will result in paralysis of upper and lower limb muscles – **quadriplegia**. Complete section at a lower level (for example, L2) would result in paralysis of the lower limb muscles – **paraplegia**. Spinal cord hemisection leads to paralysis in the limbs of the affected side only – **hemiplegia**.

ASCENDING PATHWAYS IN THE SPINAL CORD

Ascending pathways in the spinal cord relay sensory information from the peripheral sensory receptors to the higher centres in the central nervous system.

Afferent fibres entering the spinal cord terminate in the grey matter and some also send branches which ascend in the white matter. The termination of the afferent fibres within the grey matter is related to their diameter. Large-diameter afferents, such as Ia and Ib afferents terminate in the deeper laminae of the grey matter (lamina V or deeper), whereas the smaller diameter afferents, such as group III and IV afferents terminate in laminae I and II. The primary afferent fibres make synaptic connections with secondary neurones in these laminae and these secondary neurones are involved in spinal reflexes, and/or send further branches to higher centres via the ascending pathways of the white matter.

Rexed's laminae I to V make up the **dorsal horn** of the grey matter; laminae VI and VII constitute the **intermediate zone**; laminae VIII and IX make up the **ventral horn** of the grey matter. Located in these zones are six major nuclei of cell bodies:

1. The **marginal zone** is located in lamina I, and serves as a relay for pain and temperature sensation to higher centres.
2. The **substantia gelatinosa** (from the Latin, 'jelly substance') is located in laminae II and III, and integrates pain and temperature information from small diameter, unmyelinated afferents.
3. The **nucleus proprius** is located in laminae IV and V at the base of the dorsal horn and integrates sensory afferent information with descending inputs from higher centres.
4. **Clarke's nucleus** is located in the intermediate zone in lamina VII and is found only in segmental levels T1 to L2 in man. It is involved in the relaying of proprioceptive afferent information about limb position and movement to the cerebellum for processing.
5. The **intermediolateral nucleus** is also located in the intermediate zone in lamina VII, and consists of autonomic preganglionic neurones.
6. The **motor nuclei** are located in the ventral horn in lamina IX, and contain motoneurones innervating the skeletal muscles.

Figure 3.16 shows the distribution of terminations of different afferents in the different laminae of the grey matter.

There are two major ascending pathways in the spinal cord white matter – the **dorsal column–medial lemniscal system** and the **anterolateral system**. These systems relay sensory information to higher centres in order to produce a conscious awareness of physical sensation and also to participate in motor control by the higher centres.

The dorsal column–medial lemniscal system carries information concerning touch and proprioception to higher centres. As the name of this pathway suggests, there are two components to this system. The first of these – the dorsal columns – conveys information up the spinal cord to the medulla and travels ipsilaterally. Axons running in the dorsal columns originate both from branches of the primary afferent fibres and also from secondary neurones from the spinal cord nuclei. These second order axons account for about 15% of the total axons in the

Figure 3.16   Cross-section of the spinal cord showing, on the left, Rexed's laminae (I to IX) in the grey matter and the terminations of different peripheral afferent fibres in these laminae. The right of the diagram shows the location of the major nuclei of the spinal cord grey matter. It should be noted here that not all of the nuclei shown in the diagram are always present at the same segmental level of the spinal cord (e.g. Clarke's nucleus is only found at levels T1 to L2).

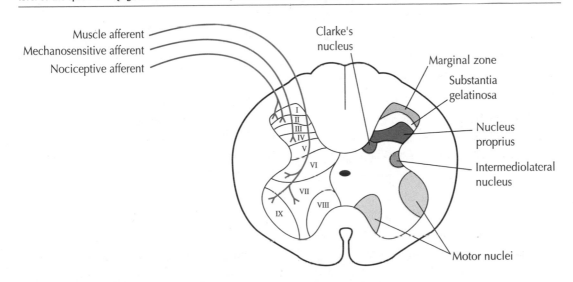

dorsal columns. Ascending fibres in the dorsal columns terminate in the dorsal column nuclei of the medulla.

As afferent fibres enter the spinal cord at different levels and start to ascend, they occupy space at the lateral portions of the dorsal columns. As new fibres enter from higher spinal segments, these push the existing fibres in the dorsal columns more medially. At higher segmental levels, the dorsal columns therefore have a somatotopic arrangement (from the Greek *soma* (body), *topos* (place)). The dorsal columns are also arranged in two distinct fascicles – the gracile and cuneate. The **gracile fascicle** lies medially and contains ascending fibres from the lower limbs (lumbar and sacral fibres). The **cuneate fascicle** lies laterally and contains ascending fibres from the upper limbs and neck (thoracic and cervical fibres).

Fibres in each of these fascicles terminate in the appropriate dorsal column nucleus in the medulla – the gracile and cuneate nuclei. Here, the ascending fibres synapse with the second-order neurones in this pathway. These second-order neurones then pass over to the contralateral side of the brainstem via the internal arcuate (arch). After crossing the midline, these fibres ascend to the thalamus via the second portion of the ascending pathway – the medial lemniscus. The medial lemniscus also has a somatotopic organization.

The thalamus basically acts as a relay station for information ascending to the cortex. Ascending fibres synapse with third order neurones in the thalamic nuclei. The ventral posterior lateral nucleus (VPLN) of the thalamus relays information from the trunk and limbs, whilst the ventral posterior medial nucleus (VPMN) of the thalamus relays information from the face.

From the thalamus, the axons of the third-order neurones ascend to the cortex via the posterior limb of the **internal capsule**.

The organization of the dorsal column–medial lemniscal system is summarized in Figure 3.17(a).

The anterolateral system conveys information concerning pain and temperature sensation and some information about crude touch to the higher centres. This system can be subdivided into three main pathways: (i) the spinothalamic, (ii) spinoreticular and (iii) spinotectal pathways.

Axons in the anterolateral system cross the midline at the level of the spinal cord, as opposed to the medulla and this can occur over several segments. The fibres travelling in the anterolateral system are always second-order axons which have their cell bodies in the marginal zone or substantia gelatinosa of the dorsal horn grey matter. The primary afferents therefore make synaptic connections with these second-order neurones in these dorsal horn nuclei. Some of these second-order axons will ascend ipsilaterally for a few spinal segments before crossing the midline, while others will cross immediately. Whereas most medial lemniscal fibres terminate in the thalamus, anterolateral fibres terminate throughout the whole of the brainstem as well as the thalamus.

The spinothalamic tract is concerned with the relay of information concerning pain to the higher centres. The spinothalamic tract is mostly concerned with 'fast' pain mediated by group III and IV fibres, whereas the spinoreticular tract is more concerned with 'slow' pain mediated by nonmyelinated group IV fibres. The spinoreticular tract also relays information to the **periaqueductal grey matter,** an area of the brain associated with pain modulation.

One other important ascending pathway is the

spinocerebellar tract. This conveys information about muscle, joint and skin proprioception to the cerebellum for integration and coordination with motor output from the cortex. This proprioceptive information is unconscious.

The organization of the anterolateral system is summarized in Figure 3.17(b).

EFFECTS OF SPINAL CORD LESIONS ON ASCENDING PATHWAYS

Lesions of the spinal cord can affect the transmission of sensory information to higher centres of the nervous system. The most dramatic effects of this can be seen when the lesions are due to severe spinal cord injury caused by trauma such as occurs in a car accident or by knife or bullet wounds. The pattern of sensory loss observed in these situations is dependent on the site and extent of the injury. For example, complete transection of the spinal cord results in a total sensory loss below the level of the transection (Figure 3.18a). The pattern of sensory loss for hemisection of the spinal cord (Brown-Séquard syndrome) is somewhat more complex, however (Figure

Figure 3.17 (a) Anatomical organization of the dorsal column — medial lemniscal system. (b) Anatomical organization of the anterolateral system. Neurones I, II and III represent the primary, secondary and tertiary neurones of these ascending pathways.

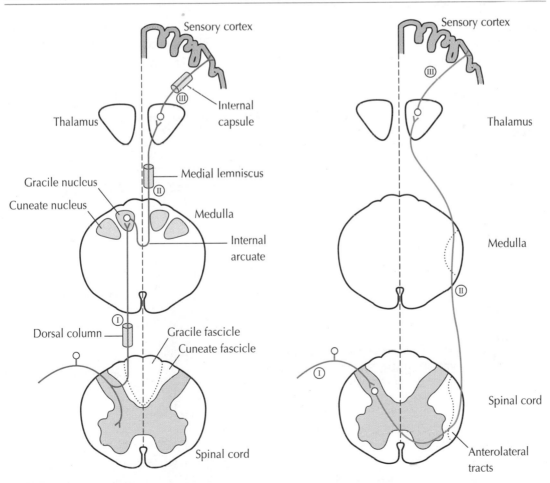

3.18b). Here, there is a loss of position and vibratory sensation and touch on the same side as the section, due to disruption of the dorsal columns on that side. There is also an accompanying loss of pain and temperature sensation on the contralateral side, due to disruption of the anterolateral pathways. Since crossing of fibres ascending in the anterolateral pathways occurs over several spinal segments, some pain and temperature fibres may ascend to a spinal level higher than the hemisection before crossing the midline. This therefore means that some contralateral pain and temperature sensation will persist in those skin areas supplied by spinal segments just below the level of the hemisection. Conversely, there may also be some ipsilateral loss of pain and temperature sensation in these same skin areas. It is therefore important to know both the level and extent of any spinal lesion when considering the accompanying sensory loss which would be a consequence of this.

Testing of the distribution of pain, temperature and proprioceptive sensation, together with a knowledge of dermatomal innervation (see p. 54) is therefore important in determining the level and nature of any spinal lesion.

Syringomyelia is a condition which affects the central canal of the spinal cord and results in the formation of cysts within the central portion of the cord. With further progression of the disease, the cysts will extend to other areas of the cord. These cysts tend to be segmentally localized, and are more common in cervical segments of the spinal cord. The pattern of sensory loss accompanying the formation of these cysts is the bilateral abolition of pain and temperature sensation from the skin supplied by the affected segments. This occurs due to the interruption of the

Figure 3.18 (a) Pattern of sensory loss with complete transection of the spinal cord. Areas supplied by nerve fibres from spinal segments below the level of the lesion experience complete loss of proprioceptive, touch, vibration, pain and temperature sensations. (b) Pattern of sensory loss following spinal cord hemisection (Brown-Séquard syndrome) on the left side. See text for details of loss of sensation. The extent of these patterns of sensory loss depends on the segmental level of the spinal cord lesion. [Adapted from Kandel ER *et al.* (1991).]

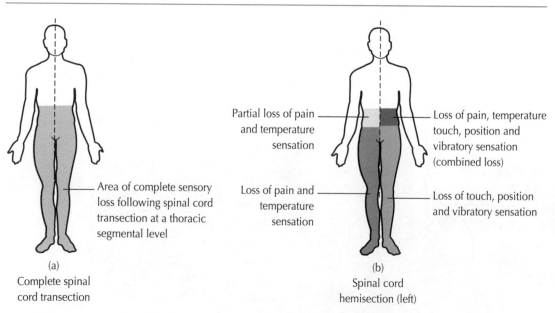

(a)
Complete spinal
cord transection

Area of complete sensory loss following spinal cord transection at a thoracic segmental level

Partial loss of pain and temperature sensation

Loss of pain and temperature sensation

(b)
Spinal cord
hemisection (left)

Loss of pain, temperature touch, position and vibratory sensation (combined loss)

Loss of touch, position and vibratory sensation

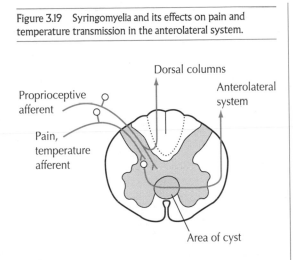

Figure 3.19   Syringomyelia and its effects on pain and temperature transmission in the anterolateral system.

second-order axons crossing the midline in the anterior commisure of the cord (Figure 3.19). Sensation above and below the level of the cyst is unaffected. Similarly, proprioceptive information is unaffected, as the dorsal columns remain intact. This pattern of sensory loss can lead to painless injury (particularly burns) to the affected skin areas, which may have serious consequences if unnoticed or left untreated.

Cortical Control of Movement

The output of the motor cortex can be influenced by several factors. Corticocortical connections allow some areas of the cortex to interact with others in order to affect the final motor output from the cortex. Area 4, the primary motor cortex, receives most of its input from area 6, the premotor cortex. Area 6, in turn, receives input from the prefrontal cortex (area 8), which is concerned with gathering visual information from the occipital cortex (areas 17, 18 and 19), somatic sensation from the parietal cortex (areas, 1, 2, 3, 5 and 7) and auditory information

from the temporal cortex. This relay of information from different cortical areas means that input from visual, auditory and other sensory receptors throughout the body can be used to integrate and guide movements in a meaningful way. The sensory input from a particular area of the body usually projects to that part of the motor cortex which controls the muscles of that body area, i.e. the afferent input to the cortex coincides with the cortical motor output.

Each cerebral hemisphere can also communicate with the opposite hemisphere via the corpus callosum — the bridge of nerve fibres which connects the halves of the brain.

The motor cortex itself is divided into six layers of cells and possesses several types of nerve cells. Two of the main nerve cell types in the cortex are the **pyramidal cells** and the **stellate cells**. The pyramidal cells are mainly responsible for the cortical output, i.e. their axons leave the cortex via the corticospinal tracts, while the stellate cells (of which there are several subtypes) represent cortical interneurones.

Groups of cells within the cortex are arranged vertically in columns of cells with similar functions. These columns form the basic functional unit within the cortex, and all cells within the same column share the same input and output connections. Horizontal connections between columns exist, and these are made via the stellate cells (Figure 3.20).

Electrical stimulation of different areas of the motor cortex demonstrates that there are areas where stimulation will produce movements of different body parts. These electrical stimulation experiments were first performed by Penfield and Rasmussen in the 1950s on patients who were undergoing brain surgery under local anaesthesia. More recent developments allow magnetic

Figure 3.20 Cell types in the cerebral cortex. Pyramidal cell axons form the corticospinal tracts. There are numerous synaptic connections between the dendrites of the pyramidal cells and the stellate cells.

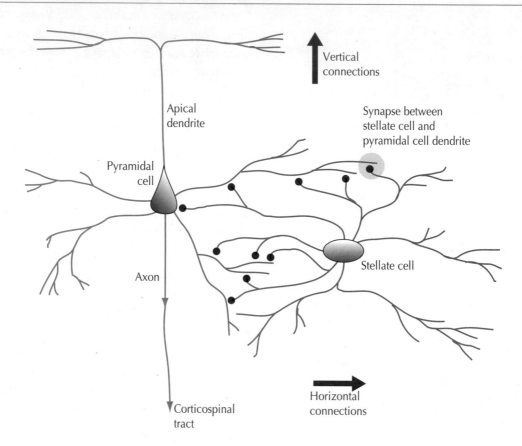

stimulation of different areas of the motor cortex in normal volunteers without the need for surgery. This allows a map of the motor cortex to be constructed which shows the areas of cortex devoted to each area of the body. This map of the motor cortex produces the **motor homunculus** (Latin *homunculus*, 'little man') as shown in Figure 3.21.

Within each area of the motor cortex devoted to each body area, the columnar arrangement of the cortex still exists with cells perpendicular to the surface being responsible for control of the same muscle groups. In the motor cortex, these col-

umns are known as **cortical efferent zones**. The nerve cells within these efferent zones receive input from either the muscle group with which that particular zone is concerned, or from an area of skin associated with the function of that muscle group. This allows modulation of motor output from the cortex based on the afferent information received by the cortical cells. This is similar to what occurs at a spinal level and, again, may in part be responsible for the modulation of motor output which can accompany proprioceptive neuromuscular facilitation techniques.

When a movement occurs by contraction of a

Figure 3.21 Cross-section through the motor cortex showing the relative proportions of cortex devoted to different body areas.

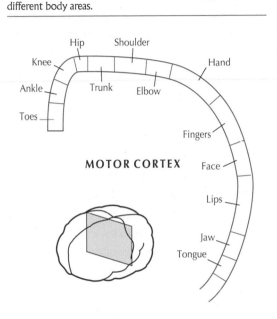

the cells of the cortex, indicating that these structures are also involved in the coordination of the muscle contraction.

Monitoring of changes in cerebral blood flow can also give indications of the role of different cortical areas in the production of movements. Increased blood flow indicates an increase in neural activity in that area. Figure 3.22 shows that when a subject is asked to perform a simple flexion movement of a finger, there is an increased activity in the primary motor cortex – area 4 (together with some increased activity in the sensory cortex as sensations accompanying the movement are produced). However, when a more complicated set of finger movements are produced, there is also an accompanying increase in activity in the premotor cortex (area 6). If the subject is asked to rehearse the movement men-

particular muscle group, it is observed that the cortical cells responsible for the control of that muscle group begin to fire about 20–50 ms before the movement starts and continue to fire during the movement. The frequency of firing of these cells is related to the amount of force produced by the muscle contraction, rather than the degree of movement produced by the contraction. Since the firing of the cortical cells occurs before the contraction begins, it would be more correct to say that the frequency of firing of the cortical cells codes for the intended force. Changes in the firing frequency of the cortical cells is related to the direction of the exerted force with some cells increasing frequency with flexion movements and others with extension movements.

It is also observed that cells in other structures of the brain, such as the basal ganglia and the cerebellum, will also increase their firing rate before

Figure 3.22 Changes in cerebral blood flow to cortical areas: (a) during performance of a simple movement task (e.g. flexing a finger); (b) during performance of a complicated movement task (e.g. finger movements accompanying playing a musical instrument); (c) during mental rehearsal of a movement task.

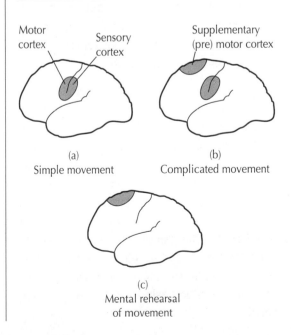

increase in activity is seen only in area 6, but not in the primary motor cortex. These patterns of activity demonstrate the coordination of different cortical areas in the production of more complicated sequences of movements.

Spasticity

The condition of spasticity develops following upper motor neurone lesions (e.g. due to stroke) or after spinal cord transection.

Spasticity is characterized by the presence of **hypertonia** (increased muscle tone) and **hyperreflexia** (abnormal, exaggerated reflex activity). The development of these is usually delayed following the initial lesion whether it occurs at the spinal or cerebral level. The characteristics of hyperreflexia have already been described on p. 73. Hypertonia is demonstrated by an increased resistance to slow, passive stretch of the muscle. This increased resistance is due to exaggerated stretch reflexes in the affected muscle. Hypertonia is observed in the flexor muscles of the upper limb and in the extensors of the lower limb (both are antigravity muscles in each respective limb).

Electromyographic recordings of muscle activity as the muscle is stretched shows that the amount of reflex activity induced in the muscle is dependent on the velocity of stretch; faster stretches induce greater reflex contraction. In spastic muscles, some degree of reflex contraction is observed at all velocities of stretch, whereas in normal muscles this is usually only evident with very fast stretches (similar to a tendon jerk). In spastic muscles, rapid stretch of the muscle may also induce **clonus** — a rapid, rhythmical pattern of contraction and relaxation in the stretched muscle.

The exaggerated stretch reflexes in spasticity may be due to alterations in the excitability of the stretch reflex, changes in the mechanical properties of the muscle tissue or a combination of both of these.

Increased excitability of the stretch reflex could be brought about by several mechanisms. The first is by increased stretch sensitivity of the muscle spindles due to increased gamma motoneurone activity. This would contract the intrafusal muscle fibres, thereby increasing the sensitivity of the annulospiral ending to imposed stretch. There is no evidence that such increases in gamma motoneurone activity are observed in spastic subjects, and this mechanism is therefore unlikely to account for the exaggerated stretch reflexes. Another mechanism is altered reflex excitability in the spinal cord due to changes in the level of pre- and postsynaptic inhibition. Decreased levels of postsynaptic inhibition would occur due to the loss of descending inhibitory inputs to the lower motoneurones. Overall, this would lead to increased excitability of the alpha motoneurones. Additionally, there may be a decrease in Ia reciprocal inhibition from antagonist muscles due to decreased Ia inhibitory interneurone excitability, again caused by a loss of descending inputs (in this case facilitatory). This decrease in reciprocal inhibition may be different for specific muscle groups in the upper and lower limbs. In the lower limb, reciprocal inhibition from an extensor muscle group such as gastrocnemius/soleus onto the motoneurones of its antagonist muscle — tibialis anterior — may be powerful. However, the reciprocal inhibition from tibialis anterior onto gastrocnemius/soleus motoneurones may be weak. Contraction of tibialis anterior would therefore be inhibited, while reflex inhibition of the powerfully contracting gastrocnemius/soleus is abolished. The reverse would be true in the upper limbs, with powerful contraction of flexors, but little or no reciprocal inhibition arising from the extensors. This specific increase in activity in the antigravity muscles may be due to some form of differential disinhibition (removal of inhibition) of these specific motoneurones in the spinal cord.

Presynaptic inhibition may also be affected in spasticity. In normal subjects, vibration of a muscle belly at about 100 Hz will cause reflex inhibition of tendon jerks. This is brought about through presynaptic inhibition of the Ia afferent terminals. In spastic subjects, this inhibition of tendon jerks by muscle vibration is lost, therefore suggesting that the degree of presynaptic inhibition in the spinal cord is reduced in spasticity. Such reduced presynaptic inhibition could account for the increased excitability of the stretch reflex.

Other postsynaptic mechanisms which could account for an increase in alpha motoneurone excitability include those mechanisms responsible for hyperreflexia which have been discussed earlier (see discussion of spinal shock on p. 73).

The principal cause of exaggerated stretch reflexes in spasticity would therefore appear to be reflex in origin.

Mechanical changes in the spastic muscle tissue could occur due to lack of voluntary use. This may lead to fibrosis of the muscle fibres and the tendons. This, in turn, will increase the mechanical stiffness of the muscle and will contribute to the overall resistance to stretch. The extent of this contribution has not been fully elucidated.

Treatment of spasticity relies to a certain extent on the use of drugs to interfere with pre- and postsynaptic inhibition in the spinal cord. Baclofen inhibits the effects of excitatory transmitter release in the spinal cord. Benzodiazepines such as diazepam (Valium) enhance presynaptic inhibition. Both of these drugs will therefore reduce the overall excitability of the alpha motoneurones. Dantrolene is another drug used to treat spasticity but which operates on the muscle itself rather than centrally. Dantrolene inhibits the release of calcium ions from the sarcoplasmic reticulum, thereby reducing the strength of muscle contraction.

Physiotherapeutic intervention may also be of use in the treatment of spasticity. While one of the goals of physiotherapy may be to restore range of movement to the spastic subject, alterations in peripheral afferent input may be able to change the relative amounts of inhibition and excitation in the spinal cord by influencing the activity of excitatory and inhibitory interneurones, or by altering the levels of presynaptic inhibition.

The Basal Ganglia and the Extrapyramidal Motor System

The term 'basal ganglia' is used collectively to describe five subcortical nuclei which are closely involved in motor control. These five nuclei are the **caudate nucleus**, the **putamen**, the **globus pallidus**, the **substantia nigra** and the **subthalamic nucleus**. These nuclei lie in the central portion of the cerebral hemispheres and in the midbrain (Figure 3.23).

The basal ganglia are involved in the initiation and control of movement, but have no direct output to the motoneurones of the spinal cord via the corticospinal tracts and, because of this, are said to form the extrapyramidal system.

The connections between the different structures comprising the basal ganglia are complicated in that there are numerous loops formed between

Figure 3.23   Section of the cerebral hemispheres showing the location of the major nuclei comprising the basal ganglia.

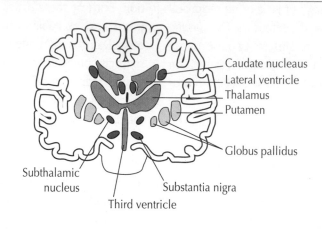

the structures and with the premotor and motor areas of the cerebral cortex. The caudate nucleus and the putamen are collectively known as the **corpus striatum** (due to their striped appearance in microscopic sections stained for myelin). These structures receive input from the motor cortex and from the substantia nigra and the thalamic motor nuclei. The corpus striatum processes this input before sending an output to the globus pallidus and back to the substantia nigra. The output from the globus pallidus then travels to the motor cortex via the thalamic motor nuclei, as well as to the substantia nigra. These connections are summarized in Figure 3.24.

The basal ganglia serve to modify the intended motor output from the cortex before this output occurs. In this respect, the basal ganglia are important in the initiation of movement. This is also suggested by the fact that the neurones of the basal ganglia begin their firing up to 800 ms before the cells of the motor cortex begin to fire. The basal ganglia are thought to *prepare* the motor cortex for the forthcoming movement by changing the balance of the excitability of excitatory and inhibitory cortical interneurones.

The connections between the different portions

of the basal ganglia are also important with regard to the neurotransmitters utilized by the different neurones in the pathways. Some of these are summarized in Figure 3.25.

The integrity of these connections and the transmitters used at each stage is important clinically. In Parkinson's disease, there is a loss or destruction of **dopamine**-containing cells of the substantia

Figure 3.24   Summary of the connections between the major nuclei of the basal ganglia.

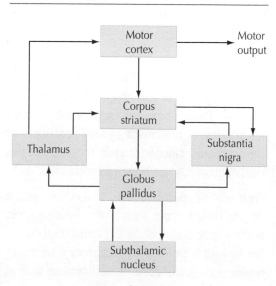

Figure 3.25 Neurotransmitters utilized in some of the connections between the nuclei of the basal ganglia (GABA = gamma-aminobutyric acid).

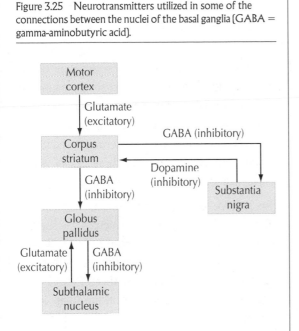

nigra, leading to a loss of the black pigmentation which gives this nucleus its name. With the loss of these **dopaminergic neurones** (i.e. neurones which exert their effects through dopamine), there is a loss of the normal inhibitory input from the substantia nigra to the corpus striatum. This, in turn, leads to a disinhibition of the corpus striatum and therefore an abnormal firing pattern of the cells in the corpus striatum and consequently in the globus pallidus. Since the globus pallidus projects to the motor cortex via the thalamus there is therefore ultimately an abnormal input from the basal ganglia to the motor cortex, resulting in abnormal motor output from the cortex. This abnormal motor output leads to the classical symptoms of Parkinson's disease, i.e. rhythmical tremor at rest, rigidity and slowness in initiation of movements (akinesia) and slowness during movements (bradykinesia).

The resting tremor first appears in the hands and fingers and is often described as 'pill-rolling' – as if the subject was rolling a small pill between thumb and forefinger. In later stages of the disease, the resting tremor may be seen to affect the lips and tongue and, in some cases, the feet. This resting tremor is usually observed to disappear on voluntary movement, although it may persist in more advanced stages of the disease.

The rigidity associated with Parkinson's disease is observed on passive manipulation of the joints and affects both flexor and extensor muscle groups. In some cases, this rigidity may be displayed as 'cog-wheel' rigidity, where some element of tremor is superimposed on the background stiffness of the muscles.

The akinesia and bradykinesia associated with Parkinson's disease can often be demonstrated by the fixed, mask-like appearance of the subject's face, reduced spontaneous blinking rate and the rather bent, shuffling gait which is observed during walking. Subjects with Parkinson's disease often experience falls which are associated with the loss of stepping reactions and protective arm reactions.

It has been estimated that these symptoms appear only if > 80% of the dopaminergic neurones have been destroyed. If > 20% of these neurones are intact, it appears that the nervous system can, in some way, compensate for the disordered motor output. Some of the symptoms of Parkinson's disease can be reversed by supplementing the reduced levels of dopamine, but since dopamine cannot cross the blood–brain barrier, the precursor L-DOPA (levodopa) is administered instead. L-DOPA is converted to dopamine within the nerve cells of the basal ganglia. Treatment with L-DOPA is not successful in all cases and may not always be long-lasting in its effects where it is successful – deterioration in response to L-DOPA may be observed in up to 40% of patients receiving the drug for more than five years. This may be partly due to a reduction in sensitivity of dopamine receptors as the damage to the basal ganglia becomes more progressive. An additional drug therapy which may be utilized is to attempt to restore the effective balance of dopamine and acetylcholine in the basal ganglia by reducing the effects of acetylcholine. This may be achieved by administering atropine or an atropine-like drug such as benzhexol. More recent research has suggested that implantation of fetal brain tissue may help to regenerate dopaminergic neurones in the substantia nigra, but this has so far been inconclusive. There are besides, certain moral and ethical implications in the use of human fetal tissue. Very recent research indicates that nerve growth factors such as glial-cell-line derived neutrophic factor (GDNF) may be able to protect and repair the dopaminergic neurones in the substantia nigra, with possible use in the treatment of Parkinson's disease.

Huntington's chorea (or Huntington's disease) is another disorder which affects neurotransmitter function in the basal ganglia. In this case, there is a reduction in the production of gamma-aminobutyric acid (GABA) in cells of the corpus striatum. Again, this leads to disordered motor output which is manifested as slowness in execution of fine movements and ataxic gait (clumsy, uncoordinated movements during walking). Irregular and involuntary face and mouth movements may also be observed. As the disease progresses, there is gradual loss of memory coupled with dementia. Huntington's disease is an inherited disorder which is dominant and can affect either sex.

The Cerebellum

The cerebellum is located at the base of the brain, and is a complex, convoluted structure which is divided into two hemispheres such that it resembles a miniature version of the cerebral hemispheres.

Generally, the cerebellum is composed of an outer cortical layer of grey matter surrounding white matter which contains three pairs of nuclei deep within. These nuclei are the **fastigial nucleus,** the **interposed nucleus** (or interpositus) and the **dentate nucleus.** It is these three nuclei which convey the output of the cerebellum.

The surface of the cerebellum is very highly folded. The folds – **folia** – run across the surface of the cerebellum forming deep fissures. Two of these fissures are deeper than the rest, effectively dividing the cerebellum into three lobes – the **anterior, posterior** and **flocculonodular lobes** (Figure 3.26).

The cerebellum is also divided into two hemispheres by a midline strip known as the **vermis** (Latin *vermis,* 'worm').

Figure 3.26 Diagrammatic representation of the surface of the cerebellum showing folds and fissures. The cerebellum is divided into three lobes – the anterior, posterior and flocculonodular lobes. The flocculondular lobe comprises the flocculus and nodule. The vermis is the midline structure which divides the cerebellum into two hemispheres.

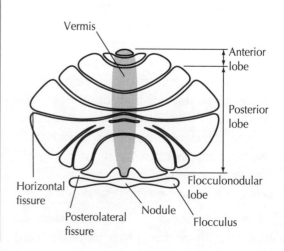

Each of the three lobes of the cerebellum receive inputs from different sources. The anterior lobe receives input from spinal cord afferents (skin, muscle, joint tendons) via the spinocerebellar tracts. The posterior lobe receives input from cortical afferents (frontal, parietal, occipital and temporal cortices). The flocculonodular lobe receives input from vestibular afferents (from the vestibular nuclei in the brainstem).

The cerebellar cortex comprises three layers of cells. The deepest of these is the **granular layer,** which contains the cell bodies of small, densely-packed cells – granule cells. Above this is a layer of large cells which provide the output from the cerebellar cortex to the deeper cerebellar nuclei. These are the Purkinje cells (named after the Czech anatomist), which form the **Purkinje layer.** The most superficial layer of the cerebellar cortex is the **molecular layer,** which contains very few cell bodies, but consists mainly of projections and dendrites from granule cells and Purkinje cells. The molecular layer does contain two types of neurones which act as cerebellar interneurones – **stellate** and **basket cells.** The organization of the cerebellar cortical neurones is shown in Figure 3.27.

Figure 3.27 Organization of neurones of the cerebellar cortex. Purkinje cells receive excitatory inputs from the climbing fibres and the granule cells. Granule cells receive excitatory input from the mossy fibres from the spinal cord and brainstem nuclei. The Purkinje cells give rise to the output from the cerebellar cortex to the deeper cerebellar nuclei, which subsequently represent the output from the cerebellum as a whole.

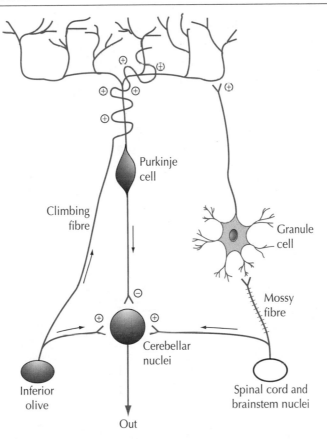

Input to these cerebellar cortical cells is from two sources. Inputs from the spinal cord and the vestibular nuclei are conveyed by fibres known as **mossy fibres** (so-called because of their many dendritic branches) which synapse onto the granule cells. The second set of inputs comes from a nucleus in the medulla – the **inferior olive**. The inferior olive itself receives input from the spinal cord and from the motor cortex and projects to Purkinje cells in the cerebellum via fibres known as **climbing fibres**. There is a one-to-one relationship between climbing fibres and Purkinje cells. The climbing fibres wrap around the Purkinje cell projections. The input from mossy fibres and from climbing fibres to the cerebellum are both excitatory. Output from the cerebellar cortex is achieved via the Purkinje cell axons. This is the only output path from the cerebellar cortex and output goes to the deeper cerebellar nuclei. Through the output from these nuclei, the cerebellum can exert descending influences on the spinal cord as well as ascending influences on the motor cortex.

In general, the **fastigial nucleus** influences proximal muscle groups, the **interposed nucleus** influences distal limb muscles and the **dentate nucleus** influences the motor cortex via projections to the thalamus.

Since the cerebellum receives inputs from the spinal cord, the motor cortex and the brainstem nuclei and also sends output to these same structures, the question might therefore be asked, what is the function of the cerebellum? The cerebellum is concerned with the planning and initiation of movement and also the moment-to-moment control of movement as it progresses. This moment-to-moment modulation of movement is brought about by cerebellar monitoring of sensory feedback from proprioceptors during the movement.

The initiation and control of movement is thought to occur in conjunction with the motor cortex and other cortical areas. This may be summarized as shown in Figure 3.28.

Recent evidence has suggested that the cerebellum may act as an array of pattern generators which control specific limb movements. The activity of these neural networks are under the control of Purkinje cells in the cerebellar cortex, and may store specific motor programs which have been

Figure 3.28   Role of the cerebellum in the planning and initiation of movement. The initial idea for a movement arises in the association areas (e.g. premotor cortex) which then signals this intention to the motor cortex and to the cerebellum. The cerebellum integrates this information with that received from the motor cortex itself and with the sensory information from the spinal cord. The cerebellum then feeds back to the motor cortex to guide the final motor output which produces the movement.

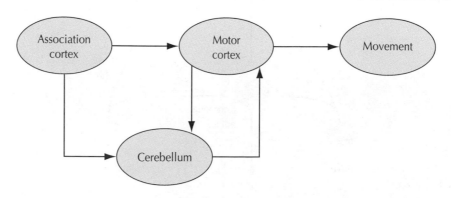

previously learned. When required, these motor programs can be recalled from memory and then carried out under the control of the cerebellar cortex.

It has also been recently suggested that the cerebellum 'predicts' the sensory outcomes of a particular movement pattern, and compares this, via peripheral afferent feedback, to the actual sensory outcome when the movement takes place.

The cerebellum may also be involved in the learning of new motor tasks and, in this respect, may therefore be involved in relearning compensatory movements during other motor disorders. This has implications for the role of physiotherapy in re-education of motor control during rehabilitation.

Cerebellar Syndrome

Lesions of the cerebellum present several types of symptoms which, collectively, are known as 'cerebellar syndrome'. These symptoms include hypotonia, ataxia, dysarthria, nystagmus and intention tremor.

The hypotonia, or decreased muscle tone, associated with cerebellar disease is due to a decreased cerebellar facilitatory input to stretch reflex circuitry in the spinal cord. A reduction in resistance to passive stretch of the limb is observed.

Ataxia is observed as an incoordination of movement, with the subject making errors in the rate, force and direction of movement. There is poor coordination of agonist and antagonist muscle activity. This can lead to the appearance of a staggering lurching gait (similar to a drunken gait), with the legs held wide apart during walking. If the subject is asked to touch his or her nose with the fingertips, there is a break down in the normal smooth movement, with the trajectory of the limb wandering considerably before the target is reached. This is known as **dysmetria** — inaccurate range and direction of movement. Ataxia is also observed when the subject is asked to rapidly rotate his or her hands at the wrist in an alternating movement. The subject is unable to maintain a steady rhythm to the movement. This is known as **dysdiadochokinesia**.

Ataxia can also affect the muscles of speech, and this is exhibited as dysarthria — jerky, slurred speech, which is sometimes so severe as to render speech unintelligible.

Nystagmus is observed as rapid, jerky side-to-side eye movements at rest, which may also be accompanied by rhythmic head movements. The subject may use more frequent, smaller eye movements (saccades) to move the direction of gaze from one position to another. Eye movements are therefore more jerky, with less smooth pursuit movements observed. Nystagmus is observed when lesions affect the flocculonodular lobe of the cerebellum.

Intention tremor is manifested as rhythmic shaking of the limbs during voluntary movement. It is thought that this tremor may, in part, be an attempt to compensate for the dysmetria which occurs during a movement. There is no tremor observed at rest as there is in Parkinson's disease.

These disorders of movement observed in cerebellar disease underline the importance of normal cerebellar function in the smooth coordination of normal motor action.

Nervous System and Motor Control: Summary

Figure 3.29 summarizes the contents of this chapter. Each box provides a summary of each of the major topics covered, and gives an overview of

Figure 3.29   Summary of the nervous system and motor control.

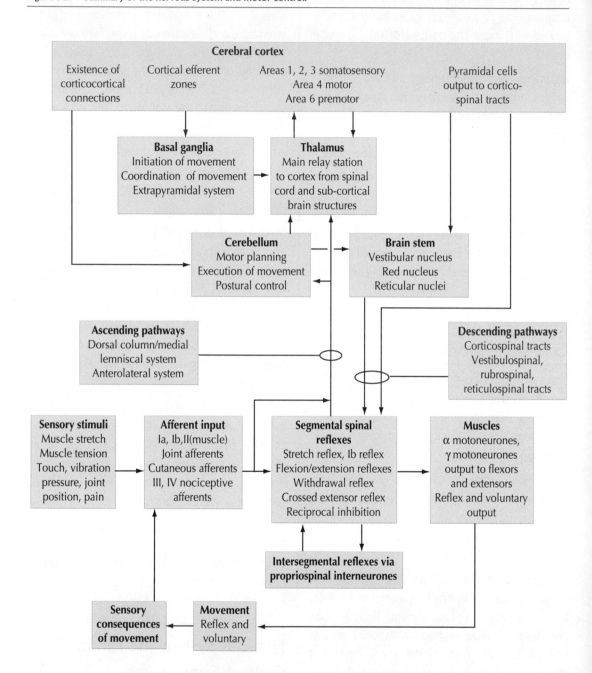

how all of these components operate as part of an integrated whole within the nervous system.

Bibliography

Baxendale, RH, Ferrell, WR (1981) The effect of knee joint afferent discharge on transmission in flexion reflex pathways in decerebrate cats. *Journal of Physiology*, 315: 231–242.

Carr, JH, Shepherd, RB, Ada, L (1995) Spasticity: research findings and implications for intervention. *Physiotherapy*, 81: 421–429.

Cohen, H (1993) *Neuroscience for Rehabilitation*. Lippincott, Philadelphia.

Granat, MH, Heller, BW, Nicol, DJ, Baxendale, RH, Andrews, BJ (1993) Improving limb flexion in FES gait using the flexion withdrawal response for the spinal cord injured person. *Journal of Biomedical Engineering*, 15: 51–56.

Kandel, ER, Schwartz, JH, Jessel TM (1991) *Principles of Neural Science*. 3rd Edition. Appleton and Lange, Connecticut.

Kiernan, JA (1987) *Introduction to Human Neuroscience*. Lippincott, Philadelphia.

Miall, RC, Weir, DJ, Wolpert, DM, Stein, JF (1993) Is the cerebellum a Smith predictor? *Journal of Motor Behaviour*, 25: 203–216.

Nicholls, JG, Martin, AR, Wallace, BG (1992) *From Neuron to Brain*. 3rd Edition. Sinauer, Sunderland, MA.

Readings from *Scientific American* (1993) *Mind and Brain*. Freeman, San Francisco.

Roberts, TDM (1995) *Understanding Balance – the Mechanics of Posture and Locomotion*. Chapman and Hall, London.

Roland, PE, Larsen, B, Lassen, NA and Skinhof, E (1980) Supplementary motor area and other cortical areas in organization of voluntary movements in man. *Journal of Neurophysiology*, 43: 118–136.

Rothwell, J (1994) *Control of Human Voluntary Movement*. 2nd Edition. Chapman and Hall, London.

Rymer, WZ, Katz, RT (1994) Mechanisms of spastic hypertonia. *Physical Medicine and Rehabilitation*, 8: 441–454.

Tomac, A, Lindqvist, E, Lin, L-FH, Ogren, SO, Young D, Hoffer, BJ, Olsen, L (1995) Protection and repair of the nigrostriatal dopaminergic system by GDNF *in vivo*. *Nature*, 373: 335–339.

Wood, L, Ferrell, WR, Baxendale, RH (1988) Pressures in normal and acutely distended human knee joints and effects on quadriceps maximal voluntary contractions. *Quarterly Journal of Experimental Physiology*, 73: 305–314.

4

The Nervous System: Pain

Peripheral Aspects of Pain
•
Central Aspects of Pain
•
Referred Pain
•
Phantom Limb Pain

Pain is the subjective sensations which accompany the activation of nociceptors. These sensations are variable in quality and can have serious effects on the physical and emotional well-being of the subject. Pain sensations can range from mild irritation to severe, intractable pain which can be beyond endurance. Despite this, pain is a necessary sensation for normal functioning of the body. It normally serves a protective function by providing information concerning the location and strength of noxious and potentially tissue-damaging stimuli.

The physiology of pain, and the potential for reducing the pain sensations has only fairly recently been investigated in any great depth. Related to this, is the psychology of pain. The influence of higher brain centres on the perception of pain can be an important tool in pain relief.

Peripheral Aspects of Pain

The types of sensory receptors responsible for the detection of painful stimuli — the nociceptors — are mostly found to be **free nerve endings**. These are nerve endings which possess no specialized accessory structures, and are found in almost all types of tissue in the body.

The nociceptors give rise to two types of afferent nerve fibre:

1. Small-diameter myelinated fibres, group III afferents, which conduct impulses at 5–30 m s^{-1},

and are usually associated with sharp, pricking pain sensations, so-called **acute** or **fast pain**. These pain sensations have a short latency and are well localized to the specific areas of the body where the stimulus has arisen. The duration of these sensations is relatively short and the pain has less emotional involvement.

2. Small-diameter nonmyelinated fibres, group IV afferents, which have a much slower conduction velocity, about 0.5–2 m s^{-1}. These fibres are usually associated with longer lasting, dull throbbing- or burning-type pain sensations, **chronic** or **slow pain**. These pain sensations have a much slower onset following the painful stimulus, and are more diffuse in their localization. Pain sensations associated with group IV activation are longer lasting and may be difficult to endure, promoting greater emotional associations, and can be accompanied by autonomic responses such as sweating, increased heart rate and blood pressure and nausea.

Both types of nociceptor are **polymodal** receptors, in that they can respond to a variety of different stimuli – mechanical, thermal and chemical. These can be light and heavy pressure, extremes of temperature, or chemical factors. All of these are stimuli which can be potentially damaging to the tissues. The nociceptors are usually inactive (silent) in non-injured tissue; indeed, some nociceptors may *never* be activated throughout a person's life. However, following tissue injury, the nociceptors increase their activity and become more sensitive to stimulation.

Chemical mediators of pain are released by damaged tissue and will activate the nociceptors. These include bradykinin, substance P, histamine, prostaglandins and 5-hydroxytryptamine (5-HT). Such chemical mediators are also released in situations such as inflammation, arthritis, coronary occlusion and ulceration.

These chemical mediators are responsible for the longer-lasting aspects of the pain once the initial physical stimulus has ceased.

A short, noxious stimulus to the skin, joints or muscles, such as might be produced if a thumb is struck with a hammer, results in a 'double' pain response. There is an initial fast component due to activation of the group III afferents by the mechanical stimulus, followed by a slower response due to activation of group IV afferents by the release of chemical mediators from the damaged tissue. The pain sensations accompanying striking of the thumb with a hammer are therefore an initial sharp pain, followed by a dull, throbbing pain.

Central Aspects of Pain

Both group III and group IV afferent fibres project to the spinal cord where they synapse (both directly and via interneurones) with neurones in the dorsal horn of the grey matter. These neurones – **transmission cells** are either involved in local spinal reflexes, or project to higher centres of the nervous system via the spinothalamic tracts. The transmission cells are therefore responsible for the relaying of peripheral information regarding pain sensation to the higher centres. The excitability of these spinal interneurones can be elevated for a considerable time (up to several hours) following activation of group IV afferents.

As well as receiving excitatory input from the primary afferent fibres, the transmission cells are also subject to an inhibitory input from interneurones arising in the substantia gelatinosa of the dorsal horn grey matter. These substantia gelatinosa interneurones (SG cells), in turn, are excited by input from large-diameter, low-threshold, mechanosensitive afferents. Therefore, activation of low-threshold mechanoreceptors whether by electrical or mechanical means will inhibit the transmission of pain signals through the transmission cell by altering the balance of excitatory and inhibitory inputs to the transmission cell (Figure 4.1).

This modulation of pain transmission by altering afferent input to the spinal cord is known as the **gate-control theory**, which was established by Melzack and Wall in 1965. This theory has important implications for the management of pain in physiotherapy. Any technique which involves the activation of large-diameter mechanosensitive afferents has the potential to modulate pain transmission in the spinal cord. Techniques such as massage, joint manipulation, traction and compression, thermal stimulation and electrotherapy all have the capability to produce sensory inputs from low-threshold afferents, which can ultimately inhibit pain transmission in the spinal cord by 'closing the gate' i.e. inhibiting transmission-cell excitability via the SG cells.

Figure 4.1   Peripheral influences on transmission of information through the transmission cells of the dorsal horn of the spinal cord grey matter. Nociceptive afferents stimulate the transmission cell (T), thereby transmitting nociceptive information to higher centres. Excitation of large-diameter mechanosensitive afferents stimulates the substantia gelatinosa (SG) cell which inhibits this transmission.

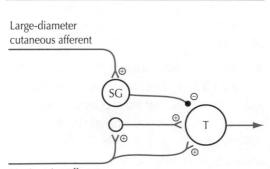

Large-diameter
cutaneous afferent

Nociceptive afferent

Transcutaneous electrical nerve stimulation (TENS) can be used to directly stimulate these afferents in an appropriate area and at an appropriate voltage which will influence pain transmission in the relevant spinal segments. Both the therapist and the patient can therefore have control over pain modulation and can adjust the levels of this at any time.

The inhibitory interneurones in the substantia gelatinosa of the spinal cord can also be influenced by descending inputs from higher brain centres. Stimulation of the grey matter which surrounds the cerebral aqueduct (periaqueductal grey matter, PAGM) and of the raphe nucleus in the medulla can produce analgesia by inhibiting pain transmission in the spinal cord. These structures possess receptors for opiates, and can be activated by drugs such as morphine. Endogenous opiates such as the enkephalins and endorphins also activate these structures to produce analgesia through descending influences on the inhibitory interneurones in the substantia gelatinosa (Figure 4.2).

The descending inputs to the spinal cord are thought to modulate activity in the inhibitory interneurones of the substantia gelatinosa by releasing monoaminergic neurotransmitters such as 5-hydroxytryptamine and noradrenaline. The action of opiates on the cells of the periaqueductal grey matter and the raphe nucleus is thought to be a suppression of the action of gamma-aminobutyric acid (GABA) (inhibitory) released by an interneurone acting on the cells. The analgesic effects of opiates are therefore brought about by a removal of normal inhibition of the descending inputs to the spinal cord.

Higher cognitive functions of the brain such as emotions can also influence pain transmission. Fear, stress and excitement can reduce, or even abolish, the feelings of pain associated with injury.

Figure 4.2   Descending influences on SG cell excitability. The periaqueductal grey matter and the raphe nucleus are normally inhibited by the action of inhibitory GABA-ergic interneurones. Opiates interfere with this inhibition, releasing the excitatory influence of these structures on the SG cells (mediated by 5-hydroxytryptamine). This therefore suppresses pain transmission in the spinal cord. T = transmission cell.

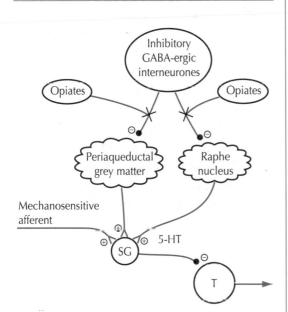

A well-known example of this is the so-called 'battlefield analgesia', where a soldier may have sustained a severe injury to a part of the body but is unaware of it until some time later, usually after the soldier has reached safety. Similar reduced responses to pain are observed in many sports, with players managing to continue while injured. This suggests that there is modulation of pain transmission brought about by the influences of higher centres, probably mediated by the PAGM and raphe nucleus (see Figure 4.2). This also has important therapeutic implications at a psychological level: a patient simply receiving attention from a therapist, regardless of the techniques being employed, may be sufficient to induce an emotional response which could modulate the pain they are feeling.

Referred Pain

Pain which arises from deep structures in the body — visceral pain — is often felt by the subject in locations which are far removed from the site of origin. Such translocation of pain sensation is known as **referred pain**. An example of this is the pain associated with anginal episodes. Here, the organ which is affected is the heart, but the pain is often described as arising in the upper chest, left shoulder and arm. Similar patterns of referred pain are seen for pain arising in other structures, such as the diaphragm and appendix.

The explanation for the pattern of referred pain lies in the pattern of convergence of afferent never fibres in the dorsal horn of the spinal cord. Dorsal horn neurones, including those which act as transmission cells, receive input from several sources which are innervated by the same spinal segments (T1–T4 in the case of the heart and left arm). These may include nociceptive input both from cutaneous areas and visceral areas (Figure 4.3).

As previously discussed, these transmission cells pass this nociceptive information to higher centres where it is perceived as pain sensation. How-

Figure 4.3   Convergence of nociceptors from different structures onto the same transmission cell (T). Input from cardiac nociceptors (arrow) is interpreted by higher centres as input from cutaneous nociceptors which impinge on the same transmission cell.

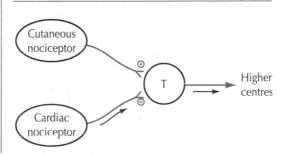

ever, the higher centres cannot distinguish the source of this information as being either cutaneous or visceral in origin since they only receive input from single transmission cells. Since peripheral input from cutaneous receptors normally predominates, this may account for the pain sensation being incorrectly ascribed to the skin rather than the visceral organ.

It is important for the physiotherapist to be aware of the possible patterns of referred pain, since the patient might describe pain as arising in a structure which has no underlying lesion, misleading the therapist as to the real source of complaint.

Phantom Limb Pain

When a limb has been amputated or the sensory nerves from a limb have been destroyed, the sensation of the limb still being present can exist in some cases (phantom limb) and, sometimes, pain referred to the missing limb can be perceived. Pain associated with a missing limb is known as **phantom limb pain**. Phantom limb pain is often described as burning, electric or cramping sensations, and may persist for many years after the loss of the limb.

The source of this phantom limb pain may be the severed ends of the peripheral nerves which were cut during the amputation or injury. This may set up abnormal patterns of discharge in the peripheral nerve fibres, particularly nociceptors, which are then relayed to higher centres and perceived as pain sensations arising in the areas these nerves formerly supplied. Additionally, there may be altered activity in the neurones of the dorsal horn associated with pain transmission. This altered activity may arise as a result of afferent

degeneration inducing postsynaptic changes in the dorsal horn neurones (see the discussion on neuroplasticity on p. 99).

Recent research has suggested a further cause of phantom limb pain. This proposes that phantom limbs and the sensations associated with them are a consequence of activity in neural networks in higher centres of the brain. These neural networks form a so-called **neuromatrix**, the structure and functioning of which may be genetically determined, and which is susceptible to inputs from peripheral structures. This neuromatrix is not localized, but is widespread throughout the brain. It provides a neural framework which underpins the subject's experience of their own body as a physical entity which 'belongs' to them. Sensory inputs from all areas of the body can manipulate and modify the activity of the neuromatrix. It has been suggested that phantom limb pain arises as a result of abnormal or absent modulating input to this neuromatrix and missing channels of output from the neuromatrix to the muscles.

Bibliography

Charman, RA (1989) Pain theory and physiotherapy. *Physiotherapy,* 75: 247–254.

Cohen, H (1993) *Neuroscience for Rehabilitation.* Lippincott, Philadelphia.

Kandel, ER, Schwartz, JH, Jessel, TM (1991) *Principles of Neural Science.* 3rd Edition. Appleton and Lange, Connecticut.

Kiernan, JA (1987) *Introduction to Human Neuroscience.* Lippincott, Philadelphia.

Melzack, R (1990) Phantom limbs and the concept of a neuromatrix. *Trends in Neuroscience,* 13: 88–92.

Melzack, R, Wall, P (1988) *The Challenge of Pain.* 2nd Edition. Penguin Books, Harmondsworth.

5

The Nervous System: Neuroplasticity

We have already discussed some of the changes in nervous system function which occur after injury. These included spinal shock, hyperreflexia and spasticity. The mechanisms which are responsible for these changes demonstrate the ability of the nervous system to modify the structure and function of its neuronal circuits following damage. Such modifications are not restricted only to the injured nervous system. Higher nervous functions such as learning and memory also rely on this adaptation of the nervous system. This ability of the nervous system to produce changes in its function is known as **neuroplasticity**.

Injury to the nervous system produces changes in its organization and function which, in some cases, can allow some degree of restoration of function. These changes reflect the **plasticity** of the nervous system. Plasticity can be defined as the capability of the nervous system to adapt or modify to imposed change. Such plastic changes can result in abnormal activity (as is seen in spasticity) or recovery of some semblance of normal function (although this is *not* the same as restoration of normal function). The adaptation and modification of the different components of the nervous system, which constitute these plastic changes, are induced by the effects of the lesions which result from the injury.

The existence of neuroplasticity challenges the older concept that the circuitry within the nervous system is 'hard-wired' — i.e. that it is not capable of adapting to change. While this might be true for certain components of the nervous system, the normal existence of plasticity can be demonstrated in the following circumstances:

- **Developmental plasticity.** This demonstrates the modification in structure and function of the nervous system during embryonic growth and development.
- **Functional plasticity.** This is the change in the adult nervous system which can be induced by an environmental input, e.g. as occurs in memory and learning.
- **Adaptive plasticity.** This is the change in normal functioning of the nervous system induced by injury or lesions to particular components of the nervous system.

It is these last two categories which are of particular use and importance to the physiotherapist. Before discussing this further, it is useful to appreciate the neuronal changes which can accompany injury to a nerve fibre. If a peripheral nerve is injured (e.g. by crushing), several things may happen which affect both the nerve fibres within the peripheral nerve or the parts of the central nervous system which those nerve fibres influence: there may be abnormal membrane excitability in the injured fibres which can give rise to irregular and unnatural patterns of action potential firing; there may be a reduced effectiveness of synaptic connections between the injured nerve fibres and postsynaptic neurones; there may also be neurone degeneration which may ultimately lead to neuronal death.

Degeneration of the nerve fibre spreads along the axon in both directions away from the site of injury. Degeneration can therefore affect both the synaptic terminals and the cell body (Figure 5.1). Degeneration of synaptic terminals in efferent, motor nerves affects the neuromuscular junction, thereby leading to muscle denervation. Degeneration of synaptic terminals in afferents

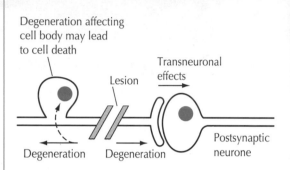

Figure 5.1 Nerve fibre degeneration following injury. Degeneration spreads in both directions along the axon from the site of injury, leading to cell-body degeneration and synaptic degeneration. Postsynaptic neurones may also be affected due to loss of normal synaptic input.

Degeneration affecting cell body may lead to cell death

Lesion

Transneuronal effects

Degeneration   Degeneration

Postsynaptic neurone

affects nerve–nerve junctions and will therefore result in changes in postsynaptic neurones. These postsynaptic effects include **supersensitivity** to neurotransmitters, **collateral sprouting** of other afferent terminals and **unmasking** of previously unused synaptic connections.

Neurotransmitter supersensitivity can be due to a number of factors, including a reduced uptake and enzymic destruction of transmitter in the synaptic cleft as a result of degeneration of synaptic terminals and an increase in the number and the sensitivity of postsynaptic neurotransmitter receptor sites (Figure 5.2).

As has been previously discussed, such supersensitivity to neurotransmitters may contribute to some of the symptoms observed in spasticity – hyperreflexia and hypertonia. However, there may be some cases where supersensitivity can be advantageous. Following reduced dopaminergic input from substantia nigra neurones to neurones in the corpus striatum of the basal ganglia in Parkinson's disease, the neurones of the corpus striatum can exhibit an increased sensitivity to dopamine. This may help to offset the effects of reduced dopamine levels in the basal ganglia, and delay the onset of the symptoms of Parkinson's

Figure 5.2 Neurotransmitter supersensitivity. Neurotransmitter released into the synaptic cleft may not be broken down enzymatically, or the re-uptake of the transmitter by the presynaptic cell may be reduced. The number of postsynaptic receptor sites for the transmitter may increase. These changes effectively increase the response of the postsynaptic cell to the neurotransmitter.

Figure 5.3 Sprouting axon collaterals from peripheral afferents can fill the synaptic vacancies left by degeneration of other axon terminals. This effectively increases the synaptic input from these peripheral afferents, thereby enhancing the response of the postsynaptic cell to this afferent input.

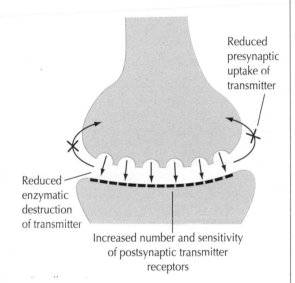

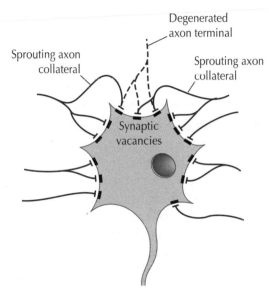

disease (it will be recalled that it has been estimated that these symptoms only appear after > 80% of the dopaminergic neurones have been destroyed, see the discussion on basal ganglia lesions, p. 85). Such increased sensitivity to dopamine may also increase the subject's responsiveness to L-DOPA.

Following synaptic degeneration, axon collaterals from unaffected neurones may sprout to fill the synaptic 'vacancies' which remain. These axon collaterals may arise from other peripheral afferent neurones, involving several spinal segments, or from descending fibres (Figure 5.3). This filling of synaptic vacancies may occur in a haphazard fashion, with axon collaterals from several diverse sources making contact with the postsynaptic cell. This **non-specific sprouting** may contribute to the abnormal reflexes seen in spasticity or following injury to the spinal cord.

A degree of **functional sprouting**, however, may occur, in which the input from the other peripheral sources, particularly those from other spinal segments which have a broadly similar function to those inputs which have been lost, may be utilized to sustain 'new' functional inputs which can be used to restore normal function to a certain extent.

The outcome of these processes of collateral sprouting is that a new *abnormal* synaptic organization has been established which will affect functional performance. Physiotherapy techniques may have a role to play in ensuring that it is the latter form of functional collateral sprouting which is achieved, by increasing appropriate afferent input to the spinal cord soon after the initial injury.

Distinct from collateral sprouting is a mechanism whereby previously-existing synapses which were not normally utilized (so-called **latent synapses**) are activated following injury or lesion, probably due to removal of inhibitory influences from other pathways. This remodelling of synaptic input therefore allows the possibility for new 'alternative' neural pathways to be opened up. This may be particularly important in the central nervous system, where regeneration of nervous tissue is impossible or limited, by enabling restructuring of important pathways following central nervous system lesions (e.g. in stroke).

Recent research, using positron emission tomography (PET), has demonstrated that in some patients with localized lesions of the corticospinal tract in the brain, there is recruitment of other accessory motor areas which are normally used for selection of movements and attention to movement, as well as a functional reorganization of the motor and sensory cortices. In other words, new motor pathways are being utilized in these patients.

Such plastic reorganization of central neural pathways has important implications for clinicians and physiotherapists. They must recognize that the potential for such reorganization exists, and that they have the ability to influence the outcome of this reorganization through appropriate therapeutic intervention.

Bibliography

Cohen, H (1993) *Neuroscience for Rehabilitation*. Lippincott, Philadelphia.

Kandel, ER, Schwartz, JH, Jessel, TM (1991) *Principles of Neural Science*. 3rd Edition. Appleton and Lange, Connecticut.

Kidd, G, Lawes, L, Musa, I (1992) *Understanding Neuromuscular Plasticity — a Basis for Clinical Rehabilitation*. Edward Arnold, London.

Rothwell, J (1994) *Control of Human Voluntary Movement*. 2nd Edition. Chapman and Hall, London.

Stephenson, R (1993) A review of neuroplasticity — some implications for physiotherapy in the treatment of lesions of the brain. *Physiotherapy,* 79: 699–704.

Weiller, C, Ramsay, SC, Wise, RJ, Friston, KJ, Frackowiak, RS (1993) Individual patterns of functional reorganization in the human cerebral cortex after capsular infarction. *Annals of Neurology, 33*: 181–189.

6

Skeletal Muscle

Skeletal Muscle Composition
•
Molecular Aspects of Muscle Contraction
•
Mechanical Aspects of Muscle Contraction
•
Energetics of Muscle Contraction
•
Contraction of Whole Muscles *in vivo*
•
Growth, Aging and Adaptability of Skeletal Muscles
•
Physiology of Skeletal Muscle Damage and Repair
•
Skeletal Muscle Fatigue

Skeletal Muscle Composition

Skeletal muscle is the largest tissue in the body and accounts for approximately 40–45% of the total body weight. This muscle mass performs a variety of functions within the body; some functions are under voluntary control while others are performed through involuntary mechanisms. The diversity of roles necessitates differences in the composition and innervation of the muscle.

Differentiation of Skeletal Muscle Fibres

Skeletal muscle can be differentiated into fibre types by a number of different methods. One of the most common is a histochemical procedure in which frozen pieces of muscle are cut into very thin sections and placed on a microscope slide. The temperature of the section is then allowed to rise to 37°C and is reacted with various chemicals in order to identify visually both structure and enzyme activities with a microscope. The most useful reaction used to differentiate skeletal muscle fibres is one which identifies the different speeds of muscle fibre contraction. The reaction is based on the principle that the speed at which a muscle contracts is dependent on its ability to release energy for the mechanical contraction. The energy is released by an enzymatic splitting of **adenosine triphosphate** (ATP) to **adenosine diphosphate** (ADP) and **inorganic phosphate** (P_i).

$$ATP = ADP + P_i$$

This splitting process is referred to as the ATPase activity. The histochemical process links this to chemicals which cause a deposit at the site of activity on the slide, thus differentiating each fibre according to ATPase activity and hence its contractile speed.

Two primary classes of muscle fibre emerge from this ATPase reaction, namely **type I** and **type II**. Functionally fibres which split ATP quickly and therefore contract quickly are termed type II fibres while those which split ATP slowly and hence contract slowly are termed type I fibres. Further chemical reactions can be carried out to divide the type II fibres into types IIA, IIB and IIC. The difference in contractile speeds between type II fibres is minimal. A section through a human muscle, which has undergone chemical reaction to demonstrate its ATPase activity, is shown in Figure 6.1.

Figure 6.1   ATP-reacted skeletal muscle identifying type I, IIA and IIB fibres.

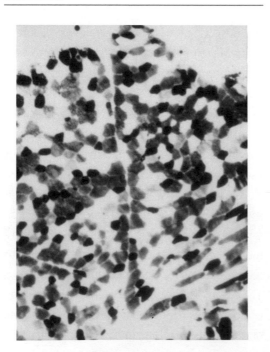

The differences in the ATPase activity of muscle fibres are due to differences in the multimolecular structure of a protein within the muscle called **myosin**. Immunological techniques using specific antibodies for components of the myosin, the **isozymes,** have been able to show that within each class of muscle fibre there is a spectrum of isozyme activity and perhaps that the classification into only three type II fibres is simplistic. Although it is possible to visualize these fibres using histochemical procedures they are much easier to differentiate using immunological procedures. In general, each muscle fibre contains only one class of myosin (type I or type II). However the proportion of the different isozymes within each class may vary thus resulting in a spectrum of contractile speeds. But because there appears little difference in the contractile speeds within the two primary classes the simple differentiation into types I, IIA, IIB and IIC tend to be used.

Although the ATPase activity of a fibre can identify contractile speeds it is also sometimes important to identify how a fibre obtains its energy. This can be carried out by biochemical assessment of the activity of an enzyme within a single muscle fibre or by histochemical technique. Classically, the enzyme used is **succinic dehydrogenase** (SDH) which is an enzyme within the mitochondria and is indicative of the fibre's ability to produce ATP by **aerobic** mechanisms (see p. 107). Thus it is possible to differentiate those fibres which have a high capacity to generate energy by aerobic means and those which are dependent to a greater extent on **anaerobic** sources. Figure 6.2 shows a section of human muscle which is reacted for SDH. This information, together with the contractile information displayed in Figure 6.1, allows muscle fibres to be profiled. The number of serially matched sections need not be

Figure 6.2   SDH-reacted skeletal muscle identifying high and low SDH activity fibres.

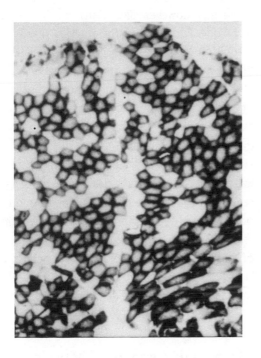

Table 6.1

Comparison of Muscle Fibre-typing Systems

ATP activity	Succinic dehydrogenase	Electrophysiology
I	High	S
IIa	High	FR
IIb	Low	FF
IIc	—	F_{int}

Percutaneous Needle Biopsy

The investigation of human skeletal muscle composition *in vivo* has been made possible by the use of the needle biopsy technique which was introduced by Bergstrom in 1962. Prior to that, information on the composition of muscles was derived from cadavers or from pieces of muscle which were removed by surgical operation. The biopsy has therefore been critical in developing the understanding of muscle metabolism in health and disease. The biopsy requires only a local anaesthetic and a small scalpel incision to allow the insertion of a needle. The only sensation felt can be likened to hitting oneself on the corner of a sharp object, i.e. a feeling of deep pressure. Ambulant patients walk, or in exercise studies subjects run or cycle, immediately afterwards. It is possible to obtain about 100–200 mg of muscle which is quite sufficient to enable detailed analysis. The biopsy needle procedure is illustrated in Figure 6.3.

The biopsy is used as a diagnostic tool for the identification of muscle pathology. Alterations in the size and distribution of fibre types occur in a variety of muscle disorders. Selective atrophy of type II fibres can frequently be found in osteomalacia (Figure 6.4), steroid therapy and metabolic disease. McArdle's disease, a deficiency in the phosphorylase system is also routinely diagnosed using histochemical techniques.

limited to only these two histochemical reactions. Sections can be reacted for capillary density as well as other enzymes. This type of profiling is referred to as histochemical profiling.

Another common method for differentiating muscle types is by **electrophysiological techniques**. By stimulating specific motor neurones and measuring the time to peak tension and the time to fatigue, it is possible to identify four types of muscle fibre: fast twitch and easily fatigued (FF), fast twitch and resistant to fatigue (FR), fast twitch and intermediate to fatigue (F_{int}) and slow twitch and resistant to fatigue (S). A twitch is the mechanical response generated by a single action potential. These methods of characterizing fibres are not directly interchangeable although it is possible to make some generalizations as detailed in Table 6.1.

Figure 6.3 (a) Components of a biopsy needle; (b) the biopsy procedure; (c) the muscle obtained after biopsy.

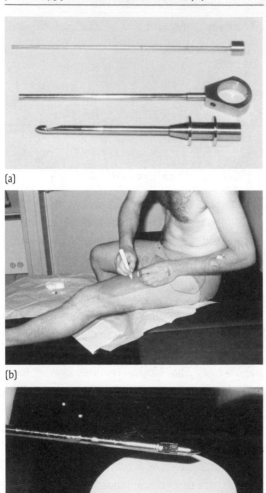

(a)

(b)

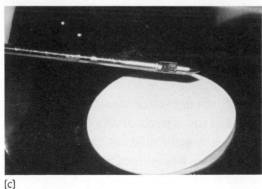

(c)

Muscle composition of healthy individuals can also be detected by biopsy. Classically, the sprinter has a high proportion of type II fibres, which are not necessarily high in SDH activity, whereas the marathon runner has a high proportion of type I fibres, which are high in SDH activity. The degree to which these muscle profiles can be altered by physical activity and training is discussed in Chapter 9.

There are, however, limitations to the biopsy technique. For example, the anterior tibialis has a total muscle fibre count of around 150 000 fibres while the biopsy routinely samples only 500 fibres. Few studies standardize for the depth or the specific spot for biopsy, because an assumption was always made that the fibre-type distribution was random throughout the muscle. However, by the 1980s, studies indicated that this was not the case. It became clear that in the deeper regions of the muscle there is an increase in the occurrence of type II fibres. Also in denervating diseases, such as motor neurone disease, groups of atrophic fibres occur alongside groupings of larger fibres and this type of irregular patterning would not necessarily be detected by biopsy.

Molecular Aspects of Muscle Contraction

The anatomical details of skeletal muscle have been presented in Chapter 1 and are reviewed here in order to allow the functional mechanisms of contraction to be considered. Skeletal muscle is composed of two principal proteins, **actin** and **myosin**. The myosin molecule, as discussed above, is responsible for splitting the ATP molecule and has been likened in shape to a golf club because of its long stem and head. The actin molecule forms a helical shape and is smaller than myosin. The arrangement of actin and myosin within the fibre give it a characteristic banding pattern when viewed microscopically, and with each set of bands arranged in repeating units called **sarcomeres**. The different bands within the sarcomere are ascribed a specific nomenclature. The arrangement of the proteins within the sar-

Figure 6.4   Section through skeletal muscle in (left) a normal subject and (right) a patient with proximal muscle weakness secondary to osteomalacia. The patient's muscle shows a severe degree of type II atrophy.

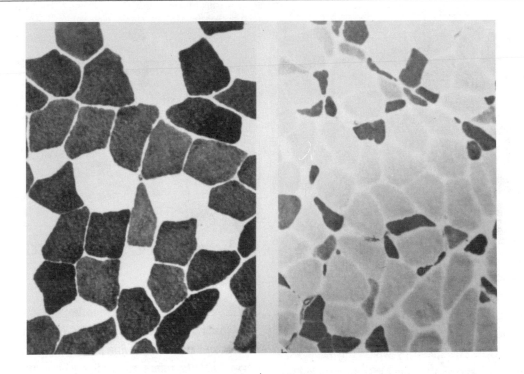

comere are displayed diagrammatically in Figure 6.5 and as seen under an electron microscope in Figure 6.6. In the region of overlap of the actin and myosin, the myosin heads are randomly attached to the actin, giving the muscle a firmness or tone.

Figure 6.5   The arrangement of the proteins, actin and myosin, within the sarcomeres of skeletal muscles and the resultant A and I banding pattern.

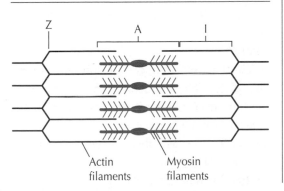

In addition to the two proteins actin and myosin there are, associated with the actin, two regulatory proteins **troponin** and **tropomyosin**. These proteins are bound together in such a way that the tropomyosin prevents the actin and myosin from binding together. However, on the muscle receiving an impulse from a motor neurone, calcium is released from the **sarcoplasmic reticulum** which is equivalent to the endoplasmic reticulum found in most other kinds of cells. The calcium binds to specific sites on the troponin and alters its shape. This in turn alters the nature of the attachment between troponin and tropomyosin. The resultant effect is that tropomyosin is pulled out of its blocking position and the actin and myosin are allowed to bind. Removal of the calcium from the troponin reverses the process. The process is presented diagramatically in Figure 6.7.

Figure 6.6   Ultrastructural micrograph of skeletal muscle identifying A band, I band, Z line, mitochondria, H-zone and T-tubules.

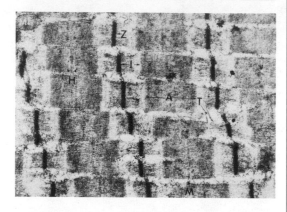

In the presence of calcium and energy, movement progresses by means of a ratchet-like motion. In this way, the I band shortens without any change in the length of the A band. This process by which skeletal muscle contracts is known as the **sliding-filament theory** and was devised by H.E. Huxley in the 1960s. The speed by which this happens, as discussed above, varies in different muscle fibres. The cyclical process by which muscle contracts and relaxes is illustrated in Figure 6.8.

Figure 6.7   The tropomyosin (TR) in (a) does not allow the myosin cross-bridge to contact the actin. When calcium (Ca^{2+}) attaches to the troponin (T) it alters its shape which in turn removes the tropomyosin from its blocking position and allows the actin and myosin to make contact (b).

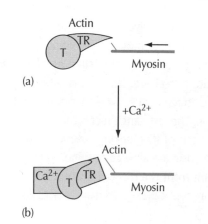

Figure 6.8   The cyclic process of muscle contraction and relaxation.
A = actin, M = myosin, Ca^{2+} = calcium, ATP = adenosine triphosphate, ADP = adenosine diphosphate, P_i = phosphate.

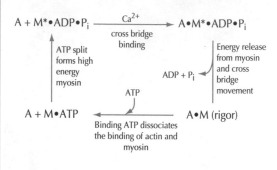

Mechanical Aspects of Muscle Contraction

The mechanical aspects of muscle contraction can be studied in a variety of ways. When contraction is looked at in the moving animal, it is termed *in vivo*. *In situ* refers to studies where muscle is examined in an anaesthetized animal preparation. Finally, the *in vitro* method is where a tissue is isolated from its environment and experiments are conducted with the tissue bathed in a physiological fluid bath. Our initial consideration of how whole muscles contract will draw on information gathered from *in vitro* animal experiments.

The mechanical response to a single action potential is termed a 'twitch'. Following this stimulus but prior to the muscle developing **tension**, defined as the force exerted on an object by a contracting muscle, a **latent period** exists during which the excitation contraction mechanisms take place. The contraction time is defined as the time from the onset of contraction to the time of peak tension and varies in the different fibre types. In type I fibres the contraction time can be 100 ms, whereas in type II fibres the contraction time can be 10 ms.

Functionally, as action potentials last only 1–2 ms, it is possible for a second stimulus to be received before the muscle has finished the previous contraction. In such cases the muscle responds again and results in an increase in muscle tension. This process is called **summation**. When the frequency of the action potentials is sufficiently high then the muscle will produce a **tetanus**. Thereafter, as action potential frequency increases, the tension produced rises until maximum tetanic tension is reached (Figure 6.9).

The maximum tetanic tension can be altered by changing the resting length of the muscle. The resting length of most muscles in the body represents the optimal length to produce maximum tension. Either side of the optimal length (i.e. either shorter or longer) and the ability to produce tension decreases. This can be explained in terms of the sliding-filament theory. Essentially, when the muscle is stretched, there are fewer opportunities for the myosin heads to make contact with the actin. In the extreme, this would mean no overlap of the actin and myosin. At lengths less than that which are optimal, the actin filaments from either end of the sarcomere over-

Figure 6.9   The response of skeletal muscle to an increased frequency of stimulation.

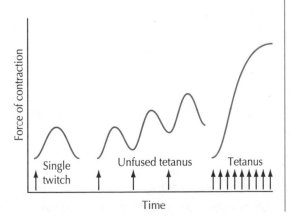

Figure 6.10   Length-tension relationship in skeletal muscle fibres, illustrating the cross-bridge relationship between the actin and myosin.

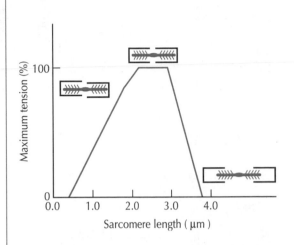

lap and interfere with the myosin interaction (Figure 6.10).

When muscle develops tension, it can either shorten or not. If the muscle does not shorten, then the contraction is termed **isometric** (Figure 6.11a). Where the muscle shortens and a load is moved, it is termed **isotonic** (Figure 6.11b). If a muscle, as it is contracting, is simultaneously being stretched, the movement is termed **eccentric**. This would be the case for the quadriceps muscle of the thigh when walking downhill or jumping from height onto the ground. Conversely, if a muscle is shortening and the lever is closing, the movement is called **concentric**.

Energetics of Muscle Contraction

The ATP which is used for the contraction of muscle is derived from two primary energy sources, carbohydrate and fat. Only when carbohydrate stores are particularly low or when exercise is particularly prolonged would protein be used as a fuel.

Figure 6.11 Methods of recording isometric and isotonic muscle contractions. (After Vander *et al.*, 1990.)

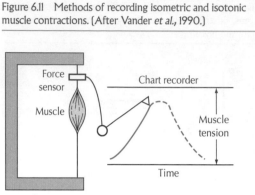

(a) ISOMETRIC CONTRACTION

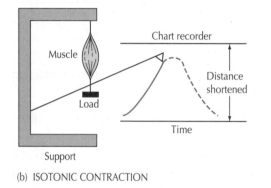

(b) ISOTONIC CONTRACTION

Carbohydrate is stored in the muscle as **glycogen**. Muscle glycogen is progressively broken down by a series of enzymatic reactions in the muscle to carbon dioxide and water. The glucose formed from its breakdown is not released into the bloodstream. During this process ATP is formed as a product of these reactions at various stages in the pathway. The enzyme phosphorylase, which is responsible for initiating the breakdown of glycogen to **glucose-6-phosphate,** is activated by an increase in the level of calcium in the cytoplasm. It has already been noted that it is also calcium which allows the combining of the actin and myosin to initiate the cross-bridge cycling of muscle contraction. It is therefore the same trigger which initiates the energy release necessary for muscle contraction that also initiates the mechanical contraction.

Glycogen is also stored in the liver and through hepatic enzymatic processes, glucose is released into the bloodstream.

The glucose-6-phosphate concentration in the muscle can be augmented by phosphorylating the glucose from the blood. In patients suffering from McArdle's syndrome, there is no activity of muscle phosphorylase, therefore, glucose from the bloodstream is the sole source of glucose-6-phosphate. The process collectively from glycogen to glucose is termed **glycogenolysis**.

The subsequent rate of breakdown of glucose to pyruvate, termed **glycolysis,** is controlled by the activity of the enzyme phosphofructokinase. The pyruvate then has two possible fates. The principal one is to enter the mitochondria and proceed through the **tricarboxylic acid** (TCA) cycle to form carbon dioxide, water and ATP. The process is dependent on a sufficient supply of oxygen and is therefore termed aerobic. When the rate of glycolysis exceeds that of the delivery of oxygen to the tissue then the pyruvate is metabolized to lactate or in some circumstances alanine. This latter process, as it occurs in the absence of oxygen, is termed 'anaerobic'. Although a large proportion of the ATP is formed from the activity of the TCA cycle (38 ATP per molecule of glucose substrate), it is possible to produce ATP solely from the glycolytic pathway (2 ATP per molecule of glucose substrate). An overview of the breakdown of glycogen to yield ATP is presented in Figure 6.12.

The average male has about 15% fat whereas a lean female has about 20% fat. The more of this vast fat store that can be utilized during exercise, the

Figure 6.12   Overview of the energy pathways for skeletal muscle.

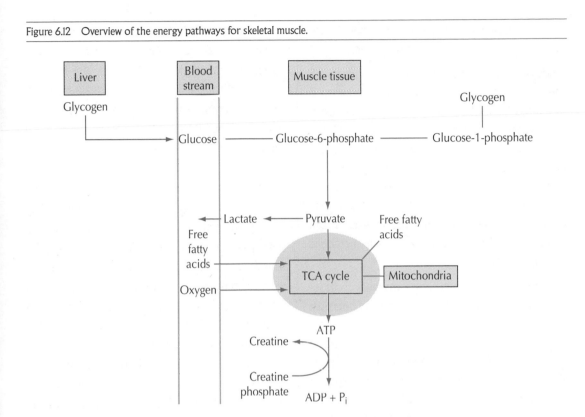

greater sparing effect on the limited glycogen stores.

Fat is stored in adipose tissue of which there are two types, **white adipose tissue (WAT)** cells and **brown adipose tissue (BAT)** cells. Fat is stored as **triacylglycerol** in these cells and in skeletal muscle. WAT cells are the long-term storage sites for fat whereas the BAT cells have a specific function related to energy balance in response to overfeeding and to increased heat production on exposure to cold. The triacylglycerols in the WAT cells and the skeletal muscle are those principally used for skeletal muscle energy. The triacylglycerol is hydrolysed to form **free fatty acids (FFA)** and **glycerol**. The FFA released from the WAT circulates in the blood associated with a plasma protein, **albumin**. On reaching the muscle tissue, the FFA is taken up by the mitochondria of the muscle and degraded to yield ATP through the TCA cycle. Similarly, the intramuscular triacylglycerol is broken down to FFA and glycerol and the FFA enters the TCA cycle. Although the energy yield resulting from the aerobic metabolism of FFA is greater (e.g. 129 ATP from 1 molecule of palmitic acid) than that from an equal amount of carbohydrate, the rate of production is slower. The excess glycerol and FFA which are not picked up by skeletal muscle are passed to the liver where the glycerol can be converted by **gluconeogenesis** to glycogen and the FFAs are released back into the bloodstream in a form called chylomicron.

In addition to the two metabolic fuels, carbohydrate and fat, there is a limited store of ATP and a slightly larger store of **creatine phosphate** within muscle. Creatine phosphate stores can replete ADP to ATP, although these stores can only maintain supplies for approximately 3–5 s and are essentially used to allow the other slower multienzyme pathways to be put in place.

Understanding of how muscle is provided with the energy it requires to function properly is facilitated by looking at the chemical processes detailed above. However, more fundamental is the understanding of how these various pathways integrate to allow the muscle to respond to different activity demands. No one pathway is used exclusively but in different situations one pathway may be dominant. This integration can be exemplified by considering muscle metabolic response to acute exercise.

In response to a demand for a maximal contraction, the ATP energy stores are brought into play. These are immediately repleted by creatine phosphate. Simultaneously, the calcium concentration of the cytosol increases and phosphorylase is activated causing the breakdown of glycogen to glucose-6-phosphate. This action raises the concentration of glucose-6-phosphate which in turn then inhibits the phosphorylation of glucose collected from the blood. It is not until the glycogen stores are low that there is a significant usage of blood glucose. Glycolysis then continues the process of energy production until pyruvate is produced. If the mitochondria are able to meet the aerobic needs of the glycolytic flux, then pyruvate will enter the TCA cycle. If the intensity of exercise is so high that the energy demands cannot be met aerobically then pyruvate is converted to lactate. The slowest of the systems, fat utilization, comes into play, particularly as the duration of exercise is prolonged and also in the aerobic recovery from exercise.

The recent development of noninvasive **nuclear magnetic resonance (NMR)** spectroscopy units large enough to accommodate whole limbs is greatly enhancing our knowledge about fuel utilization with different functional demands. Use of

in vivo NMR offers the advantage of being non-invasive and has the advantage over other forms of radiography as it does not involve any form of ionizing radiation. Thus atoms containing naturally occurring, nonradioactive elemental isotopes such as ^{31}P, ^{13}C and ^{1}H can be used to trace metabolites. ^{31}P NMR is used to study concentrations of ATP, creatine phosphate and inorganic phosphate. It can also indirectly measure pH. The results arising from NMR experiments differ slightly from those derived from biopsy, this is perhaps because there is no delay in preparing the muscle for assay after biopsy. Clearly further work is required to determine the true values for these and other metabolites. A typical scan from an NMR is presented in Figure 6.13. One disadvantage of this technique is that it is not possible to distinguish cell specific characteristics, i.e. differentiate between the metabolic profiles of the different fibre types. However, the full potential of NMR spectroscopy has yet to be developed with the possibility of it being used to measure lactate by ^{1}H NMR and of glycogen and glucose levels by ^{13}C NMR.

Positron emission tomography (PET) is another technological advance that offers great potential for studying regional blood flow and metabolism. This system is based on short half-life isotopes such as ^{11}C and ^{82}Rb which emit positrons when they decay. When a positron-emitting isotope is injected into the circulation supplying a tissue, then the isotope will flow where the blood flows. PET does have the disadvantage of needing a radioactive injection of isotope; however, the half-life of the isotopes commonly used is only minutes. So far, the technique has concentrated on heart and brain metabolism but the potential for work in studying skeletal muscle blood flow is enormous.

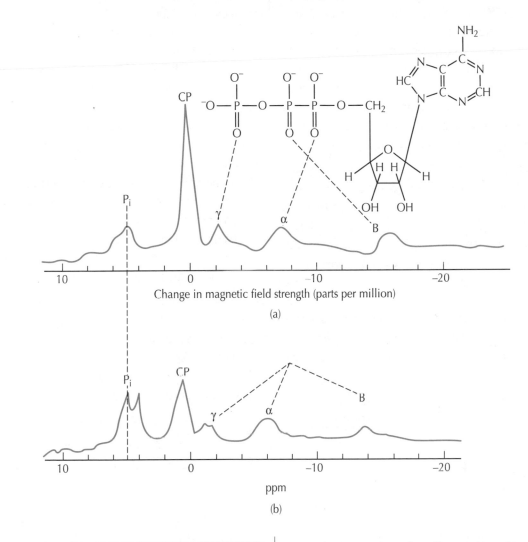

Figure 6.13   Topical NMR phosphate spectrum from a human forearm before (a) and after (b) fatiguing isometric exercise. The area under each peak is proportional to the concentration of free phosphate increase and the levels of creatine phosphate (CP) and ATP decrease. In addition, the phosphate peak splits and shifts to the right. (After Nunnally *et al.,* (1983) Macmillan, New York.)

Contraction of Whole Muscles *in vivo*

Although studies of *in vitro* muscle provide a great deal of information, the properties of isolated muscle do not always reflect those of *in vivo* muscle. One reason for this is that the muscles work across a system of levers. A contracting muscle only produces a pulling action, drawing the bones to which it is attached toward each other. This movement is termed **flexion**. In contrast, the opening up of the angle of a joint is termed **extension**. This latter movement requires an additional muscle working antagonistically to the muscle which has closed the joint. Therefore groups of muscles that work across a joint are known as **agonists**. *In vitro,* muscle would produce a maximum isometric tension at the length that the muscle is at full extension. However, maximal tension during elbow flexion is generated at 90°. In addition, the forces generated in a linear model of isolated muscle do not mirror those forces generated when the muscles are working in a lever system (Figure 6.14). Also, the tension of the muscle can be added to, *in vivo*, when external tension is applied. If the supporting contractile mechanisms cannot bear this additional external tension, then injury ensues.

Clearly, within the whole muscle, the force generated is the composite force of many muscle fibres. The greater the number of fibres involved, the greater the tension development. It has already been discussed that muscle is not homogeneous and that the speed of contraction varies. It was also noted that in order to gain maximum diversity of muscle function, it is necessary to innervate the muscles differentially. The systematic recruitment of muscle fibres dictates the tension development of the whole muscle fibre. The abil-

ity of type I fibres to develop force does not differ greatly from type II fibres when expressed as per unit of cross-sectional area. However, the size of the motor unit innervating the two types of fibre does vary. The type I fibres are innervated by small, low-threshold, slowly conducting motor nerves, whilst the type II fibres are innervated by large higher threshold, fast conducting motor nerves. In general, glycogen depletion will be highest in the type II fibres when high intensity work is carried out. Conversely, the primary fibre involved in low intensity work is the type I fibre. When the activity is prolonged there is a progressive recruitment of the type IIa fibres. At exhaustion, all motor units will have been involved. In reality, the differences are not as discrete as would appear from the model but rather there is a continuum of thresholds for activation.

Functionally therefore, it is clear that not all muscle fibres within a muscle are recruited at the same time for any one action and it is this facility that allows human skeletal muscle to work over a range from delicate movements to extremely powerful contractions.

Figure 6.14 In the body, muscles act across bone levers so that the force exerted will usually be different from the force of muscular contraction. (After Brooks and Fahey, 1985.)

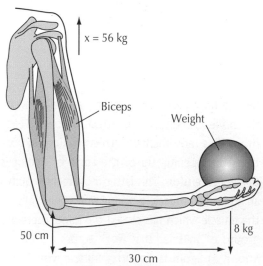

Figure 6.15 Diagram illustrating that there is a point at which increasing the girth of the muscle does not produce a linear increase in the force produced.

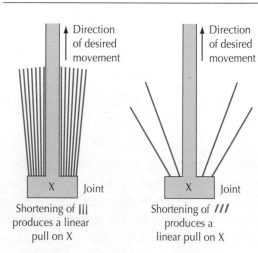

Figure 6.16   CAT-scan of quadriceps of (a) a lean individual and (b) an individual carrying a degree of fatty tissue around the thigh.

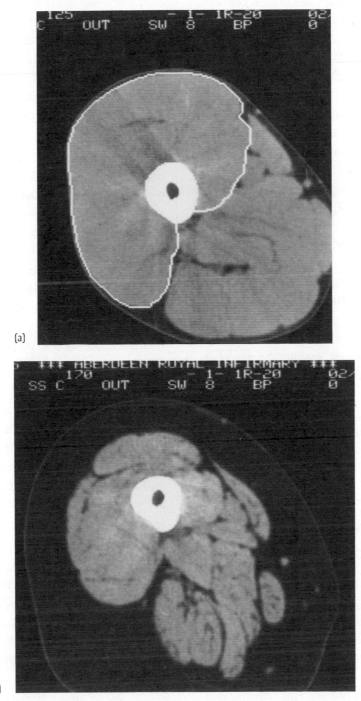

(a)

(b)

Muscle size is also another important determinant of the force of muscle contraction. The greater the number of cross-bridges connecting actin and myosin, the greater the tension the muscle is able to produce. Basically, the bigger the muscle the greater the contractile force, although there is a finite size beyond which the full benefits of the increase in tissue cannot be realized because of an increased angle of pennation (Figure 6.15). Measurement of muscle size can now be accurately measured using **computerized axial tomography (CAT)** scan (Figure 6.16) or more recently through the safer **magnetic resonance imaging (MRI)** which uses the same principles as NMR. Simpler techniques of measuring the size of the muscle by measuring its circumference have now repeatedly been shown to be invalid because of the complexities of estimating the amount of fat. There are, however, reports of multiple peripheral measures which do correlate with the CAT-scan data. These measures would appear to be muscle specific and therefore it would be necessary to ensure that the equation used to calculate muscle size was derived from a validated study that was concerned with the muscle being investigated.

Growth, Aging and Adaptability of Skeletal Muscle

Prepubertal Development

Fetal muscle does not develop to a stage that can be differentiated into fibre types. Progressively, up to about one year of age, fibres become differentiated. Few studies have investigated the fibre type composition of the young primarily due to the ethical considerations associated with the use of the needle biopsy in children and as yet NMR studies have not produced detailed analysis. However, the available evidence would suggest that there is a dominance of type I fibres and the undifferentiated IIC fibres in early to mid-childhood. Within the limited type II population there is also a dominance of type IIA rather than IIB. This would suggest a skeletal muscle profile which was aerobically based with a low ability for fast contraction.

Fibre number would not appear to alter with development and is therefore thought to be genetically predetermined. Growth occurs by increasing the size of the fibres proportionally to body dimensions. Linear growth occurs by increasing the number of sarcomeres on the distal ends of the myofibrils. The cross-sectional size of the fibres at one year is in the range 500–600 µm (Aherne et al., 1971), whereas in adults there have been reports of fibres being anything between 2500–10 000 µm (Costrill et al., 1976).

Gender Differences

There is little difference, in the speed or strength characteristics of muscle, between the genders before puberty. However, the hormonal changes associated with puberty cause significant changes in the profile of the skeletal muscle.

The cross-sectional area of the female whole muscle is normally less than that of males with a consequent weaker force generation. There is some evidence to suggest that this is due to fewer muscle fibres rather than a reduced size of the individual muscle fibres (Saltin and Gollnick, 1983). This would imply that the potential for strength increase is always greater in males than in females as normally fibre number cannot be altered. No difference appears the percentage of different fibre types between males and females but in females the type I fibres are larger than the type II. Functionally, therefore, more of the total muscle is operating within the characteristics of type I fibres. This histochemical data is borne out by other studies where the time to reach 70% of maximum leg force, termed 'force-time', is approximately twice as long in females as males.

Biochemical evidence is also able to identify differences between men and women in that when matched for similar relative intensities of work women will tend to utilize fat stores to a greater extent than men.

In general, therefore, females are predisposed to low-intensity, long-duration activities. There is much statistical evidence within the sports literature that endorses this view.

Aging

Changes associated with aging in skeletal muscle have been confounded by the decrease in physical activity that accompanies it. However, it is clear that the muscle strength and power increases associated with normal growth and maturation, levels out and begins to decline during middle age and diminishes progressively with advancing age and senescence. Longitudinal studies report 1.8% and 2.8% decline per annum in muscle strength measured in men and women, respectively, between the ages of 70 and 75 years. Functionally, the loss in strength is critical with a large proportion of the older population reported to have limb strengths that hamper normal daily activity.

Functional tests measuring 65–84-year-old men's and women's abilities to raise themselves from a 42-cm high chair with their arms folded would indicate that 100% of men and 95% of women should be able to accomplish this in 1.8 and 2 s respectively. This height equates to the British Standards Institute recommendation for the height of a toilet pedestal. However, there is difficulty in some of this age group, particularly women, to step up onto a 50-cm step. This height of step is not uncommon in public transport.

The decline in muscle strength is most likely to be due to a decline in the size of the muscle, together with a reduction in the amount of active tissue by a progressive replacement by fat and connective tissue.

It would also appear that the reduction in the size of the muscle is not solely due to muscle atrophy but to a reduction in the number of fibres. The magnitude of the reduction in muscle fibres during adult life has been estimated to be around 33–50%. Two different phenomena may account for the loss of muscle fibres with age. They may become injured and because **satellite cells**, which are intimately involved in the repair of damaged muscle, lose the ability to proliferate with age and the repair process of the muscle cell is limited. Alternatively, fibres could be lost through the denervation of muscle fibres.

Differences occur in the mechanism by which muscles are recruited. Beyond 60 years it would appear that the number of motor units are about half that of youth. This is partially counteracted by an increase in the size of the motor units. This functional compensation must be due to re-innervation, of denervated muscle fibres, by sprouting from healthy adjacent nerve axons. The implication of these changes would suggest a diminution of fine motor control in the older person. There is parallel evidence of muscle fibre-type grouping with aging although the extent to which this occurs varies in different muscles.

The incorrect widespread belief that there is a selective loss and **atrophy** of type II fibres has essentially been explained by limitations in the needle biopsy technique. Autopsy work has demonstrated that both type I and type II fibres are equally susceptible to the aging process.

Exercise can offset some of the atrophy and subsequent loss in muscle strength but, as at least some of that loss is due to a diminished regenerative capacity of muscle tissue, there is an inevitable loss of muscle tissue and thus function.

Alongside the loss of muscle strength, aged muscle has been shown to have an altered metabolic profile. There exists a reduced capacity to regenerate ATP and aerobically performed tasks are also reduced because of an inability of the cardiovascular system to deliver oxygen and a reduction of the capacity of the mitochondria to utilize the oxygen. The cumulative consequence of these alterations is an impaired ability for prolonged muscular activity.

Adaptability of Muscle to Changes in the Pattern of Stimulation

It is a consistent observation that if a type I muscle fibre is innervated by a nerve which normally innervates a type II fibre then conversion of the type I fibre to a type II fibre takes place. The converse is also true. Chronic electrical stimulation of the motor nerves mimicking the pattern of the opposite nerve will produce similar conversions.

Chordotomy, which produces electrical silence of the nerves, effects a conversion of type I fibres to type II fibres. This would suggest that the maintenance of type I properties depends on chronic electrical activity. Experimental chordotomy is like spinal cord section in humans resulting from accidents. In such patients all fibres in the paralysed muscle react as type II fibres. Also, in **hemi-**

plegia there is an increase in the percentage of type II fibres on the affected side.

Electrical stimulation of muscle is a commonly used and well-substantiated strategy that physiotherapists use to augment strength in patients with muscle weakness as well as a technique to restore function to paralysed muscle. The mechanisms by which electrical stimulation restores strength, however, appear to be different from that achieved by voluntary activation of muscle. Evidence for this lies in the observation that strength gains are possible using neuromuscular electrical stimulation (NMES) in patients at training intensities as low as 25% of maximum voluntary contraction (MVC). No such parallel evidence is available from volitional exercise. This observation only seems to apply to patient studies. In healthy subjects NMES has similar effects to volitional exercise. However, the disparity may be due to methodological differences.

The different pattern of recruitment with the two types of innervation may partly explain the difference in muscle response. In volitional isometric contractions it is clear that the smaller motoneurones are activated first whereas with NMES the nerve fibre is activated at or near the motor endplate, resulting in activation of all motor units. In addition, the afferent input from the cutaneous stimulation results in inhibition of the type I fibres and an excitatory input to type II fibres. Further histochemical evidence and fatigue studies suggest that NMES does not 'train' the aerobic fatigue-resistant type I fibres but preferentially selects the type II fibres.

Studies on paralysed muscle where computers have been used to control movements of paralysed limbs in **paraplegia** and **quadriplegia** have increased quadriceps strength by two- and three-fold within only a few months. Some individuals paralysed for 6–8 years have been able to develop leg strength comparable to normal individuals. There does not appear to be any definitive answer as to the nature of the contractile response of the muscles of these patients to this type of stimulation.

These data illustrate the **plasticity** of adult skeletal muscle. Whether or not stimuli such as exercise are sufficient to alter the major contractile properties of skeletal muscle is explored further in Chapter 9.

Physiology of Skeletal Muscle Damage and Repair

Muscle strains appear to occur with the highest frequency in muscles that cross two joints and in those muscles with the highest proportion of type II muscle fibres. In addition, eccentrically exercised muscle appears to be predisposed to pain.

Muscle can be injured as a result of intrinsic or extrinsic factors. Damage to the blood vessels will normally occur and the consequent result is a **haematoma**. This will cause an increase in pressure and resultant pain and loss of function. If the injury has resulted in damage to the fascia then the haematoma may develop outwith the muscle. This external type of haematoma tends to cause less pain and is therefore less intrusive on muscle function.

Muscle repair is initiated by an invasion of macrophages within 24 h. After the initial inflammatory reaction is minimized, circulation must be enhanced to aid recovery. However, the timing of the introduction of therapy is difficult because the therapist is unaware when recovery has sufficiently progressed. New technologies, as will be seen later, would indicate that the recovery process is longer than has been assumed in the past.

The macrophage cells rapidly form fibroblasts and a collagen precursor is produced which gradually forms scar tissue. Because of the noncontractile nature of the collagen, the scar tissue does not contribute to the contractile function of the muscle but does allow the undamaged muscle to perform its function.

The capacity for skeletal muscle to regenerate has allowed for the development of techniques for the transplantation of muscle from one site to another. When a muscle is removed surgically, severing all nerve, blood and tendon connections the muscle degenerates before it regenerates. The degeneration is specific to the muscle cells. The satellite cells survive and trace a course which is similar to that of embryological muscle fibres. Although functionally these muscles do regenerate, they are impaired in terms of mass, strength and endurance. The training and timing of training associated with transplant is critical to the final performance of the muscle.

At present, muscle transplantation is most frequently used to improve the appearance of individuals after facial injuries, myopathies or for improving locomotion of patients with lower limb disorders.

The type of muscle damage described above is a fairly extreme result of injury. Less-severe muscle damage or muscle soreness, however, is a more common experience. This type of damage occurs after physical effort. The intensity of that effort could be minimal but if it exceeds that which is normally performed then it falls into the category of overuse. Therefore muscle soreness can result in an elderly person from walking a short distance whereas similar soreness in an athlete would take a much more severe exercise stress.

Soreness can be immediate or delayed. Immediate discomfort may be due to increased metabolites affecting free nerve endings or may result from ischaemia of the muscle tissue. Whatever the cause, this type of muscle soreness is short-lived. In contrast, **delayed onset muscle soreness (DOMS)** normally results 24–48 h after unaccustomed physical activity and will take 5–7 days to subside. The severity of DOMS differs with different exercise regimens. Eccentric muscle contractions produce the greatest degree of DOMS, with isometric and concentric contractions producing progressively less. After isometric work, DOMS is maximized at 24 h whilst concentric and eccentric peaks occur later at 48 h. Exercises working over a joint range that involves near maximal lengthening of the active muscle produces the highest levels of DOMS. The speed of the contraction does not appear to influence DOMS.

The particular agents causing DOMS have not been specifically identified. Lactic acid, although almost certainly a cause of acute pain after intense exercise, cannot satisfactorily explain DOMS. Another potential cause, the production of spasms in muscle has also been negated. A theory which does have considerable support is one that proposes the soreness results from damage to the connective tissue. This is evidenced by experiments identifying the predominant site of muscle soreness as occurring at the musculotendinous junction. Also elevated urinary excretion of hydroxyproline, which is a breakdown product of connective tissue, parallels muscle soreness.

Magnetic resonance imaging (MRI), based on the same principles as NMR has been tremendously powerful in identifying compositional changes of skeletal muscle which are subclinical. It is more powerful than the more traditional CAT-scan and ultrasound. Also, of course, it is nonionizing.

The results from MRI have progressed the debate around the underlying pathology of DOMS. Experiments exercising ankle plantar flexion have associated DOMS with a marked alteration in the medial head of gastrocnemius. MRI has also been able to identify an occurrence of perifascial fluid collections within a few days of injurious exercise; these are similar to the occurrence with strains and recede concurrent with resolution of symptoms. Abnormal signals from the injured muscle can be detected using MRI up to 80 days after the event, i.e. long after the symptoms have disappeared. The ability to detect the muscle injury for that length of time explains at least in part why muscle that has sustained an injury is susceptible to further injury beyond that time when, using other techniques, it appeared completely healed. MRI is still a relatively new technique in its application to skeletal muscle injury but lends itself well to further understanding of muscle repair mechanisms.

Although the specific processes underlying DOMS are unclear, there has been much work carried out on practices which could potentially alleviate muscle soreness. The effectiveness of stretching, ultrasound treatment and **transcutaneous electrical nerve stimulation (TENS)** is yet to be fully endorsed with contradictory evidence being available in the literature. Equally, the use of light exercise or massage is difficult to interpret due to the large number of variables used in producing the DOMS and the subjective scales used to classify the degree of pain and soreness. A rationale for thinking the application of ice might be used to alleviate DOMS was based on the known ability of removing heat to reduce inflammation associated with injury. It was thought logical to assume that ice might prove useful. However, ice does not seem to reduce muscle soreness.

In summary, therefore, currently the best mechanism for the treatment of DOMS is preventative, i.e. not to expose the muscle to excessive unfamiliar exercise but to progressively train the muscle to cope with the increased load.

Skeletal Muscle Fatigue

Although a great deal has been learned about the muscle fatigue process over recent years, the precise cause is not yet fully understood. This may be due, in part, to the fact that no one factor is responsible. Also, the cause of fatigue depends on the nature of the activity, and the individual's nutritional state, physical state and age.

Fatigue can be defined as the inability to maintain a required or expected power output. Power output is dependent on the neural input to a muscle as well as the intrinsic properties of the muscle itself.

The **Setchenov phenomenon,** named after its investigator, provides some evidence for central neural fatigue. Setchenov was able to demonstrate that recovery from fatigue is improved if a diverting activity is performed. In addition, central fatigue can be demonstrated by exposing the CNS to metabolic factors such as hypoglycaemia induced through prolonged exercise and ammonia produced with maximal exercise. It has also been suggested that the ratio of types of amino acids is altered with long-term exercise and this in turn can affect motivation and mood. These central effects could have implications for clinical assessment of patients.

Experimentally, involvement of the CNS can be excluded by stimulating the muscle directly. Such experiments suggest that fatigue in healthy individuals primarily occurs at the periphery beyond the neuromuscular junction. However impaired electromechanical activation is seen in patients with myasthenia gravis and some forms of myotonia.

As ATP is the sole source of direct energy for muscle, a depletion in this substrate must be considered a contributing factor in the fatigue process. During high intensity voluntary isometric contraction, blood flow is restricted and therefore the primary sources of fuel to replenish the ATP are creatine phosphate and anaerobic glycolysis. The rate of resynthesis of ATP from glycolysis and creatine phosphate declines at a rate similar to the loss in force production and it is possible to speculate that this is the cause of fatigue in this type of intense exercise. It is also clear that resynthesis is slower in the type II fibres with little or no change in the type I fibres thus suggesting that the capacity of the type II fibres to replenish their ATP is the limiting factor.

In parallel with increases in lactate during high-intensity exercise, venous ammonia concentrations also increase, particularly in type II fibres. A reduction in the concentration of blood ammonia appears to delay the onset of fatigue and increase duration of intense exercise. Ammonia is also linked with dysfunctional states such as epileptic seizures, mental confusion and altered neuronal excitability.

If high-intensity exercise is prolonged, then there is a concomitant decrease in muscle pH caused by an elevation of lactate. However, the likelihood of a decrease in pH being the primary cause of fatigue is remote as the recovery of force output in muscle occurs before the pH has returned to normal and more closely relates to the regeneration of creatine phosphate.

In long-term exercise, fuel utilization is still thought to be the primary cause of fatigue but

Figure 6.17   A series of slides reacted for (from left to right) ATP, glycogen and SDH at pre-exercise, post 25 miles and 50 miles. Although the animal was exhausted at 50 miles and a large number of the fibres are completely depleted of glycogen there are at least three fibres which look to be still full of glycogen fuel.

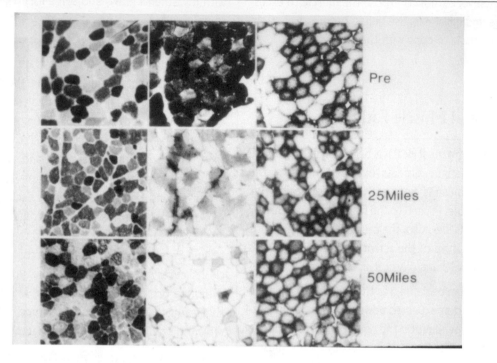

because the intensity is low, the replenishment of ATP is met sufficiently from aerobic processes. Fatigue therefore occurs progressively as the glycogen stores are utilized. This depletion can be fibre-type specific so that an athlete can be fatigued and exhausted whilst still retaining glycogen in adjacent muscle fibres. Figure 6.17 illustrates progressive glycogen depletion in a horse galloping over 50 miles.

Accumulation of calcium ions within the mitochondria has also been linked with muscle fatigue, as the accumulation can cause uncoupling of the energy production process. These changes are noted most significantly in conditions of rhabdomyolysis.

Bibliography

SKELETAL MUSCLE COMPOSTITION

Billeter, R, Heizman, CW, Howard, H, Jenny, E (1981) Analysis of myosin light and heavy chain types in single human skeletal muscle fibres. *European Journal of Biochemistry*, 116: 389.

Brooke, MH, Kaiser, KK (1970) Muscle fibre types. How many and what kind? *Archives of Neurology* 23: 369.

Buchtal, F, Schmalbuich, H (1970) Contraction times and fibre types in intact human muscle. *Acta Physiologica Scandinavica*, 79: 435.

Burke, RE, Edgerton, VR (1973) Motor unit properties and selective involvement in movement. *Exercise and Sports Sciences Review*, 31.

Curleso, RG, Nelson, MB (1975) Needle biopsies in infants for diagnosis and research. *Development Medicine and Child Neurology*, 17: 592.

Edwards, RHT (1981) Human muscle function and fatigue. *Human Muscle Fatigue: Physiological Mechanisms*, R Porter and J Whelan (eds), pp. 1–19. Pitman, London.

Edwards, RHT, Young, A, Wiles, C (1980) Needle biopsy of skeletal muscle in the diagnosis of myopathy and the clinical study of muscle function and repair. *New England Journal of Medicine*, 302: 261.

Elder, GCB (1977) The heterogeneity of fibre type populations in human skeletal muscle. *Medicine and Science in Sports and Exercise,* **9**: 64.

Eriksson, PO, Eriksson, A, Ringquist, M, Thornell, LE (1980) The reliability of histochemical fibre typing of human necropsy muscle. *Histochemistry,* **5**: 193.

Henriksson-Larsen, KB, Lexell, J, Sjostrom, M (1983) Distribution of different fibre types in human skeletal muscles. I. Method of preparation and analysis of cross-sections of whole tibialis anterior. *Histochemical Journal,* **15**: 167.

Jennekens, FGI, Tomlison, BE, Walton, JN (1971) Data on distribution of fibre types in five human limb muscles. An autopsy study. *Journal of Neurological Sciences,* **18**: 111.

Lexell, JD, Downham, D, Sjostrom, M (1983) Distribution of different fibre types in human skeletal muscle. A statistical and computational model for the study of fibre type grouping and early diagnosis of skeletal muscle fibre denervation and reinnervation. *Journal of Neurological Sciences,* **61**: 301.

Lexell, J, Downham, D, Sjostrom, M (1984) Distribution of different fibre types in human skeletal muscles. *Journal of Neurological Sciences,* **65**: 353.

MOLECULAR ASPECTS OF MUSCLE CONTRACTION

Brooks, G, Fahey, TD (1985) *Exercise Physiology,* Ch. 19, p. 377. Macmillan, New York.

Carlson, FD, Wilkie, DR (1974) *Muscle Physiology.* Prentice-Hall, New Jersey.

Vander, AJ, Sherman, JH, Luciano, DS (1990) *Human physiology* (5th edn.), Ch. 11, p. 283, McGraw-Hill, New York.

MECHANICAL ASPECTS OF MUSCLE CONTRACTION

Vander, AJ, Sherman, JH, Luciano, DS (1990) *Human physiology* (5th edn.), Ch. 11, p. 283, McGraw-Hill, New York.

ENERGETICS OF MUSCLE CONTRACTION

Berbus, G, Gonzales de Suso, JM, Alonso, J (1993) ^{31}P-MRS of quadriceps reveals quantitative differences between sprinters and long-distance runners. *Medicine and Science in Sports and Exercise,* **25**(4): 479.

Koretsky, AP, Williams, DS (1992) Application of localised NMR to whole organ physiology in the animal. *Annual Review of Physiology,* **54**: 799.

Mccully, KK, Kakihira, H, Vandenborne, K, Kent-Braun, J (1991) Non-invasive measurements of activity induced changes in muscle metabolism. *Journal of Biomechanics,* **24** (suppl.): 153.

Newsholme, EA, Leech, AR (1973) *Biochemistry for the Medical Sciences.* John Wiley, Chichester.

Newsholme, EA, Start, C (1973) *Regulation in Metabolism.* John Wiley, Chichester.

Sapega, AA, Sokolow, DP, Graham, TJ, Chance B (1987) Phosphorus nuclear magnetic resonance: a non-invasive technique for the study of muscle bioenergetics during exercise. *Medicine and Science in Sports and Exercise,* **19**(4): 656.

CONTRACTION OF WHOLE MUSCLES *IN VIVO*

Burke, RE, Tzairis, P (1977) The correlation of physiological properties with histochemical characteristics in single muscle units. *Annals of the New York Academy of Science* **301**: 144.

GROWTH, AGING AND ADAPTABILITY OF SKELETAL MUSCLES

Aherne, W, Ayyar, DR, Clarke, PA, Walton, JN (1971) Muscle fibre size in normal infants, children and adolescents *Journal of Neurological Science* **14**, 171–182.

Allied Dunbar National Fitness Survey (1992) A Report on Activity Patterns and Fitness Levels. Commissioned by the Sports Council and Health Education Authority.

Aniansson, A, Sperling, L, Rundgten, A, Lehnberg, E (1983) Muscle function in 75 year old men and women: a longitudinal study. *Scandinavian Journal of Rehabilitation Medicine* **9**: 92.

Costill, DL, Daniels, J, Evans, W *et al.* (1976) Skeletal muscle enzymes and fibre composition in male and female track athletes. *Journal of Applied Physiology* **40**, 149–154.

Delitto, A, Snyder-Mackler, L (1990) Two theories of muscle strength augmentation using percutaneous electrical stimulation. *Physical Therapy* **70**: 158.

Drinkwater, BL (1984) Women and exercise: physiological aspects. *Exercise and Sport Sciences Reviews,* **12**: 21.

Dubowitz, V (1988) Responses of diseased muscle to electrical and mechanical intervention. *Plasticity of the Nervous System,* Vol. 138, p. 240. Ciba Foundation Symposium, John Wiley, Chichester.

Essen, B, Jansson, E, Henriksson, J (1975) Metabolic characteristics of fibre types in human skeletal muscle. *Acta Physiologica Scandinavica,* **95**, 153.

Fleckenstein, JL, Shellock, FG (1991) Exertional muscle injuries: magnetic resonance imaging evaluation. *Topics in Magnetic Resonance Imaging,* **3**(4): 50.

Green, HJ, Fraser, IG, Ranney, DA (1984) Male and female differences in enzymes activities or energy metabolism in vastus lateralis muscle. *Journal of Neurological Sciences,* **65**: 323.

Malone, TR, Sanders, B (1993) Strength training and the athletic female. *The Athletic Female,* AJ Pearl (ed.), p. 169. Human Kinetics, Champaign, Illinois.

Milner-Brown, HS, Miller, RG (1988) Muscle strengthening through electrical stimulation combined with low resistance weights in patients with neuromuscular disorders. *Archives of Physical Medical Rehabilitation,* **69**: 20.

Nygard, E, Hede, K (1986) Physiological profiles of the male and female. *Exercise Benefits, Limits and Adaptations,* D MacLeod *et al.* (eds), p. 289. E & FN Spon, London.

Petrofsky, JS, Le Donne, DM, Rinehart, JS, Lind, AR (1976) Isometric strength and endurance during the menstrual cycle. *European Journal of Applied Physiology,* **35**, 1.

Physical Activity and Ageing (1988) *American Academy of Physical Education Papers*, No. 22, Human Kinetic Books, Champaign, Illinois.

Saltin, B, Gollnick, PD (1983) Skeletal muscle adaptability: significance for metabolism and performance. In: *Handbook of Physiology*, section ID: skeletal muscle (ed. LD Peachey). Oxford University Press, New York.

Skelton, DA, Greig, CA, Davies, JM, Young, A (1994). Strength, power and related functional ability of healthy people aged 65–89 years. *Age and Ageing* **23 (5)**: 371.

Young, A, Stokes, M, Crowe, M (1985) The size and strength of the quadriceps muscle of old and young men. *Clinical Physiology*, **5**: 145.

PHYSIOLOGY OF SKELETAL MUSCLE DAMAGE AND REPAIR

Appell, HJ, Soares, JM, Duarte, JA (1992) Exercise, muscle damage and fatigue. *Sports Medicine*, **13**(2): 108.

Ciccone, CD, Leggin, BG, Callamaro, JJ (1991) Effects of ultrasound and trolamine salicylate phonophoresis on delayed-onset muscle soreness. *Physical Therapy* **71**(9): 666.

Cleak, MJ, Eston, RG (1992) Delayed onset muscle soreness: mechanisms and management. *Journal of Sports Science*, **10**(4): 325.

Donnelly, AE, Clarkson, PM, Maughan, RJ (1992) Exercise induced muscle damage: effects of light exercise on damaged muscle. *European Journal of Applied Physiology*, **64**(4): 350.

Evans, WJ, Cannon, JG (1991) The metabolic effects of exercise-induced muscle damage. *Exercise in Sport Sciences Reviews*, **19**: 99.

Hasson, S, Mundorf, R, Barnes, W *et al.* (1990) Effect of pulsed ultrasound versus placebo on muscle soreness perception and muscu-

lar performance. *Scandinavian Journal of Rehabilitation Medicine*, **22**(4): 199.

Henriksson-Larsen, KB, Lexell, J, Sjostrom, M (1983) Distribution of different fibre types in human skeletal muscles. I. Method of preparation and analysis of cross-sections of whole tibialis anterior. *Histochemical Journal*, **15**: 167.

Nurenberg, F, Giddings, CJ, Stray-Gunnersen, J (1992) Imaging guided muscle biopsy for correlation of increased signal intensity with ultrastructural change and delayed onset muscle soreness after exercise. *Radiology*, **184**(3): 865.

White, TP, Villancci, JF, Morales, PG (1982) Influence of physical conditioning on autografted skeletal muscle. *Medicine and Science in Sports and Exercise*, **13**(2): 81.

SKELETAL MUSCLE FATIGUE

Bergstrom, J (1962) Muscle electrolytes in man. *Scandinavian Journal of Clinical Laboratory Investigations*, **14**(suppl): 1–60.

Bigland-Ritchie, B, Furbush, F, Woods, JJ (1986) Fatigue of intermittent submaximal voluntary contractions: control and peripheral factors. *Journal of Applied Physiology* **61**: 421.

Edwards, RHT (1971) Percutaneous needle biopsy of skeletal muscle in diagnosis and research. *Lancet*, **2**: 593.

Hultman, E, Greenhaff, PL (1991) Skeletal muscle energy metabolism and fatigue during intense exercise in man. *Sci Progress Edinburgh*, **75**: 361.

Mutch, BJ, Banister, EW (1983) Ammonia metabolism in exercise and fatigue: a review. *Medicine and Science in Sports and Exercise*, **15**: 41.

Sahlin, K (1992) Metabolic factors in fatigue. *Sports Medicine* **13**(2): 99.

7

The Cardiovascular System

Introduction
•
Body Fluids and Their Components
•
Blood Cellular Components
•
The Heart
•
Blood Vessels
•
Cardiovascular Responses

Introduction

In its simplest form, the function of the cardio-vascular system can be said to be to provide a system of transport for oxygen and nutrients *to* the tissues for all aspects of cellular metabolism and for the removal of carbon dioxide and cellular waste products *from* the tissues. This function is provided by a pump — the heart, together with a system of tubes (the blood vessels) — which allows transport of materials either in the fluid contained within the vessels or carried in the cells of the blood. The pumping power of the heart must be strong enough to ensure that blood is supplied to even the most distant tissues. The organization of the smallest blood vessels is normally such that no cell in any tissue is further than 80 μm from a blood vessel, thereby ensuring that all cells receive an adequate supply of oxygen and nutrients.

The general organization of the cardiovascular system is outlined in Figure 7.1.

Body Fluids and Their Components

Water and Plasma

Before components of the cardiovascular system are dealt with, it is important to first secure an understanding of the normal composition and

Figure 7.1 A schematic diagram, showing the general arrangement of the cardiovascular system, with the heart and pulmonary and systemic circulations. RA = right atrium, RV = right ventricle, LA = left atrium, LV = left ventricle.

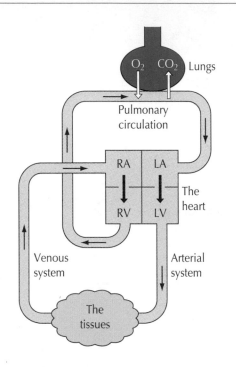

distribution of the fluids in the body and their volumes.

The most abundant constituent of the body's composition is **water**. Water accounts for about 60% of the total body weight in humans. The actual amount of water present in any one individual is variable, however, and depends to a certain extent on the body fat composition. Since lipids are highly hydrophobic, fatty tissue contains very little water and therefore an obese individual may contain as little as 40% total body weight as water, while a lean individual may contain as much as 80% total body weight as water.

The normal water content of the body is very carefully regulated, both by hormonal and circulatory mechanisms, some of which will be covered in more detail later (p. 147). It is useful at this

stage, however, to introduce the concept of **water balance**. This basically proposes that water losses in urine, sweat, from the respiratory tract and in the faeces are normally balanced by water intake from drinks and food and from water produced by metabolism (metabolic water).

The total body water can be divided into two main components — water within cells (**intracellular fluid**) and water outside cells (**extracellular fluid**). Intracellular fluid accounts for approximately two-thirds of the total body water with extracellular fluid comprising the other one-third. In addition, the extracellular fluid can be further subdivided into **interstitial fluid** (fluid between the cells) and **plasma** (fluid found within the circulatory system). Interstitial fluid makes up approximately 80% of the extracellular fluid, with plasma making up the remaining 20%. The distribution of water between these two compartments of the extracellular fluid can vary and depends on the balance of forces pushing fluid *out* of the circulation and *into* the interstitial compartment and forces pushing fluid *into* the circulation *from* the interstitial compartment. The nature of these forces and the balance between them and how this is important in normal fluid regulation will be dealt with later (p. 149). It will also be seen how imbalances in these forces can lead to oedema in tissues.

Actual volumes for these different fluid compartments are summarized in Figure 7.2. Fluid exchange between the two compartments of the extracellular fluid takes place at the level of the very smallest blood vessels (the **capillaries**). The capillary membrane acts as a sieve-like barrier to the movement of particles from one side of the membrane to the other. Very small particles, such as water, ions and the smaller organic molecules are therefore free to pass across this barrier. Larger particles such as proteins are, however,

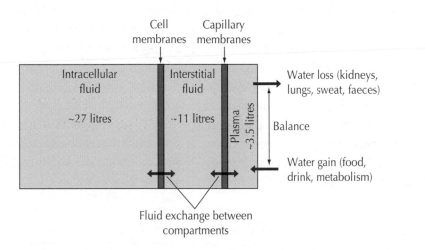

Figure 7.2 The distribution of fluid volume between the body fluid compartments. Two-way arrows indicate exchange of fluid between different compartments across the cell membranes or capillary membranes. One-way arrows indicate fluid intake (water gain) or excretion (water loss).

restricted in their movement across the membrane and are therefore retained in the plasma. The main difference in the composition of interstitial fluid and plasma is therefore the protein content. The concentrations of different constituents of the two compartments of the extracellular fluid are summarized in Table 7.1, together with values for intracellular fluid.

It is important to have an appreciation of the differences in these components in the different fluid compartments as this has implications for such things as nerve activity, muscle activity, blood function, volume regulation for cells and tissues and cellular absorption of nutrients. Even slight alterations in the composition of each compartment can have important consequences for the normal functioning of these body systems. For example, an increase in plasma potassium concentration – **hyperkalaemia** – can produce abnormal contraction of cardiac muscle cells leading to fibrillation, which may be fatal.

Table 7.1

Major Cations and Ions in Body Fluids

Ion	Concentration (mmol l^{-1})		
	Plasma	Interstitial fluid	Intracellular fluid
Cations			
Na^+	150	144	10
K^+	5	5	160
Mg^{2+}	2	2	28
Ca^{2+}	3	3	Variable*
Anions			
Cl^-	110	114	3
HCO_3^-	24	28	10
$Protein^-$	17	4	65
PO_4^{3-}	2	2	100
SO_4^{2-}	1	1	20

* Dependent on intracellular Ca^{2+} stores and intake from extracellular fluid.

Antigens and Antibodies

An antigen is any molecule which has the ability to activate a specific immune response. Viruses, bacteria, fungi and parasites, pollen grains, blood cells from a mismatched transfusion (see p. 130) or cells from an organ transplant all have properties which render them antigenic.

Antibodies are specific proteins that are produced in response to a specific antigen, and are referred to as **immunoglobulins** (Ig). There are five classes of immunoglobulin — IgA, IgD, IgE, IgG and IgM. The antibody molecules all conform to a basic structure of four polypeptide chains (two light chains and two heavy chains) linked by disulphide bonds into a Y-shaped molecule. At the exposed end of each light chain there is a variable portion which can be altered in response to different antigens. The remainder of the chains are referred to as the constant regions, although these differ slightly between each class of antibody.

Antibodies contribute to the body's defence mechanism by inactivating or destroying foreign substances in a number of different ways. The antibodies do not directly destroy antigens but identify them for attack by other elements of the immune system. One important function of the antibodies is to activate the **complement system,** an elaborate system of plasma proteins and enzymes, which can directly attack and destroy the antibody–antigen complex. The complement system is a group of approximately twenty proteins which is normally found in an inactive state in the body. Following activation, complement enhances the body's defence mechanisms. Complement can increase the permeability of the cell membranes of some bacteria, causing the release of its internal contents. This can set up chemical gradients which attract phagocytes to the area.

Interferon is a group of proteins which are important in defending against invading viruses. Interferon is released from cells infected with a virus, and signals neighbouring cells to produce antiviral proteins rendering them resistant to infection, thus preventing further viral replication in other cells.

The **human immunodeficiency virus (HIV)** which can cause **acquired immune deficiency syndrome (AIDS)** attacks a specific population of circulating T-lymphocytes called T4 lymphocytes. The time taken for this population of cells to be reduced to a level that weakens the body's defences against infections can range from two to ten years. Over that time, there is a progressive collapse of the immune system allowing normally non-fatal infections to become life-threatening. AIDS victims are particularly susceptible to respiratory conditions such as pneumonia and tuberculosis, diarrhoea and shingles, as well as a host of other bacterial and fungal infections.

Blood Cellular Components

Plasma, as discussed above, forms the fluid component of the blood. Blood as a whole, however, also contains cellular components or the **formed elements of blood**. These formed elements include **red blood cells, white blood cells** and **platelets**.

Red Blood Cells

The blood volume of an adult human is about 5 litres, accounting for approximately 6–8% of total body weight. Per litre, blood contains about 0.45 litre red blood cells in males (45%) and approximately 0.42 litre in females (42%). This value is known as the **haematocrit**. The actual number of red blood cells in a sample of 1 μl of blood is about 5×10^6 in males and 4.5×10^6 in females.

The red blood cells — also known as **erythrocytes** — have the appearance of flattened, biconcave discs and are about 7 μm in diameter and about 2.2 μm thick (Figure 7.3). The cells do not possess

Figure 7.3   A red blood cell (top), with a cross-section (bottom) showing biconcave shape of the cell.

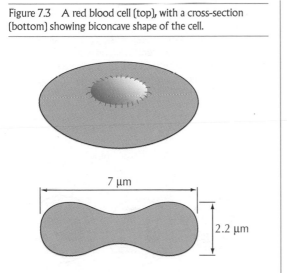

7 μm

2.2 μm

a nucleus, this having been lost during the early maturation of the cell. The shape of the red blood cell provides an increased surface area through which the respiratory gases can diffuse. The diameter of the red blood cell is similar to the diameter of the smallest of the capillary blood vessels. The easily deformable red blood cells therefore sometimes have their shape distorted in order to pass through the capillaries.

The main function of the red blood cells is to transport oxygen and carbon dioxide in the blood to and from the tissues. This is achieved by the presence of **haemoglobin** within the red blood cells (Chapter 8).

Since red blood cells are anucleate, they have no mechanism for repair of cellular damage and therefore have only a limited life span in the circulation. Red blood cells remain in the circulation for about 120 days, when they are subsequently destroyed in the spleen and within the circulation by specific white blood cells. This means that approximately 1% of the total number of red blood cells is destroyed each day. Since red blood cells are continuously being destroyed, this must normally be balanced by the number of red blood cells being synthesized and released into the circulation in order to maintain a roughly constant number of circulating red blood cells.

Red blood cells are produced in the red bone marrow of the bones of the chest, base of the skull and upper arms and legs by a process known as **erythropoiesis**. In this process, large, nucleated bone marrow cells — the **proerythroblasts** — divide until they become immature erythrocytes, gradually acquiring haemoglobin as they do so. The amount of haemoglobin in these cells steadily increases and the nucleus becomes smaller and eventually disappears (Figure 7.4). This mature red blood cell then enters into the circulation via the rich capillary supply of the bone marrow.

The whole process is under hormonal control, the hormone responsible being **erythropoietin**. This hormone is produced mainly in the kidneys. Normal levels of the hormone in the circulation maintain the routine rate of formation of red

Figure 7.4   Erythropoiesis, showing the stages of maturation of the red blood cell (erythrocyte).

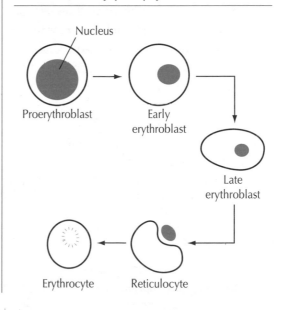

Nucleus

Proerythroblast   Early
                           erythroblast

                                    Late
                                    erythroblast

Erythrocyte   Reticulocyte

blood cells. The rate of synthesis of the hormone may be increased, however, in situations where a sustained decrease in oxygen supply to the tissues occurs (e.g. due to haemorrhage, reduced cardiac efficiency or reduced atmospheric oxygen content at high altitudes). The increased production of erythropoietin stimulates an increased synthesis of red blood cells in the marrow, thereby enhancing the oxygen-carrying capacity of the blood as a whole. In the past, some athletes used to employ this mechanism by training for a period at high altitudes to allow their haematocrit to increase in response to low atmospheric oxygen. They would then completely replace their blood by transfusion, keeping the high haematocrit blood in storage to be retransfused for use to enhance their performance at a later time. It is unclear whether this technique of so-called 'blood doping' did, in fact, enhance the performance of the athletes who used it, but the technique is now illegal in sporting events.

White Blood Cells

White blood cells (or leukocytes) form part of the defence mechanism of the body. They are of various types and include *neutrophils, eosinophils, basophils* (each type so named because of the way it reacts with different types of stain in histological preparations), *lymphocytes* and *monocytes* (Figure 7.5). These different cell types can be divided into two basic divisions – the **granulocytic** and the **non-granulocytic**. Granulocytic cells include the neutrophils, eosinophils and basophils; non-granulocytic cells include lymphocytes and monocytes.

GRANULOCYTES

Granulocytes are so named because their cytoplasm has a granular appearance on microscopic

Figure 7.5   The different types of white blood cell. Eosinophils, neutrophils and basophils are collectively known as granulocytes due to the presence of irregular granules in the cytoplasm. These granules contain enzymes and inflammatory factors such as histamine and heparin. Monocytes and lymphocytes are non-granulocytic cells.

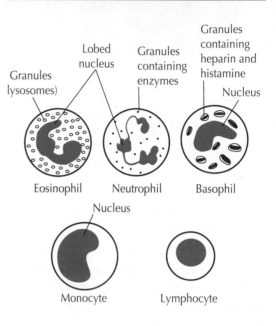

examination. The granulocytes include those which have multilobed nuclei, the **polymorphonuclear granulocytes**. **Neutrophils, eosinophils** and **basophils** are all polymorphonuclear granulocytes. Eosinophils are phagocytic cells which increase in number during allergic reactions and during parasitic infections. Basophils do not display much phagocytic activity. The granules of these cells contain **heparin** (an anticoagulant) and **histamine** (a chemical mediator involved in inflammatory responses). These cells are involved in the general immune response to foreign (non-bacterial) materials. Neutrophils are the most abundant of the white blood cells, accounting for about 50–60% of all white blood cells and about 90% of all polymorphonuclear cells. These cells are actively motile, and rapidly gather at any site of infection or tissue damage. The granules of these cells are packed with enzymes involved in phagocytic activity. The neutrophils are capable of ingesting many types of particulate material, including microorganisms. The neutrophils are attracted to the site of infection by chemotaxis.

NON-GRANULOCYTIC CELLS

Monocytes are non-granulated cells which, as well as being found in the blood, are also located in the connective tissue and in body cavities. They form part of the **reticuloendothelial system** (mononuclear phagocytic system) which is involved in defence mechanisms utilizing phagocytic activity in the body. These cells are capable of crossing the capillary wall and entering the connective tissues.

Lymphocytes are produced in the bone marrow and migrate to different lymphoid tissues to mature and differentiate. Those which mature in the thymus gland are referred to as **T-lymphocytes**, while those that remain in the bone marrow are the **B-lymphocytes**. They are also, respectively, commonly called T- and B-cells.

T-lymphocytes have the ability to bind and engage directly invading pathogens through two subpopulations of cells – the **cytotoxic T-lymphocytes** and the **helper T-lymphocytes**. This defence response is known as **cell-mediated immunity**. B-lymphocytes produce proteins, known as **antibodies**, which bind to invading pathogens and destroy them. This defence mechanism is known as **humoral immunity**.

The immune response to the invading pathogen involves both T-lymphocytes and B-lymphocytes. However, there are differences in the relative importance of the roles of these two cell types. In general, if the invading microorganism is a bacterium, B-lymphocytes will have a greater influence, as bacteria multiply extracellularly. Viruses, however, invade and affect cell function from the inside, by altering the genetic information in the cell and so T-lymphocytes have a greater role in viral infections.

Both types of lymphocyte have the ability to become 'memory' cells which arise due to exposure to antigens in the blood and which can memorize for the future the identity of the particular antigen which stimulated their production. A subsequent exposure of the body to that particular antigen will result in a rapid proliferation of these cells as part of the immune response to counteract any deleterious effects.

Blood Groups

All cells contain proteins on their surface which identify them as being native to the body. If these cells are transplanted to another individual, the recipient's immune system would recognize these cells as being foreign and would activate the immune system to destroy them. These surface proteins therefore act as antigens when introduced into a different body. The particular antigens present on the surface of the red blood cells are used as the basis of blood typing.

Red blood cells from an individual carry a particular type of antigen on their surface. If these red blood cells are transfused into an individual of a different blood type, they will interact with antibodies in the recipient's plasma which will cause clumping of the red blood cells – **agglutination**. These antigens are therefore sometimes referred to as **agglutinogens**.

Blood is grouped according to the presence or absence of agglutinogens on the surface of the red blood cells. Several types of red blood cell agglutinogens are important in blood grouping. The best known of these is the **ABO system**, based on the presence or absence of two agglutinogen types, A and B. If the red blood cells possess the A agglutinogen on their surface, the blood is classified as **type A blood**. If the red blood cells have the type B agglutinogen on their surface, the blood is classified as **type B blood**. It is also possible to have neither the A or B agglutinogen on the surface of the red blood cells, and this blood type is classified as type O. It is also possible for the red blood cells to possess both the A *and* B agglutinogens on their surface, giving rise to type AB blood.

The body does not normally produce antibodies against a particular antigen until it has been exposed to that antigen. However, this is not the case with regard to the blood group agglutinogens. Depending on blood type, there are antibodies present in the plasma capable of binding to the specific agglutinogens. These natural antibodies are termed **agglutinins**. An individual with type A blood will have agglutinins against the type B agglutinogen (anti-B), while an individual with type B blood has agglutinins against the type A agglutinogen (anti-A). Type AB blood has no agglutinins present in the plasma, while type O blood has both A and B agglutinins (Figure 7.6).

In blood transfusions, care must be taken to ensure that the correct blood type is given to the recipient in order to prevent any immunological response or agglutination from occurring. While the ABO system is the most common for typing blood, there are many other inherited blood group systems. A further means of grouping blood is by the presence or absence of the **Rhesus (Rh)** agglutinogen, named after its discovery in Rhesus monkeys. An individual with the Rh agglutinogen on the surface of their red blood cells is classed as having Rh-positive blood, while a subject without the Rh factor is regarded as being Rh-negative. The Rh grouping differs in that a subject without the Rh factor does not normally have naturally occurring agglutinins against it in

Figure 7.6   The ABO system of blood grouping. The four main blood types are shown (A, B, AB and O). See text for details.

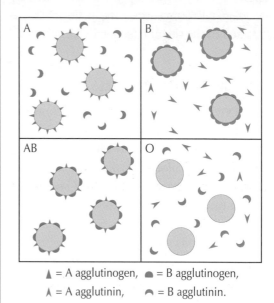

▲ = A agglutinogen,   ● = B agglutinogen,
⋏ = A agglutinin,   ⌒ = B agglutinin.

their plasma. However, Rh-negative subjects exposed to Rh-positive blood will respond by producing the appropriate agglutinins against the Rhesus agglutinogen. Obviously this can happen in mismatched blood transfusions, but it can also occur during pregnancy. Since blood groups are inherited, it is possible that one parent may have Rh-positive blood and the other Rh negative. If a mother is Rh negative and the developing child is Rh positive from the father, the mother will produce antibodies against the developing child's blood type. This does not normally cause a problem, as the exposure usually only occurs around the time of birth. However, if the mother's exposure to the fetal blood is earlier, for example due to some trauma, the maternal antibodies can cross the placenta and enter the fetal circulation destroying the red blood cells. This is known as **haemolytic disease of the newborn**. Similarly, problems can develop during subsequent pregnancies with Rh-positive children. It is possible to circumvent these problems by giving the mother an injection of anti-Rh agglutinins within 48 hours after the birth of the first child. These bind to the fetal blood cells preventing them from stimulating the mother's immune system into producing substantial quantities of anti-Rh agglutinins.

Platelets and Coagulation

Blood, as well as containing red and white blood cells, also contains small fragments of cells originally found in the bone marrow (megakaryocytes). These small fragments of the megakaryocytes are known as **platelets** or **thrombocytes**.

Platelets are found in concentrations of about 250 million per millilitre of blood. Platelets are smaller than the blood cells, having an average diameter of about 3 μm. Platelets, like red blood cells, do not possess a cell nucleus and consequently only have a lifespan of between 5 and 9 days. After this time, the platelets are destroyed in the spleen and liver.

Platelets are important components in the process of **blood clotting,** or **coagulation.** This process occurs in order to prevent loss of blood and the stopping of bleeding after injury or damage to a blood vessel. This process as a whole is known as **haemostasis.**

Under normal circumstances, platelets do not aggregate with each other or adhere to the walls of the blood vessels. This is due to the presence of **prostacyclin,** a prostaglandin, which is produced by the endothelial cells of the blood vessel walls. Prostacyclin prevents platelet aggregation and therefore prevents the initiation of clot formation in non-injured blood vessels.

Damage to the wall of a blood vessel exposes the collagen fibres of the tunica externa to the blood (see p. 143). It is this exposure to collagen fibres

that causes platelets to aggregate, adhering to the site of collagen exposure. When platelets adhere to collagen, this triggers the release of secretions from the platelets. These secretions include **thromboxane A_2** (a prostaglandin derivative). Thromboxane A_2 causes a local vasoconstriction and also causes the platelets themselves to become stickier, causing them to clump with other platelets, which also become sticky and so on in a positive feedback loop. As this process continues, so a platelet plug is eventually formed at the site of vessel damage.

As well as inducing platelet aggregation, the chemicals that are released from the platelets on contact with the exposed collagen in the vessel walls also cause the activation of plasma clotting factors. These plasma clotting factors are necessary components of the normal mechanism of blood clotting.

The conversion of blood to a solid gel-like plug — the clot — is related to the conversion of the plasma protein **fibrinogen** to **fibrin.** This conversion is catalysed by an enzyme present in the plasma, **thrombin.** The conversion reaction involves several small, negatively-charged polypeptide fragments splitting off from the fibrinogen molecule. This leaves a large molecule which has a high degree of attraction for other similar molecules. These molecules then join end to end and side by side to form a large, insoluble, fibrous molecule which is fibrin.

The long fibrin molecules form a meshwork at the site of injury to the blood vessel. Other plasma components such as cells and platelets become entangled in this meshwork, so adding to its overall strength. It is this fibrous meshwork, together with the platelet plug described above, which constitutes the blood clot.

The protein fibrinogen is always present in the

plasma under normal conditions. Since clots are only formed in response to injury, this must mean that the enzyme, thrombin, which converts fibrinogen to fibrin, must normally be absent from the plasma. In fact, thrombin is itself formed from an inactive precursor, **prothrombin**. Prothrombin is synthesized in the liver and is normally present in the blood. During clot formation, prothrombin is enzymatically converted to thrombin which can then go on to catalyse the conversion of fibrinogen to fibrin.

The question which arises from the above account is, what catalyses the conversion of the inactive prothrombin to the active thrombin? The answer is that it is catalysed by an active enzyme, which itself is formed from an inactive precursor. The enzyme which catalyses this reaction is itself also formed from an inactive precursor, and so on. This therefore represents a reaction sequence which involves a **cascade** of plasma clotting factors,

each of which is normally inactive until converted to an active form by a previous active factor in the sequence (Figure 7.7). The whole sequence of reactions in the cascade is triggered by damage either to the blood vessel wall caused by risk factors such as atherosclerosis (see later) or cigarette smoking, or by damage to tissue cells close to the blood vessels.

Damage to the blood vessels may expose collagen in the vessel wall. When plasma comes into contact with this collagen, the activation of the first factor in the sequence is triggered. The first factor in the cascade is known as **Hageman factor**.

Damage to cells close to the blood vessels releases a protein – **thromboplastin** – from the surface of the damaged cells. This activates one of the clotting factors at a later stage in the cascade pathway.

Initiation of coagulation by damage to blood vessels is known as the **intrinsic pathway**, since

Figure 7.7   Diagrammatic representation of the cascade process of coagulation. No specific names are given to the plasma clotting factors; they are referred to simply as factor A, B, C. The inactive form of each clotting factor is normally found in the plasma, until it is converted to the active form by a previous active factor in the cascade. Calcium ions, platelets and vitamin K are necessary cofactors for some of the stages in this process.

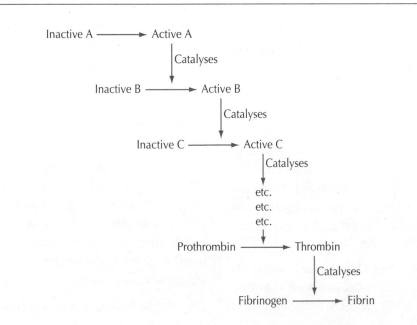

it involves a direct interaction with clotting factors in the blood. Coagulation initiated by damage to the cells is known as the **extrinsic pathway,** since it follows an indirect route initially external to the plasma. As the extrinsic pathway triggers a clotting factor at a later stage of the cascade, there are fewer steps involved than for the intrinsic pathway.

Other cofactors are also necessary for coagulation to proceed normally. These include calcium ions, phospholipids produced by the platelets and vitamin K (which is necessary for the normal synthesis of some of the clotting factors in the cascade sequence).

Damage to blood vessel walls can sometimes occur without any specific injury to the blood vessel. This may be as a result of cigarette smoking or due to lipid deposits on the inner surface of the vessel. In such circumstances, blood clots may form inside the vessel (**thrombosis**). In many cases, the clot will dissolve due to the action of a plasma enzyme (**plasmin**). However, in other cases, the clot may travel in the circulation to eventually occlude a blood vessel. If the occluded vessel is an artery, then the blood supply to a vital organ will be impaired (**ischaemia**). This is especially important if the blocked artery is supplying an area of tissue which does not receive any additional arterial supply (collateral circulation).

If this occurs in the blood supply to the heart muscle, this can therefore lead to myocardial ischaemia, with reduced cardiac efficiency. If the affected area is large enough, the myocardial cells will die (**myocardial infarction**). Such reduced efficiency of the myocardial tissue may be sudden and dramatic, causing a 'heart attack'. Ischaemia in respect of the heart is further discussed on p. 154. If the affected area is relatively small, the effects of reduced efficiency are less prominent and sometimes only seen on exertion. These effects include shortness of breath, tightness in the chest and pain (sometimes quite severe) in the chest, left arm and shoulder, jaw or neck (**angina pectoris**).

If the blocked artery supplies an area of the brain, the cells of this area will rapidly die (they have a low capacity for survival without an adequate oxygen supply). This can severely affect the normal function of this brain area (e.g. motor or sensory performance, speech, memory). Such an occurrence is referred to as a **cerebrovascular accident (CVA)** or **stroke**.

The Heart

Cardiac Cycle

The heart is a muscular pump comprising four chambers (two atria and two ventricles). These four chambers basically act as a double pump — one half responsible for pumping blood to the lungs (the **pulmonary circulation**) and the other pumping blood to the rest of the body (the **systemic circulation**).

During a complete cardiac cycle, the right atrium receives blood returning from the body via the great veins. Most of the blood in the atrium then flows passively from the atrium to the right ventricle, with the final residual volume of atrial blood being actively pumped into the ventricle by atrial contraction. The right ventricle then contracts and pumps blood via the pulmonary artery to the lungs where the blood becomes oxygenated (see Chapter 8). This oxygenated blood then returns to the left atrium via the pulmonary veins, and is subsequently passed to the left ventricle by the combination of passive draining and active atrial contraction, described above. The left ventricle then contracts and pumps the oxygenated blood out to the tissues of the body via the aorta (Figure 7.8). The period of ejection from the heart chambers is termed **systole**, while the period of filling in the chambers is termed **diastole**.

During a normal, resting cardiac cycle, atrial systole lasts for about 0.1 s and atrial diastole for about 0.7 s. In contrast, ventricular systole lasts for about 0.3 s and ventricular diastole for about 0.5 s. These figures are based on a total cardiac cycle time, at rest, of 0.8 s, giving a resting heart rate of 75 beats per minute.

Cardiac Valves

The flow of blood within the different chambers of the heart is unidirectional, and this is achieved by the presence of valves made up of connective tissue between the atria and the ventricles and between the ventricles and the arteries.

The atrioventricular valves ensure that, when the ventricles contract, blood is not pushed back into the atria by the force of the ventricular contraction. The right atrioventricular valve consists of three flaps of connective tissue — the **tricuspid valve**. The left atrioventricular valve has only two flaps — the **bicuspid valve** (also known as the **mitral valve**).

There are small tendons (the **chordae tendinae**) which connect the flaps of the valves to small muscles on the inside surface of the ventricles, the **papillary muscles**. When the ventricles contract, the valves are pushed shut by the pressure of the blood inside the ventricles. The papillary muscles also contract at this time, pulling on the chordae tendinae which prevents the valves from turning inside out into the atria.

The valves between the ventricles and the arteries leaving the heart consist of three crescent-shaped flaps, the **semilunar valves**. These prevent backflow of blood from the aorta and the pulmonary artery into the ventricles once they have relaxed.

Cardiac Muscle Cells

As the flow of blood between the chambers of the heart is complicated, this would be difficult to achieve if there were not some degree of coordination between the contraction of the different chambers. This coordination occurs during he cardiac cycle due to the nature of the conduction of electrical impulses throughout the heart muscle tissue. Heart muscle (**myocardium**) behaves like any other muscle tissue in that it contracts after depolarization of the cell membrane. Cardiac muscle cells, however, are substantially smaller than skeletal muscle cells and are much more numerous within the cardiac muscle tissue. In order for any one chamber of the heart to contract in a coordinated manner, these cardiac muscle cells must contract at more or less the same time. If there was a random contraction of the

Figure 7.8   Cross-section of the heart showing the direction of flow of blood within the chambers (arrows).

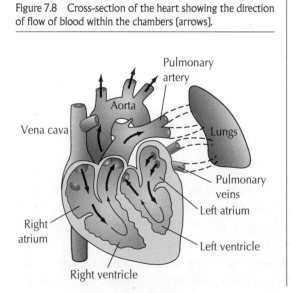

cells, there would be no strong contraction of the heart chamber and blood would not be forcefully ejected from the chamber. Coordination of contraction is therefore of vital importance. The structure of the myocardium is such that the cardiac muscle cells are functionally connected to each other via thickenings of the cell walls known as **intercalated discs** (Figure 7.9). These form a mechanical and electrical connection between adjoining myocardial cells and ensure that all cells in the tissue form a **functional syncitium**, i.e. they behave as one cell. This therefore enables the ventricles, for example, to produce a coordinated contraction as the wave of excitation (deplorization) spreads over the whole of the tissue.

CARDIAC RHYTHMICITY

The steady rhythm of the heart beat is maintained by the inherent rhythmicity of the myocardial cells (if single myocardial cells are dissected free in an experimental preparation they will still continue to beat at their own built-in rhythm) and by the action of a **pacemaker region** of the myocar-

dial tissue which can override the rate of this inherent rhythm and drive the beating rate of the whole heart.

The pacemaker region is situated at the junction between the superior vena cava and the right atrium and is known as the **sinoatrial (SA) node**. This region of the myocardium generates a wave of depolarization which spreads over the atria to reach a second pacemaker region which lies at the bottom of the right atrium close to the septum which separates the two atria (the **atrioventricular node**). This node is responsible for the spread of excitation to the ventricles and also produces a delay in this wave of excitation which allows the atria to complete their contraction before the ventricles begin to contract. The myocardial action potential is substantially different from that seen in skeletal muscle fibres due to differences in the ionic mechanisms which generate it (Figure 7.10a).

Since the ventricles are substantially larger than the atria, there exists a series of specialized myocardial cells which are responsible for conducting the wave of depolarization to different parts of the ventricles. These conducting fibres are known as the **bundle of His** (or **atrioventricular bundle**) which conducts the wave of excitation to the top portion of the interventricular septum. The bundle then branches to form the left and right bundles which further subdivide to form conduction fibres, the **Purkinje fibres**. It is these Purkinje fibres which finally transmit the wave of depolarization to the myocardial cells (Figure 7.10b).

CARDIAC CONTRACTILITY

The spread of electrical activity throughout the heart can be picked up by electrodes located on the surface of the body. When this electrical signal is subsequently amplified and displayed, it is known as the **electrocardiogram (ECG)**. Figure

Figure 7.9 Cardiac muscle cells. Like skeletal muscle cells, these are striated, although considerably smaller in length. Adjacent cardiac muscle cells make electrical and mechanical connections with each other via the intercalated discs. Cardiac muscle cells are autorhythmic; they contract spontaneously with their own built-in rhythm.

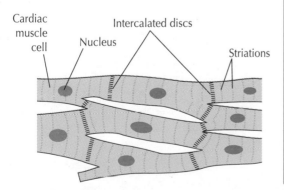

Cardiac muscle cell · Nucleus · Intercalated discs · Striations

Figure 7.10   (a) A cardiac muscle action potential (ventricular cell). This has a considerably longer duration than a skeletal muscle action potential. The depolarization phase (i) is due to rapid influx of sodium ions into the cell due to the opening of gated sodium channels in the cell membrane. The prolonged plateau of depolarization (ii) is due to slow inward leakage of calcium ions into the cell through gated calcium channels. Repolarization (iii) is due to outward movement of potassium ions due to the opening of gated potassium channels. (b) Conduction of excitation throughout the heart tissue. The wave of depolarization, initiated at the sinoatrial node (SA) spreads over the atria, eventually reaching the atrioventricular node (AV). The wave of depolarization is conducted deep into the ventricular tissue via the bundle of His, the right and left bundle branches and the Purkinje fibres. (c) The electrocardiogram, showing one complete cardiac cycle at rest (see text for details of individual waves).

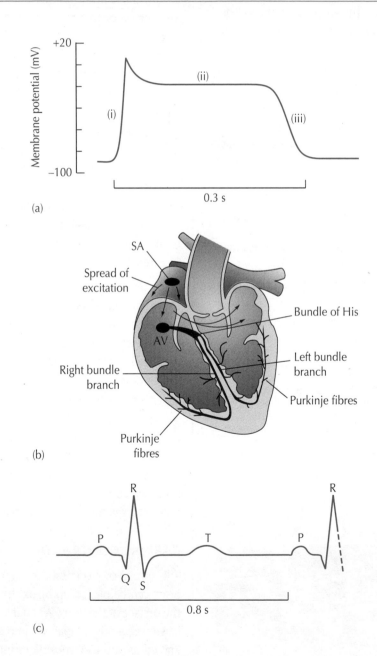

7.10(c) shows the basic shape of a typical resting electrocardiogram. Each of the waves on the ECG correspond to different components of the heart's electrical activity during the cardiac cycle. The **P-wave** represents depolarization of the atria; the **QRS complex** represents depolarization of the ventricles; the **T-wave** represents repolarization of the ventricles (atrial repolarization is masked by the QRS complex). Changes in the shape of the ECG can be used clinically to diagnose abnormalities in cardiac function.

At rest, the sinoatrial pacemaker drives the heart to contract at a rate of about 70–75 beats per minute. This rate, however, is subject to control by various external influences such as the autonomic nervous system, circulating hormones and exercise. The action of the sympathetic nervous system and the hormone noradrenaline increase the heart rate as well as increasing the strength of contraction (**contractility**) of the heart muscle. The parasympathetic nervous system decreases the heart rate and contractility. The sinoatrial node is normally subject to a background tonic level of parasympathetic activity which holds the heart rate at a lower level. If the main parasympathetic nerve to the heart (the vagus nerve) is surgically cut, the resting heart rate increases due to the removal of this background parasympathetic influence.

Each contraction of the left ventricle at rest pumps about 70 ml of blood out into the circulation. This volume of blood ejected per beat of the heart is known as the **stroke volume**. At the end of systole, a certain volume of blood remains in the heart (the **end-systolic volume**). This is usually about 80 ml. During the cardiac cycle, therefore, the volume in the heart at rest varies from about 150–80 ml. These volumes, however, can be affected by changes in venous return and strength of cardiac contraction. Given a resting heart rate of 70 beats per minute and a resting stroke volume of 70 ml per beat, the **cardiac output** (heart rate × stroke volume) can be calculated to be 4900 ml per minute, approximately 5 litres per minute.

The heart is a variable pump and its output can be altered to accommodate changes in demand for oxygen and nutrients. The normal resting cardiac output of about 5 litres per minute can therefore be adjusted by altering the two components which determine this — heart rate and stroke volume. Increases in either, or both, of these factors will obviously increase cardiac output.

Heart rate can be altered by the actions of the autonomic nervous system and therefore any factor which influences autonomic activity will ultimately have an effect on heart rate. One such controlling factor is located in the medulla of the brainstem (the **cardiovascular control centre**) which includes a cardioaccelerator region which serves to increase sympathetic output, thereby influencing the sinoatrial node to increase heart rate and therefore cardiac output. Such an alteration in cardiac output, since it stems from a controlling centre external to the heart itself, is known as **extrinsic regulation**.

Alterations in stroke volume can also occur to produce changes in cardiac output. This can be in the form of extrinsic regulation, wherein an increase in sympathetic activity will produce an increase in the contractility (strength of contraction) of the heart muscle. The heart will therefore eject a greater volume of blood per beat. Alterations in stroke volume can also be attributed to factors which originate within the heart itself. Such regulation of cardiac output is known as **intrinsic regulation**. The normal stroke volume of about 70 ml per beat can be increased to as much as 140 ml per beat in non-athletes and, in some cases, to ⩾ 200 ml per beat in trained athletes.

Intrinsic alterations in the stroke volume are principally caused by changes in the volume of blood returning to the heart from the veins (the venous return). An increase in venous return to the heart causes an increase in the volume of blood pumped out by the heart in each beat. Thus, the heart responds to the amount of blood flowing in to ensure that a corresponding amount is pumped out again. This is known as the **Frank–Starling mechanism** or **Starling's law of the heart**.

The explanation for Starling's Law is best dealt with by referring to the original experiments carried out by Frank on isolated frog heart in 1895 and Starling on isolated dog heart in 1914. In these experiments, an isolated heart was used to measure the pressure of the fluid inside the heart during contraction. This was done with the aorta tied off so that the fluid would not leave the heart during contraction (**isovolumic contraction**). This experiment was performed with different starting volumes (end-diastolic volumes) inside the ventricles. Pressure generated when the heart contracts at each of these starting volumes was then measured. The pattern of these pressure changes is shown in Figure 7.11(a). This shows that as the end-diastolic volume increases, the pressure generated by contraction initially increases to a peak level, and then declines as the starting volume is increased further.

The pressure generated by the contraction of the heart reflects the stroke work performed by the cardiac muscle fibres. The explanation for this shape relies on a knowledge of the microscopic structure of the cardiac muscle fibres. As the end-diastolic volume in the heart increases, so the cardiac muscle fibres are stretched. As in skeletal muscle, this allows for a more favourable degree of overlap between the contractile proteins in the

muscle fibres and so produces a greater strength of contraction. However, as the end-diastolic volume increases further and the cardiac muscle fibres are therefore stretched further, the amount of overlap between the contractile proteins will decrease, leading to a decrease in the force of contraction of the muscle fibres.

If this experiment is then repeated, but this time allowing the fluid to leave the heart during contraction, the pattern of pressure and volume changes shown in Figure 7.11(b) is obtained. Here, the pressures which are generated by contraction are much lower, since the fluid is allowed to be ejected in this experiment. The accompanying reduction in fluid volume is also seen here.

The importance of these two graphs becomes more evident when they are superimposed on each other, as shown in Figure 7.11(c). Figure 7.10(a) shows the pressure that *could* be generated by the heart under artificial conditions and is depicted by the upper curve in Figure 7.11(c). Figure 7.11(b) shows the pressure that is actually generated when the heart contracts and fluid is ejected and this is shown as the lower curve in Figure 7.11(c). The difference between these *possible* and *actual* pressures is represented by dP. The magnitude of dP represents the possible energy, or force, that is therefore available to the heart muscle to do the work of actually ejecting the fluid from the heart. The greater the value of dP, the greater the force of ejection and therefore the greater the stroke volume of the heart.

Figure 7.11(c) concentrates on typical resting heart volumes. If the initial end-diastolic volume is increased, the pattern of pressure changes obtained is shown in Figure 7.11(d). Here it can be seen that dP is now higher than that observed in Figure 7.10(c). This, therefore, means that a greater force can now be produced when the

Figure 7.11 (a) Changes in ventricular pressure after contraction at different end-diastolic starting volumes. These pressures are measured without allowing fluid to be ejected from the ventricle. As end-diastolic volume initially increases, the pressure generated on contraction also increases. Further increases in end-diastolic volume produce a decline in the pressure generated upon contraction. (b) Pressure–volume loop, showing the changes in ventricular pressure and volume during a complete cardiac cycle as the ventricle contracts and fluid is allowed to be ejected. OP = opening pressure for the aortic valve; this pressure must be exceeded by ventricular pressure before fluid can be ejected. IC = isovolumic contraction; pressure initially increases but volume remains constant until the opening pressure has been exceeded. E = ejection phase; opening pressure has now been exceeded and fluid can leave the ventricle as indicated by the decrease in volume. IR = isovolumic relaxation; pressure has now fallen below the opening pressure and the aortic valve is closed; pressure continues to fall, but with no change in volume. F = filling phase; volume now increases from that at the end of ejection (end-systolic volume, ESV). The volume at the end of the filling phase is the end-diastolic volume (EDV). (c) Superimposition of curves (a) and (b). dP represents the difference in pressures between what is possible to achieve by ventricular contraction and what is actually achieved. The magnitude of this pressure difference represents the possible energy which is available for the heart muscle to do work in pushing the blood out of the ventricle. (d) Effect of increased end-diastolic volume. This has now moved the pressure–volume loop on to a portion of the ventricular pressure curve which gives a greater value of dP. There is therefore a greater amount of energy available to do work and so a greater volume is ejected from the ventricle. This matches cardiac output (ejection) with venous return (end-diastolic volume), so that the heart will eventually return to normal operating volumes as seen in (c).

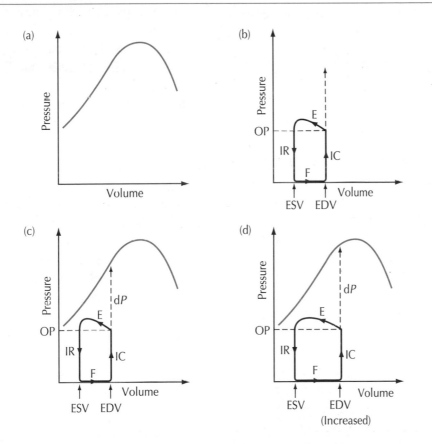

heart contracts, thereby ejecting a greater volume of fluid from the heart.

The initial volume in the heart may be altered by an increased venous return (**preload**) or by an increased resistance to outflow from the heart caused by arterial constriction raising arterial pressure (**afterload**). This mechanism, therefore, ensures that in the normal heart, the stroke volume matches the inflow from venous return, or ensures a sufficient strength of contraction to overcome increased arterial pressure. The Frank–Starling mechanism also ensures that the volume output of both ventricles remains matched.

It will be observed that if the initial starting volume is increased even further the force available for ejection (dP) will decrease as the operating volume of the heart moves on to the downslope of the upper pressure curve. This means that despite a higher end-diastolic volume, there will be less blood ejected from the heart. The heart will therefore gradually become more congested with blood, leading to **congestive heart failure**.

Further, if the initial volume is lower than normal, due to a reduced venous return for example, there will also be a reduction in the available ejection force and, again, this could be of pathological significance.

During one complete cardiac cycle there are therefore changes in volume and pressure in the left heart and the aorta, together with other mechanical and electrical events (see Figure 7.12). Immediately before contraction, left ventricular pressure is low (about 5 mmHg). The volume inside the ventricle at this stage is at its highest level (about 150 ml). When the ventricular muscle contracts, intraventricular pressure increases as the blood inside the chamber is compressed. When the pressure exceeds that of the aorta (about 80 mmHg), the aortic valve opens allowing blood to rush out of the ventricle and into the aorta. Until this point, the volume inside the ventricle remains constant (**isovolumic contraction**). When the aortic valve opens and blood leaves the ventricle, this is the **ejection phase** of the cardiac cycle.

During the ejection phase the intraventricular volume decreases from 150 ml to about 80 ml,

giving a stroke volume of about 70 ml at rest, while the pressure in the ventricle and the aorta increase to about 120 mmHg (ventricular pressure always remaining slightly higher than aortic pressure during this phase). As the ventricle relaxes, the intraventricular pressure drops. When it drops below the aortic pressure, the aortic valve closes and blood no longer leaves the ventricle (**isovolumic relaxation**).

During the ejection phase, the walls of the aorta are stretched by the large volume of blood leaving the left ventricle. Due to the elasticity of the aortic wall, when the ventricle relaxes and ejection stops, the pressure in the aorta does not drop suddenly but declines only slowly from the systolic pressure of 120 mmHg to about 80 mmHg at the end of diastole. The rapid closure of the aortic valve sends a pressure wave through the blood in the aorta and this is seen in the aortic pressure curve as the **dicrotic notch**.

When the ventricles are relaxed, and intraventricular pressure falls below that in the atria, the atrioventricular valves open allowing blood to flow from the atria to the ventricles. This is the **filling phase** of the cardiac cycle. The majority of ventricular filling is a passive process with blood trickling from the atria into the ventricles. The latter part of the filling phase sees the final few millilitres of blood being pumped into the ventricles by active atrial contraction. The pressures generated in the atria by contraction are much lower than in the ventricles, reaching about 10–15 mmHg.

The activity of the different heart chambers is coordinated by the electrical activity of the pacemakers and the spread of electrical excitation throughout the myocardium. Figure 7.12 also shows the relationship of the different waves of the electrocardiogram to the events described above.

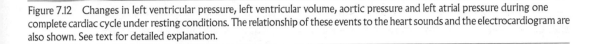

Figure 7.12   Changes in left ventricular pressure, left ventricular volume, aortic pressure and left atrial pressure during one complete cardiac cycle under resting conditions. The relationship of these events to the heart sounds and the electrocardiogram are also shown. See text for detailed explanation.

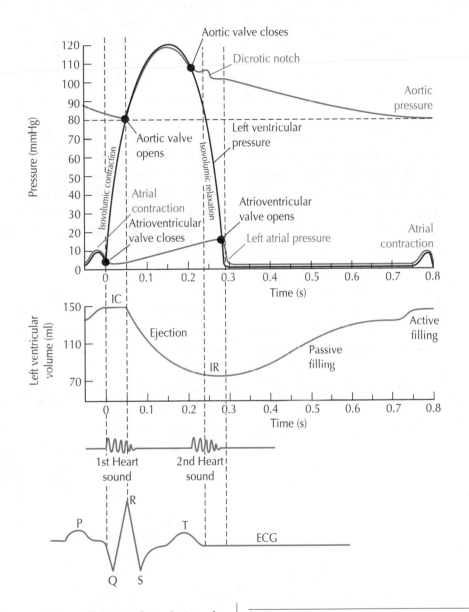

The closure of the different valves during the cardiac cycle can be heard as the **heart sounds** using a stethoscope. The first heart sound is due to the closure of the atrioventricular valves, while the second heart sound is due to closure of the aortic valve.

Blood Vessels

While the heart is the pump which pushes blood out to the tissues of the body, the blood vessels are the means by which this blood is actually conveyed to the tissues. It has already been seen that blood leaves the heart via the aorta. The aorta subsequently branches into the large **arteries** which distribute blood to the major regions of the body — head, thorax, upper limbs, abdomen, lower limbs, etc. These major arterial branches subdivide further, forming smaller and smaller arterial vessels and eventually the smallest of these (the **arterioles**). The arterioles further branch to form the smallest of the blood vessels (the **capillaries**). The capillaries form an extensive network of vessels within the tissues, and it is these vessels which are responsible for the final delivery of oxygen and nutrients to the cells of the tissues and for the uptake of carbon dioxide and waste products from the cells. As the capillaries leave the tissues they supply, they begin to reunite to form larger vessels which begin the process of returning the blood to the heart. The first of these vessels are the **venules**. From the venules, blood then passes on to the **veins** to

finally return to the heart via the great veins — the superior and inferior vena cavae.

The amount of branching and reuniting of vessels that occurs throughout the vascular system means that there are substantial differences in the diameter of the different types of blood vessels. Figure 7.13 shows the range of vessel diameters throughout the system together with the changes in the total cross-sectional area in each part of the circulation. As can be seen, even though the individual diameter of the capillaries is extremely small, because of their large number making up the capillary bed in the tissues, the total cross-sectional area of the vessels at this level of the circulation is extremely large, thereby giving a large surface area for gas exchange, nutrient delivery and waste removal.

The basic structure of the arterial and venous blood vessels is essentially similar, with variations in relative dimensions occurring throughout the system.

Figure 7.13   Blood vessel diameters (top) and the total cross-sectional area of these vessels (bottom) throughout the vascular system. Total cross-sectional area is seen to increase as vessel diameter decreases due to the larger number of these smaller vessels. (Note: vessel diameters are not drawn to scale.)

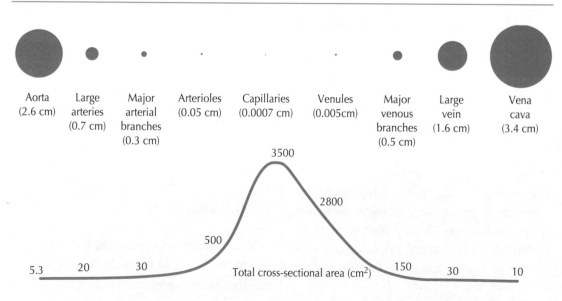

The walls of the blood vessels are composed of three main layers, or tunicae (Figure 7.14). The inner layer (**tunica intima**) is composed of the endothelial cells which form the inner lining of the vessel, together with a layer of elastic connective tissue (elastin). The middle layer (**tunica media**) is composed mainly of smooth muscle with, again, some elastin. The outer layer (**tunica externa**, also sometimes known as the **tunica adventitia**) is composed of connective tissue, mainly collagen and elastin.

Arteries

The aorta and the larger arteries bear the brunt of the pressure of the blood as it is ejected from the heart. The structure of the walls of these larger arterial vessels is ideally suited to cope with this in that they contain large amounts of elastic connective tissue. These vessels are, therefore, able to stretch to accommodate the large change in volume as the blood leaves the heart. Stretching the elastic fibres in the wall of the arteries effectively stores potential energy which is subsequently used to maintain the flow of blood through the arteries when the heart is relaxed during diastole. This also ensures that the flow of blood in the arteries is less pulsatile, giving a smoother pressure wave in these vessels.

The smaller arteries are less elastic and have a greater proportion of smooth muscle in their walls. In effect this makes these vessels somewhat less distensible and they can provide a resistance to the flow of blood, thereby influencing blood pressure. This resistance to blood flow can be increased by contraction of the smooth muscle causing vessel narrowing (**vasoconstriction**) or can be reduced by relaxation of the smooth muscle causing the diameter of the vessel to increase (**vasodilation**).

The arterioles are the smallest of the arterial vessels which branch to eventually form the capillaries. Vasoconstriction and vasodilation of the arterioles is important in the control of blood flow to the capillary beds. In addition, rings of smooth muscle (**precapillary sphincters**) surrounding the smallest of the arterioles leading to the capillary beds, are also important in determining the amount of blood flow to a particular capillary bed.

Capillaries

The capillaries are the smallest of the blood vessels (diameter about 7 μm) and it is here that the exchange of gases, nutrients and waste products between the plasma and the cells takes place. Each capillary vessel is approximately 1 mm long, and the high degree of branching which occurs within the capillary bed ensures that every cell in the

Figure 7.14 Cross-section through a generalized blood vessel. Relative dimensions of the different layers vary throughout the vascular system.

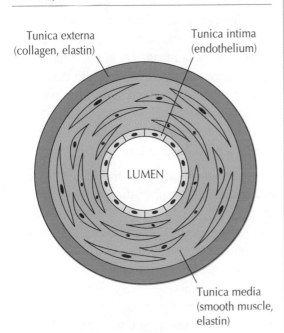

Tunica externa
(collagen, elastin)

Tunica intima
(endothelium)

LUMEN

Tunica media
(smooth muscle, elastin)

tissue is located within 60–80 µm of a capillary vessel.

The structure of the capillaries is different from that of the arteries and veins (Figure 7.15). Capillary walls are only one endothelial cell thick, with no smooth muscle or connective tissue. The endothelial cells are squamous and interlock to form the capillary wall along the length of the vessel.

Where adjacent endothelial cells are tightly joined together, they are said to be **continuous capillaries**. These capillaries allow the transfer of gases and nutrients which are small molecules (e.g. glucose), but hold back the larger molecules such as proteins. These continuous capillaries are found in tissues such as muscle, the brain and the lungs.

Other types of capillaries have wide pores (about 0.1 µm diameter) in the cells of the capillary wall. The pores are covered by a thin layer of mucoprotein which effectively forms a diaphragm barrier over the pore. These are known as **fenestrated capillaries** and can allow larger substances to pass from the plasma to the interstitial fluid. Fene-

strated capillaries are mostly found in the gut and in the kidneys.

One further type of capillary has an even greater degree of 'leakiness' than the fenestrated capillaries. These capillaries have gaps between the adjacent endothelial cells of the capillary wall which are large enough to allow much larger molecules to pass through. These vessels are known as **discontinuous capillaries** and are found in the liver, spleen and bone marrow. The gaps between the cells in these capillaries are not normally large enough to allow red blood cells to pass through.

Veins

After the blood has passed through the capillary bed, it then enters the venous circulation to be returned to the heart. The pressure in the blood vessels at this stage of the circulation is now very low (about 5–10 mmHg). Such low pressures are ineffective on their own to enable blood to be successfully pushed back to the heart, especially from the lower limbs where the effects of gravity on the pooling of blood has to be overcome. Due to the increased distensibility of the veins caused by relatively low amounts of elastic tissue and smooth muscle, blood can collect, or pool, in the veins under the action of gravity. The return of blood to the heart (venous return) must therefore be assisted in some way.

One distinctive feature of the venous vessels, which does not occur in the arterial system, is the presence of valves in the lumen of the veins. These valves prevent the backflow of blood once it has been moved towards the heart, i.e. they ensure unidirectional flow in the venous system. Contraction of skeletal muscles surrounding the veins compresses the blood within the vessels, pushing this blood along the length of the ves-

Figure 7.15   General structure of a capillary blood vessel. Several adjacent endothelial cells are shown making up the capillary wall.

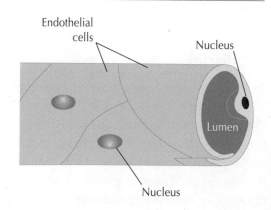

sel, the valves ensuring that the direction of flow is towards the heart. Skeletal muscle action is therefore important in assisting the venous return (Figure 7.16).

Failure to ensure an adequate venous return by assistance from skeletal muscle contraction is responsible for many instances of fainting, especially on hot days when a large volume of peripheral blood supply has been diverted to the skin for cooling purposes.

Blood Pressure

The blood flowing through the vessels of the circulation exerts a pressure on the walls of these vessels. This pressure varies throughout the circulation and is dependent on the diameter of the vessels and the amount of blood flowing through them (Figure 7.17). The diameter of the blood

Figure 7.17   Variations in blood pressure throughout the circulatory system. The major arterial vessels maintain a systolic pressure of about 120 mmHg and diastolic pressure of 80 mmHg at rest. As the vessels become smaller and the relative amount of blood flowing through each vessel decreases, the systolic and diastolic blood pressures also decrease. At the level of the capillaries and the veins, the pulsatile variations in pressure during systole and diastole are no longer observed. The pressure in the venous vessels returning to the heart are very low. Mean blood pressure is shown by the black line.

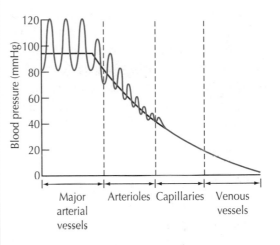

vessels determines the resistance to flow — the smaller the diameter, the greater the resistance to flow. These changes in resistance also alter the flow of blood through the vessels — decreased diameter (vasoconstriction) decreases blood flow, while increased diameter (vasodilation) increases blood flow.

The arterioles have the ability to alter their diameter by virtue of the smooth muscle in their walls and therefore are capable of altering both flow and resistance through the circulation. The smooth muscle is subject to a background, tonic level of contraction, allowing the vessel diameter to be decreased by an increased amount of contraction, or increased by a reduced amount of contraction.

The sum of all of the resistance provided by the

Figure 7.16   The effects of skeletal muscle contraction on blood flow within the venous system. Backflow of blood within the veins is prevented due to the presence of the venous valves. Skeletal muscle contraction compresses the veins pushing the blood through the valves towards the heart. When the muscles relax, backflow is again prevented by the valves. This system ensures a one-way flow of blood within the low-pressure venous system.

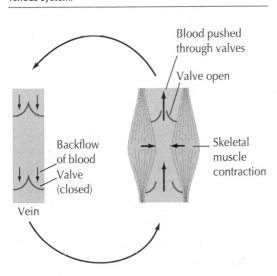

blood vessels in all organs and tissues of the body is known as the **total peripheral resistance**. Since the arteries and veins are large blood vessels, they do not contribute greatly to the total peripheral resistance. However, the arterioles are the major regulator of total peripheral resistance due to their ability to alter diameter. Peripheral resistance and blood flow are the two major determinants of arterial blood pressure. Since blood flow is determined by the cardiac output, arterial blood pressure can therefore be given by [total peripheral resistance × cardiac output]. Variations in either arteriolar diameter (controlling peripheral resistance) or cardiac output (controlling blood flow) will thus alter arterial blood pressure.

Normal arterial pressure at rest fluctuates from about 120 mmHg during systole to about 80 mmHg during diastole. A useful figure for comparison of blood pressures is the **mean arterial pressure (MAP)**:

$$\text{MAP} = \text{diastolic pressure} + \tfrac{1}{3}(\text{systolic pressure} - \text{diastolic pressure}) \qquad (1)$$

Using the above values for systolic and diastolic pressures, this gives a mean arterial pressure of 93 mmHg.

MEASUREMENT

Arterial blood pressure can be measured by several means. These include **auscultation** and **palpation**. In both cases, a **sphygmomanometer** is used. Here the brachial artery is compressed by inflating a cuff placed over the upper left arm. The cuff is inflated to a pressure above systolic blood pressure, thereby completely closing the artery. The pressure of the cuff is monitored by a small manometer which is connected to the cuff.

In auscultation, a stethoscope is placed over the brachial artery at the crook of the elbow below the cuff. The pressure in the cuff is then gradually released. When the cuff pressure is just lower than systolic pressure, blood in the brachial artery will suddenly push through, opening the artery. The flow of blood in the artery at this point is extremely turbulent, and as the blood collides with the arterial wall, this can be heard as sounds through the stethoscope. These are the **Korotkoff sounds**. The pressure at which the first Korotkoff sound is heard is the systolic blood pressure. The pressure in the cuff is then further decreased. At first, the sounds become slightly louder but then suddenly become very faint before disappearing. The pressure at which this occurs is the diastolic blood pressure.

There are many commercially-available blood-pressure machines which use this principle, by employing a microprocessor to detect the Korotkoff sounds picked up by a microphone placed within the inflatable cuff. The machine then uses a digital display to indicate the systolic and diastolic pressures. Pulse pressure (the difference between systolic and diastolic pressures) and heart rate are also sometimes displayed.

There are no set guidelines for indicating a *normal* blood pressure. Figures of 120 mmHg over 80 mmHg measured at rest are useful reference points, but not everyone who deviates from these values would be deemed to have abnormal blood pressure. High blood pressure (**hypertension**) is usually associated with resting diastolic pressures of >100 mmHg. Resting systolic pressures >140 mmHg also usually indicate hypertension. Prolonged hypertension can have serious consequences. There is an increased general strain on normal cardiac performance, leading to enlargement of the heart and reduced cardiac efficiency. Small blood vessels are also more prone to rupture, especially in the brain, which will lead to strokes.

CONTROL

Arterial blood pressure can be controlled by nervous and hormonal mechanisms and by regulation of total blood volume.

Nervous control of blood pressure relies on autonomic reflexes to detect changes in normal blood pressure and instigate appropriate action by smooth muscle effectors in the arterioles. Variations in blood pressure are detected by **baroreceptors** (sensory pressure receptors) located in the carotid sinus and in the aortic arch. These are stretch receptors which respond to distension of the walls of the carotid artery or aorta. The amount of tension in the wall is related to the pressure in the vessel (**Laplace's law**).

An increase in arterial pressure causes the baroreceptors to increase their firing of action potentials which are then transmitted from the carotid sinus and aortic arch to the central nervous system via Hering's nerve and the vagus nerve, respectively. Decreased blood pressure causes a decrease in firing frequency.

The cardiovascular control centres in the central nervous system are located in the medulla. The **vasoconstrictor centre** is responsible for increasing the sympathetic output to the smooth muscle cells of the arterioles. If blood pressure increases beyond normal levels, the increased firing of baroreceptors acts to inhibit the sympathetic output from the cardiovascular centres in the medulla, thereby inhibiting vasoconstriction in the arterioles and reducing heart rate and heart contractility. Additionally, there will be an increased output from the parasympathetic **vagal centre**, adding to the effects of decreased sympathetic output. The overall effect of these changes is that blood pressure will be reduced due to decreased peripheral resistance *and* decreased cardiac output, counteracting the original

increase. These autonomic reflexes therefore operate by negative feedback.

Similarly, decreases in blood pressure are also detected by the baroreceptors which will decrease their firing rate. This acts through the cardiovascular centres to increase arteriole vasoconstriction and increase heart rate and contractility to restore blood pressure. Additionally, the increased sympathetic output from the cardiovascular centres acts on the **adrenal medulla**, causing noradrenaline and adrenaline to be released into the circulation, enhancing the sympathetic effects on arteriole vasoconstriction.

Long-term changes in blood pressure can sometimes induce adaptation in the discharge of the baroreceptors and their role in maintenance of normal blood pressure may be reduced. The long-term regulation of blood pressure therefore must rely on additional hormonal mechanisms and on alterations in blood volume.

If an increase in blood pressure is sustained, there is an increase in the amount of fluid excreted by the kidneys — as much as eight times normal urine output can be achieved for a 50-mmHg rise in mean arterial pressure. This reduces the plasma volume which, in turn, will reduce the venous return to the heart. Cardiac output will therefore be reduced, bringing blood pressure back to normal levels. If blood pressure falls below normal, fluid excretion by the kidneys is reduced, increasing plasma volume and cardiac output and so increasing blood pressure.

Additional hormonal mechanisms include the **renin–angiotensin system** which comes into play when arterial pressure falls to very low levels. Decreased renal blood flow stimulates the release of renin from specialized cells in the kidney. Renin catalyses the production of angiotensin I in the plasma, which is converted to angiotensin II by a converting enzyme in the lungs. Angiotensin II is an extremely powerful vasoconstrictor and will therefore help to restore blood pressure to normal.

Release of **antidiuretic hormone** (also known as **vasopressin**) from the hypothalamus in response to low plasma volume will help to restore this by increasing the reabsorption of water from the kidney tubules, and will also induce arteriolar vasoconstriction.

Increased sympathetic output will also affect venous tone by causing contraction of the little amount of smooth muscle present there. This will raise venous pressure, thereby increasing venous

return by pushing more blood back to the heart. The increase in venous return will increase the cardiac output (Frank–Starling mechanism, see p. 138) and so will increase blood pressure.

The factors responsible for the regulation of normal blood pressure are summarized in Figure 7.18.

Fluid Movement from Capillaries to the Interstitial Space

The balance of hydrostatic pressures and osmotic pressures inside the capillaries and those in the interstitial spaces of the tissues is important in the

---

Figure 7.18   Factors influencing the normal regulation of blood pressure (ADH = antidiuretic hormone; NA = noradrenaline).

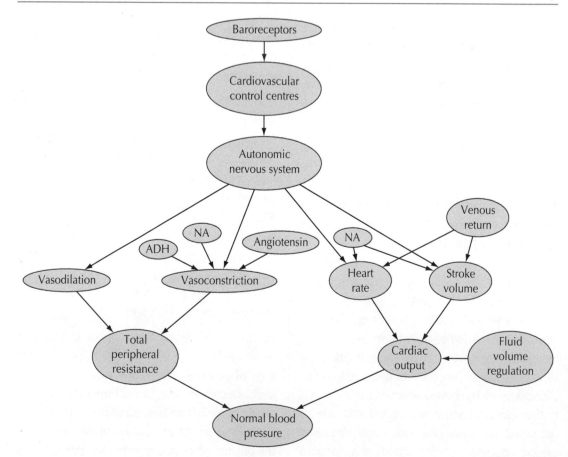

normal regulation of tissue fluid volume. Any disturbance to this balance can lead to alterations in the distribution of fluid between these two compartments, causing tissue swelling (**oedema**). Where the lymphatic system is involved, this is called **lymphoedema**.

At the arterial end of the capillaries, the blood pressure (hydrostatic pressure) is around 35 mmHg, whereas at the venous end of the capillaries this falls to around 15 mmHg. This blood hydrostatic pressure tends to push fluid out of the capillaries and into the interstitial spaces. However, this outward movement would tend to be resisted by the hydrostatic pressure of the interstitial fluid itself, which would push fluid back into the capillaries. This pressure is extremely low, however, and can essentially be ignored.

Since fluid can leave the capillaries but large particles such as proteins cannot, there is a relatively high osmotic pressure within the capillaries as a result of the high protein content with respect to that of the interstitial fluid. This is known as the **colloid osmotic pressure**. This colloid osmotic pressure tends to draw fluid back in to the capillaries, therefore resisting the outward force of the hydrostatic pressure. The colloid osmotic pressure of the interstitial fluid, which tends to draw fluid out of the capillaries, is relatively small due to the low protein content, being only 1–2 mmHg. The high protein content of the plasma, however, means that the plasma colloid osmotic pressure, tending to draw fluid into the capillaries, is relatively high (about 25 mmHg).

There is therefore a combination of forces which tend to favour movement of fluid out of the capillaries: the blood hydrostatic pressure (BP) and the interstitial fluid colloid osmotic pressure (IOP). There is also a combination of forces which tend to favour movement of fluid into the capil-

laries: the interstitial fluid hydrostatic pressure (negligible) and the blood colloid osmotic pressure (BOP). The balance of these forces is different at the arterial and venous ends of the capillaries.

At the arterial end of the capillaries, the balance is given by:

$$(BP + IOP) - BOP = (35 + 2) - 25 = 12 \text{ mmHg} \tag{2}$$

There is therefore a net outward pressure, or **filtration pressure**, at the arterial end of the capillaries.

The situation at the venous end of the capillaries is given by:

$$(BP + IOP) - BOP = (15 + 2) - 25 = -8 \text{ mmHg} \tag{3}$$

There is therefore a net inward pressure (given by the negative value), a **reabsorption pressure**, at the venous end of the capillaries.

Taking the capillaries overall, there is therefore filtration of fluid into the interstitial space at the arterial end of the capillaries. Some of this filtered fluid is reabsorbed back into the capillaries at the venous end. However, since the filtration pressure is greater than the reabsorption pressure, the overall tendency is for fluid to leak out of the capillaries and into the interstitial space. The majority of this fluid is returned to the circulation via the **lymphatic vessels**. These are a system of vessels similar in structure to veins (they also possess valves) and generally following the same path of the venous blood vessels. The lymphatic vessels also carry lipids which have been absorbed by the gut, and contain large numbers of lymphocytes from the lymph nodes. The lymphatic vessels eventually return their contents (**lymph**) to the circulation via the lymphatic ducts to the subclavian veins, and so back to the heart. Skeletal muscle contraction, together with the presence of valves in the lymphatic vessels, helps to propel the lymph along the course of the vessels back to the heart.

OEDEMA AND LYMPHOEDEMA

In some clinical situations, the normal balance of filtration and reabsorption pressures is upset, causing an increase in the volume of interstitial fluid which is formed. This increase in interstitial fluid volume leads to tissue swelling (oedema). Oedema may be due to hypertension or increased venous pressure (causing an increase in capillary hydrostatic pressure), increased capillary permeability, decreased blood colloid osmotic pressure due to loss of plasma proteins (for example, due to malnutrition, renal disease or burns) or blockage of lymphatic vessels.

Lymphatic blockage leading to lymphoedema can occur due to congenital abnormalities in the structure of the lymphatic vessels, or as a secondary problem associated with removal of the lymph glands, postradiation fibrosis from deep X-ray therapy or from blockage due to the presence of a tumour.

Treatment of lymphoedema by complex decongestive therapy involves the use of a combination of containment garments, compression pumps, massage, graduated bandaging and exercise in order to attempt to mobilize the increased volume of interstitial fluid into the lymphatic vessels.

Control of Regional Blood Flow

The 5 litres per minute of the resting cardiac output is distributed differently to different organs (Figure 7.19). Figure 7.19 also shows the maximum blood flow to each organ. The blood

Figure 7.19   Resting and maximal blood flows to different organs. Note that the blood flow to the kidneys remains relatively constant, while that to exercising skeletal muscle can increase by a large amount.

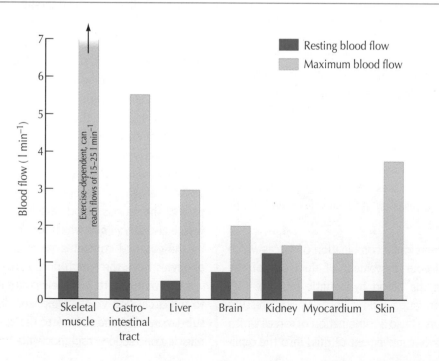

flow is carefully regulated in response to the demands of the organ for oxygen and nutrients in the blood. Increased activity in a particular organ will increase the metabolic rate of the cells, thereby increasing the need for a greater supply of oxygen and fuel molecules, as well as the need for removal of waste products. These waste products of metabolism (**metabolites**), together with low PO_2 and high PCO_2, are thought to produce relaxation of the smooth muscle in the walls of the arterioles supplying the capillary bed of the tissue. This causes vasodilation, increasing blood flow to those cells which require oxygen and fuel molecules.

Neural influences can also affect the distribution of blood flow to organs. For example, the increased sympathetic output which accompanies exercise and preparation for exercise acts on alpha-receptors on the smooth muscle of the arterioles supplying skeletal muscles, causing vasodilation. The blood flow to the active muscles is therefore increased in preparation for, and in response to, exercise.

Cardiovascular Responses

Exercise

Exercise induces several acute responses in the cardiovascular system. These include an initial, anticipatory response before the exercise has commenced, plus changes during the actual exercise. The majority of these responses are as a result of increased sympathetic output and decreased parasympathetic output from the cardiovascular centres in the medulla.

Cardiac output is increased in response to increased demand for oxygen, directly propor-

tional to the severity of the exercise. This is achieved by increasing heart rate and cardiac contractility (increasing stroke volume). Heart rate can increase to $\geqslant 200$ beats per minute in maximal exercise, while stroke volume can increase to 210 ml per beat. The extent of such changes in these parameters is dependent on the severity of the exercise and the overall physical fitness of the individual, and the above values for maximal heart rate and stroke volume apply to élite athletes rather than average subjects.

A large proportion of the cardiac output (up to 88% in maximum exercise) is diverted to the exercising muscle cells, with a concurrent decrease in blood flow to other areas of the body such as the gastrointestinal tract, kidneys and liver. Blood flow to the brain is kept constant no matter the severity of the exercise.

The increase in cardiac output which accompanies exercise produces an increase in arterial blood pressure. This mainly affects the systolic pressure, as the larger volume of blood is pumped out into the arteries during ventricular contraction. Diastolic pressure is only slightly affected since peripheral resistance is not altered much during exercise. Although there is a degree of vasoconstriction in the vessels of the gut and kidney, for example, this is offset by the vasodilation of the skeletal and cardiac muscle blood vessels.

Aging

The consequences of aging on the cardiovascular system are complex and involve a considerable amount of interaction between different factors. It is also difficult to separate the true effects of aging from those other effects which may be due to disease in an elderly subject. For a more detailed account, readers should consult the excellent review by Folkow and Svanborg (1993).

CARDIAC EFFECTS

In general, there is a degeneration of cardiac tissue with age. This leads to decreased efficiency of the myocardium, reduced elasticity and increased fibrosis of the cardiac valves.

There is very little change in resting heart rate with age. It remains between 60 and 80 beats per minute. However, with exercise, the maximum heart rate which can be achieved progressively decreases after about 25 years of age. This may partly be attributed to increased stiffness of the ventricular walls, which increases the time required for ventricular filling during diastole. There may also be a general decrease in sympathetic activity with age which would affect the stimulation of the sinoatrial pacemaker, thereby reducing heart rate.

There may also be a decrease in cardiac contractility with age, which may in turn be associated with a poor cardiac blood supply. This, therefore, produces a decrease in stroke volume, especially with increased demand on the heart during exercise.

Cardiac output on the whole is therefore reduced with age, and this is especially evident when the system is placed under stress as in exercise.

VASCULAR EFFECTS

In the peripheral blood vessels, there is a general loss of elasticity with age, due to degeneration of the elastic layers within the blood vessel walls and a general build-up of non-distensible collagen fibres. The consequence of this is that the major arterial vessels cannot accommodate the volume of blood ejected by the heart as easily as in younger, more elastic vessels. Systolic arterial blood pressure will therefore be increased. This presents a degree of afterload on the left ventricle, and may induce some enlargement of the left ventricle (hypertrophy). A further complication is that higher systolic pressures will place greater stress on the now less-distensible blood vessel walls, increasing the risk of vessel rupture and damage to the endothelial lining of the vessel wall. This, in turn, may promote the formation of atherosclerotic plaques and thromboses in these vessels.

Atherosclerosis and Coronary Heart Disease

Atherosclerosis is a condition in which deposits of fatty streaks are laid down in the arterial walls, causing a decrease in arterial diameter. It has been estimated that atherosclerosis variously affects the majority of the adult population of the Western world.

The fatty streaks in themselves are not considered to be too dangerous. However, they can lead to the development of raised **atherosclerotic plaque** formations in the artery wall. These plaques can in turn lead to *severe* arterial narrowing and also a predisposition to the formation of blood clots.

There is substantial evidence linking certain lipoproteins and cholesterol in the plasma to plaque formation. Normal plasma cholesterol concentrations are regarded as being < 5.3 millimoles per litre. Higher levels than this represent varying degrees of risk, and the importance of other blood lipid concentrations must also be considered. The European Atherosclerosis Society published guidelines in 1988 on how these different risk categories are designated (Table 7.2).

Cholesterol is transported in the plasma as **lipoproteins**. There are several different types of

Table 7.2

Risk Categories for Atherosclerosis Based on Blood Lipid Levels. Adapted from the Policy Statement of the European Atherosclerosis Society (1988)

Treatment group	A	B	C	D	E
Serum cholesterol (mmol l^{-1})	5.2–6.5	6.5–7.8	< 5.2	5.2–7.8	> 7.8
Serum triglyceride (mmol l^{-1})	< 2.3	< 2.3	2.3–5.6	2.3–5.6	> 5.6
Comment	Moderate risk	Dietary advice recommended	Hypertriglyceridaemia (possibly due to obesity or diabetes)	Combined hyperlipidaemia	Severe hyperlipidaemia

lipoproteins, but there are two of significance when considering the development of atherosclerosis. These are **high-density lipoproteins (HDLs)** and **low-density lipoproteins (LDLs)**.

The first step in the formation of an atherosclerotic plaque is some form of damage to the arterial wall. This damage most likely occurs to the endothelial cells of the tunica intima (see p. 143) and is caused by one or more of risk factors such as cigarette smoking, poor diet (high saturated fat intake), stress, lifestyle and social factors. The damage is most likely to occur at bends or forks in the artery as these are the places where changes in the direction of blood flow can cause abnormal stresses in the tissues of the arterial wall. This damage to the arterial wall increases the permeability of the endothelial lining, and therefore plasma and platelets can enter the tunica media. There are two effects of this:

- The platelets aggregate within the tunica media and release **mitogenic agents** which cause proliferation and growth of the smooth muscle cells of the tunica media (p. 143).
- The smooth muscle cells of the tunica media now become exposed to the plasma and a much higher concentration of LDL-cholesterol than normal. This LDL-cholesterol is then taken up by the smooth muscle cells by combining with

specific LDL receptors on the smooth muscle cell surface. The smooth muscle cells therefore become overloaded with cholesterol and are now referred to as **foam cells**.

The proliferating smooth muscle cells, overloaded with cholesterol, then begin to migrate from the tunica media to the tunica intima. As they do so, they also begin to synthesize collagen, elastin and mucopolysaccharides. This, therefore, initiates the formation of a fibrous layer on the intimal wall (the atherosclerotic plaque). Lipids and cholesterol in the plasma also build up on this fibrous layer, and so become incorporated into the plaque.

A single atherosclerotic plaque on its own is not particularly dangerous. However, several plaques distributed over a small section of an artery can cause an irregularity of the arterial lumen, thereby increasing the possibility of damage to the wall and also increasing the risk of clotting within the artery. Taken together, these factors can lead to significant narrowing of the artery, with serious consequences for normal functioning of the tissue which is supplied by that artery.

The cardiac muscle cells receive their blood supply via the coronary arteries. A decrease in the diameter of the coronary arteries will consequently lead to a decrease in the blood supply to cardiac muscle cells.

If, in addition to narrowing of the coronary arteries, there is also a blood clot in the vessels, there is the additional risk of complete blockage of the arteries (**coronary occlusion**). In this situation, there will be a complete failure of the blood supply to the area of myocardium which they supply, resulting in a failure of contractile activity in that area (a 'heart attack'). If the occluded artery is large, the percentage area of myocardium which is affected will also be large (Figure 7.20a). A tissue with a reduced blood supply is said to be ischaemic. If the ischaemia is prolonged, the affected tissue area will eventually die. The tissue survival time in ischaemia is different for different tissues. Heart muscle can survive about fifteen minutes of ischaemia. After this, the damage is irreversible and the myocardial tissue dies. If the subject survives this initial trauma, the dead myocardial tissue is eventually replaced with scar tissue and the resulting area is a myocardial infarction.

In order to maintain myocardial activity as close to normal as possible, it is important that the area of dead tissue is kept to a minimum. Myocardial areas which receive a **collateral blood supply** (i.e. a blood supply from more than one arterial source) will be affected by coronary occlusion to a lesser extent. The area of tissue which receives collateral circulation may receive some of its blood supply from other, non-occluded arteries and does not become fully ischaemic, but **hypoxic** instead. This area is known as the **grey zone**, where blood flows to the myocardial cells but not in adequate amounts to fully meet the oxygen demands of the tissue (Figure 7.20b).

If the subject survives the initial heart attack, the collateral circulation to the grey zone will develop, and the blood supply can begin to return towards normal.

In severe cases, it may be desirable to bypass the affected coronary artery in order to maintain an

Figure 7.20 (a) Diagrammatic representation of the effects of coronary artery occlusion on the blood supply to the myocardium. The larger the occluded artery, the greater the area affected. (b) Diagrammatic representation of the effects of collateral circulation on the blood supply to the myocardium. The shaded area represents a portion of myocardium which receives its blood supply from two major coronary arteries. If one of these arteries becomes occluded, this shaded area will still have a reasonable blood supply. It will therefore become hypoxic rather than fully ischaemic.

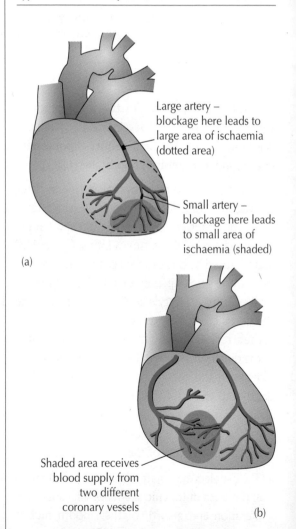

Large artery – blockage here leads to large area of ischaemia (dotted area)

Small artery – blockage here leads to small area of ischaemia (shaded)

(a)

Shaded area receives blood supply from two different coronary vessels

(b)

adequate blood supply to a particular region of the myocardium. A **coronary artery bypass graft** (**CABG**) involves using pieces of the saphenous vein or mammary artery to bypass the diseased segments of the coronary arteries.

It should be noted that atherosclerosis affects any of the vessels in the body and, consequently, the normal functioning of other organ systems such as the brain and kidney can also be affected.

Bibliography

Berne, RM, Levy, MN (1992) *Cardiovascular Physiology,* 6th Edition. Mosby, St Louis.

European Atherosclerosis Society (1988) The recognition and management of hyperlipidaemias in adults: a policy statement of the EAS. *European Heart Journal, 9*: 571–600.

Folkow, B, Svanborg, A (1993) Physiology of cardiovascular aging. *Physiological Reviews, 73*: 725–764.

Gravanis, MB (1993) *Cardiovascular Disorders – Pathogenesis and Pathophysiology.* Mosby, St Louis.

McArdle, WD, Katch, FI, Katch, VL (1994) *Essentials of Exercise Physiology.* Lea and Febiger, Philadelphia.

Rowell, LB (1993) *Human Cardiovascular Control.* Oxford University Press, Oxford.

8

The Respiratory System

General Structures

The cells of the body need a constant supply of oxygen in order that they can metabolize fuel molecules to provide energy in the form of adenosine triphosphate (ATP). As the oxygen is used up, so the metabolic reactions produce carbon dioxide, which subsequently is removed from the body.

The respiratory system, in conjunction with the cardiovascular system, enables oxygen from the atmosphere to be delivered to the blood and hence to the metabolizing tissues, and allows the removal of carbon dioxide from the body to the atmosphere.

The respiratory system consists of the respiratory passages, or airways, and the lungs. These structures lie in the thorax and their basic anatomy is shown in Figure 8.1. The upper respiratory tract consists of the mouth, the throat (**pharynx**), the voice box (**larynx**) and the windpipe (**trachea**). The lower respiratory tract comprises the airways – the **bronchi** and smaller air passages – and the lungs themselves.

Air enters the lungs via the trachea, which subsequently branches into the right and left bronchi, each supplying one lung. Each primary bronchus

Figure 8.1   Basic anatomy of the lungs and associated structures.

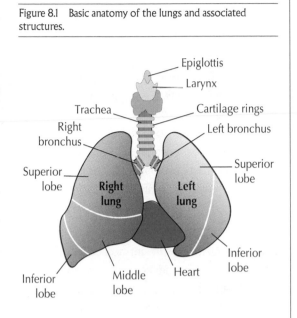

Figure 8.2   The respiratory tree. Branching of the airways leads to more numerous and smaller passageways; only one branchline is illustrated here. Exchange of gases between the air and the blood only occurs in the airways of the respiratory zone.

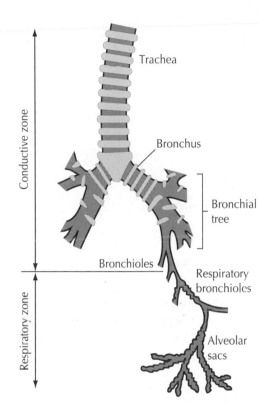

further subdivides to form the bronchial tree, consisting of terminal bronchioles, respiratory bronchioles and the alveolar sacs. The respiratory tree can be divided into two main zones — the **conductive zone**, responsible for moving air into and out of the lung, and the **respiratory zone**, which is involved in the processes of gas exchange (Figure 8.2).

Respiratory Tract

The Upper Respiratory Tract

The nose and mouth serve as the entry point to the respiratory passages. The structure of the nasal passages creates a turbulent airflow which causes the air to come into contact with the moist tissues which line these passages. The air entering the respiratory passages is therefore warmed and moistened. Hairs within the nasal passages also

serve to filter foreign particles from the incoming air.

The airways of the upper respiratory tract are lined with a specialized epithelium consisting of ciliated pseudostratified columnar cells, with mucus-secreting goblet cells (Figure 8.3). The cilia of the columnar cells beat unidirectionally so that the mucus is removed from the airways. This has a protective function, ensuring that any foreign particles (e.g. dust, dirt, bacteria) become entrapped in the mucus, and are removed from the respiratory system.

The walls of the larynx and trachea contain hyaline cartilage which helps to hold these structures

Figure 8.3 Epithelial lining of the upper respiratory tract. This is a pseudostratified columnar epithelium with cilia and goblet cells. Mucus, produced by the goblet cells, lies on a layer above the cilia of the columnar cells. Ciliary movement ensures that the mucus is transported upwards, out of the respiratory tract. Not all of the columnar cells reach the surface of the epithelial layer and cell nuceli are located at different levels. This gives the epithelium the appearance of being layered; however, all cells do make contact with the basement membrane, making this a pseudostratified, rather than true stratified, epithelium.

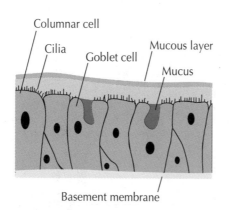

Columnar cell

Cilia

Goblet cell

Mucous layer

Mucus

Basement membrane

open, while maintaining some flexibility. In the trachea the cartilage forms 'C'-shaped rings, which can be felt by running the fingers up and down the skin overlying the trachea.

A tracheostomy is an artificial airway which is indicated when obstruction of the airway occurs above the level of the larynx. The obstruction may be due to oedema, crush injury or a tumour. A skin incision is made and the trachea is cut open below the cricoid cartilage and the patient then breathes through a metal or plastic tube inserted into the opening. As the tracheostomy bypasses the upper airways, this means that incoming air bypasses some of the body's own mechanisms for humidification of air and defence systems against airborne particles.

The Lower Respiratory Tract

The bronchi divide repeatedly into smaller and smaller airways, and as they divide the amount

of cartilage present in the walls diminishes until, in the smallest (terminal) bronchioles, there is no cartilage present.

The bronchiole walls, however, do contain smooth muscle which is under the control of the autonomic nervous system. Activity in the sympathetic branch of the autonomic nervous system causes smooth muscle relaxation in the airways and therefore dilatation, while activity in the parasympathetic branch causes smooth muscle contraction and therefore airway constriction.

Bronchodilatation and bronchoconstriction are also dependent on the intracellular concentrations of cyclic adenosine monophosphate (cAMP) and cyclic guanosine monophosphate (cGMP) in the smooth muscle cells, both of which are intracellular chemical messengers. Bronchodilator drugs, such as salbutamol, act directly on beta-receptors on the smooth muscle cells and act to increase the intracellular levels of cAMP which then leads to bronchodilatation. Anticholinergic drugs block the effect of acetylcholine on the smooth muscle cells, reducing the intracellular levels of cGMP, thus enhancing bronchodilatation.

The terminal bronchioles branch to form the respiratory bronchioles, part of the respiratory zone which leads into the lung tissue. The walls of these respiratory bronchioles do not possess smooth muscle, but instead have a layer of elastic connective tissue.

The Lungs

The lungs lie on either side of the heart and are surrounded by the **pleural membrane**. The pleural membrane consists of two layers — an outer layer attached to the wall of the thorax, and an inner layer covering the lung tissue. Between these two layers is a potential space — the pleural cavity — which contains a lubricating fluid secreted by the membranes. This fluid reduces the friction which occurs during inflation and deflation of the lungs, between the two layers of the pleural membrane.

Each lung is divided into lobes, with each lobe receiving a division of the primary bronchus. The right lung has three lobes (superior, middle and inferior) while the left lung has two (superior and inferior) (see Figure 8.1). Each lobe is further subdivided into lobules which are separated from each other by connective tissue.

The respiratory bronchioles enter the deepest portion of the lungs, and in turn divide to form several **alveolar ducts**, containing numerous **alveolar sacs** comprising clusters of individual **alveoli** (Figure 8.4). The alveoli are the main site of gas exchange between the inspired air and the blood. Each alveolus is about 0.25–0.5 mm in diameter, and there are about 150 million of these in each lung, giving a total surface area for gas exchange of about 60–80 m^2.

In the alveoli, the epithelial lining has now completely changed to that of a simple squamous epithelium which is only one cell thick. This lies in close conjunction with the endothelial cells lining the blood capillaries associated with each alveolus (Figure 8.5). This ensures that there is only a very thin barrier — about 0.5 μm — to the diffusion of gases from the alveolus to the capillary and vice versa.

The alveoli and respiratory bronchioles form the majority of the mass of the lung. Given that this is a collection of a large number of very small, roughly spherical chambers, and due to the surface tension effects of the fluid lining the alveolar walls, considerable forces develop which would tend to cause the alveoli to collapse. This collapsing force is counteracted by the presence of **surfactant**. This is a complex mixture of phospho-

Figure 8.4   An alveolar sac, showing clusters of individual alveoli arising from a respiratory bronchiole. Each alveolus is in close association with the capillary blood vessels.

Figure 8.5   The alveolar–capillary junction. The diagram shows a capillary in cross-section, together with a red blood cell, on the right. The thin barrier of the alveolar epithelial cells is shown to the left. A thin layer of interstitial space, containing some connective tissue, separates the two cells.

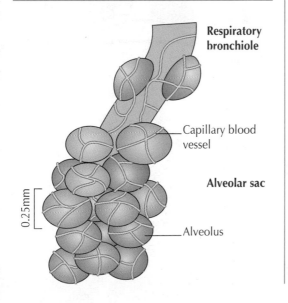

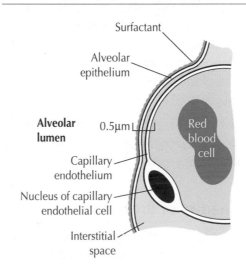

lipids which is secreted by **type II alveolar cells** (also known as **septal cells**) and which has a detergent action which lowers the surface tension within the alveoli.

Respiratory distress syndrome results from a deficiency in surfactant production. Insufficient surfactant leads to **atelectasis** (alveolar collapse) due to problems of inflation of alveoli, and the risk of alveolar collapse during expiration. The surfactant system does not mature until about 35 weeks gestation, but will begin to produce surfactant 36–48 hours postpartum irrespective of gestational age. However, mechanical ventilation of the neonate may be required immediately following birth.

Also associated with the alveolus are **alveolar macrophages**. These cells are wandering scavengers which help remove dust and other particles that have managed to reach the alveolus from the outside environment via the inhaled air.

Blood Supply to the Lungs

The right and left pulmonary arteries carry deoxygenated venous blood from the right ventricle of the heart to the respiratory portions of the lungs. The pulmonary blood vessels divide until they form the capillary vessels which are closely associated with the alveoli and which participate in gaseous exchange. These latter unite to eventually form the pulmonary veins which return the oxygenated blood to the heart.

The cells of the lung tissue receive their own blood supply via the bronchial arteries, which are direct branches of the aorta.

Mechanics of Breathing

Breathing, or **pulmonary ventilation**, is achieved by air being drawn into, and expelled from, the

lungs as a result of pressure changes brought about by movements of the chest wall and the diaphragm. Air moves into the lungs when the pressure inside the lungs is less than that in the outside atmosphere and, similarly, air moves out of the lungs when the pressure inside the lungs is greater than the atmospheric pressure. Breathing in is termed **inspiration** or **inhalation**, and breathing out is termed **expiration** or **exhalation**.

The principal muscle of breathing is the diaphragm, a dome-shaped muscle forming the floor of the thoracic cavity. Immediately prior to inspiration, the diaphragm is relaxed and is curved upwards into the thoracic cavity (Figure 8.6a). At

Figure 8.6   (a) Expansion of the thoracic cavity due to contraction of the diaphragm (arrow) causes the lungs to expand from their resting volume (solid lines) to a greater, inflated volume (dashed lines). (b) Contraction of the intercostal muscles causes the rib cage to move upwards and outwards.

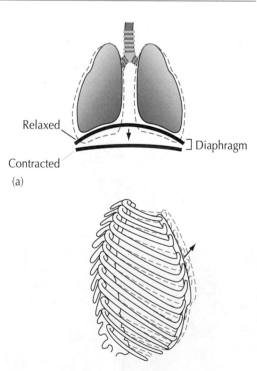

the start of inspiration, the diaphragm contracts and flattens, thereby increasing the volume of the thoracic cavity. This increase in volume reduces the intrathoracic pressure. At the same time, the **intercostal muscles** of the chest wall also contract, causing the chest wall to expand upwards and outwards (Figure 6.6b). This further increases the volume of the thoracic cavity, adding to the reduction in intrathoracic pressure.

The movement of the diaphragm and the chest wall reduces the intrathoracic pressure to a level below atmospheric pressure. Since the lungs are open to the atmosphere, the drop in intrathoracic pressure draws air into the lungs causing them to expand. This movement of air into the lungs will continue as long as there is a pressure gradient from the atmosphere to the lungs.

Deflation of the lungs during expiration is usually a passive process brought about by elastic recoil of the expanded lung tissue and chest wall. This elastic recoil raises the intrathoracic and intrapulmonary pressure so that the pressure gradient is now from the lungs to the atmosphere, and air will move out of the lungs. In some situations (e.g. voluntary hyperventilation, playing a wind instrument, singing), deflation of the lungs can be assisted by activity in the respiratory muscles, particularly the abdominal muscles.

Pneumothorax, or air in the pleural space, results from rupture of either the parietal or visceral pleura. This may occur as a consequence of external trauma, such as penetrating injuries, or internal trauma, such as rupture of a bulla. Air in the pleural space leads to a loss of the normal intrapleural subatmospheric pressure, and causes the lung to deflate. Treatment, by insertion of an intercostal drain, restores the subatmospheric pressure and aids re-expansion of the lung tissue.

Compliance

The ease with which the thoracic wall and the lungs can be expanded is termed **compliance.** Compliance is defined as the volume change of the lungs per unit pressure. The greater the compliance, the easier the expansion of the lungs and the thorax. The lower the compliance, the more the lungs and thorax will resist expansion. The compliance of the lungs is related to both the elasticity of the lung tissue and to the surface tension, and anything which interferes with these factors will affect compliance. For example, the compliance of the lungs will be increased in emphysema, where there is a loss of elastic tissue in the walls of the lung tissues. Conversely, compliance will be reduced in pulmonary oedema, where surface-tension effects prevent adequate inflation of the lungs.

Airway Resistance

The air that passes through the airways does not pass totally unimpeded; the walls of the different airways offer resistance to the flow of air. During inspiration, the stretch exerted on the lung tissues by the expansion of the thorax acts to increase the diameter of the major airways. This reduces the resistance to the flow of air through these airways. As an experiment, try breathing through a drinking straw while pinching the nose closed, and compare this with normal breathing. The straw has a much smaller diameter than that of the trachea, and so offers a greater resistance to the flow of air into the lungs. This therefore increases the effort of breathing.

In life, the diameter of the airways can be altered by neural, physical and chemical stimuli. Neural regulation of airway diameter is achieved primarily by the parasympathetic branch of the autonomic nervous system, where stimulation of the smooth muscle in the airway walls results in airway constriction. Sympathetic activity can also act to relax this smooth muscle, thereby dilating the airways. Chemical mediators such as histamine, released in response to an allergic reaction can cause smooth muscle contraction and hence airway narrowing. Physical alterations in airway diameter are most commonly the result of disease or injury. For example, a blow to the front of the neck may physically dislodge the cartilage which holds the trachea open, resulting in the collapse of the trachea and so increasing resistance to flow. The condition of cystic fibrosis results in an excessively viscous mucus secretion which is difficult to remove from the air passages and which, by its presence, narrows the airways. Airway narrowing with its accompanying increase in airway resistance has implications for the normal ventilation of the lungs and has effects on lung function. These effects will be discussed below (p. 176–177).

Lung Volumes

The normal resting lung volume varies between about 2.5 and 3 litres with each breath. This variation of about 500 ml is termed the **tidal volume**. The tidal volume may vary due to such factors as exercise or voluntary changes in depth of breathing. At rest, the **respiratory frequency** is usually between 12 and 15 breaths per minute. Tidal volume multiplied by respiratory frequency gives the **total minute ventilation** and, at rest, this is normally between 6 and 7.5 litres per minute. Increases in either tidal volume, respiratory frequency, or both will obviously increase the minute ventilation, thereby increasing the delivery of oxygen to the blood.

Of the 500 ml of air drawn into the lungs at rest, only about 350 ml comes into contact with the respiratory portion of the lung tissue. The remaining 150 ml is in the conducting airways and therefore does not participate in gas exchange. This 150 ml is termed the **anatomical dead space**. *Alveolar* ventilation, therefore, is equivalent to 350 ml × 12 inhalations per minute = 4.2 litres per minute.

At the end of every normal breath, the lungs are not completely empty. There is a volume of gas still present in the lungs – the **functional residual capacity** – which amounts to about 2.5 litres. This volume is not stagnant, but is continually replenished and refreshed with each breath.

At the end of a normal tidal breath, it is possible to exhale still further. Through the maximum contraction of all the expiratory muscles a further 1.5 litres can be expired. This is termed the **expiratory reserve volume**. Even after this maximum expiration, there is approximately 1 litre of air still left in the lungs. This is the **residual volume**. The residual volume and the expiratory reserve volume make up the functional residual capacity.

Similarly, at the end of a normal inspiration, it is possible to further increase the amount of air taken in by further contraction of the inspiratory muscles. In doing so, approximately 3 litres of air can be further inspired – the **inspiratory reserve volume**. This volume, plus the tidal volume, comprises the **inspiratory capacity**.

The sum of the inspiratory reserve volume + tidal volume + expiratory reserve volume equals the **vital capacity**, which is the maximum volume of air which a subject can expire after a maximum inspiration. This volume is normally about 4–5 litres. The **total lung capacity** is equal to the vital capacity + residual volume and is usually about 6 litres.

These values for the different lung volumes are

Figure 8.7 Trace showing changes in normal lung volumes in litres. V_T = tidal volume; ERV = expiratory reserve volume; IRV = inspiratory reserve volume; VC = vital capacity; RV = residual volume; FRC = functional residual capacity.

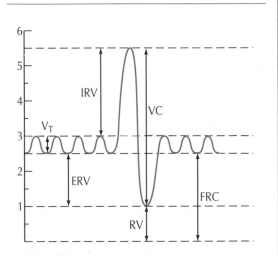

approximate and vary from subject to subject. The actual volumes depend on such factors as sex, age and body frame size.

Figure 8.7 summarizes these lung volumes. Some can be measured using a **spirometer**. This is basically a floating cylinder or wedge filled with air from which a subject can breathe. As the subject breathes in and out, the floating cylinder will move up and down. By attaching a pen to this cylinder and allowing it to trace a path on a rotating drum, the changes in lung volumes associated with the breathing movements can be measured (Figure 8.8).

The spirometer can also be used to measure changes in lung volumes during forced expiration. Here, the subject makes a maximum inspira-

Figure 8.8 General principles of spirometry. The subject breathes from gas contained within the floating cylinder. Inspiration causes the cylinder to move downwards, while expiration will cause it to move upwards. These movements can then be recorded using a pen to trace a path on paper attached to a rotating drum. Several variants of this system are available, including a floating wedge rather than a cylinder, and utilizing computer technology to record the respiratory movements.

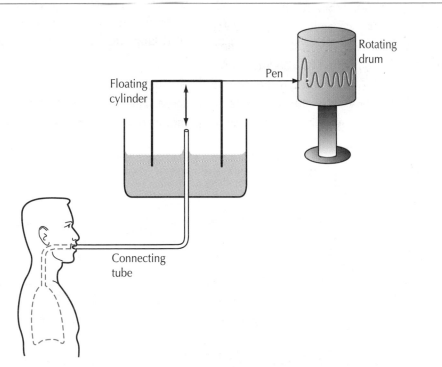

tion followed by a forced maximum expiration. The subject exhales as completely as possible. This type of test is used clinically to identify problems in lung function, and a number of important parameters can be measured from such a test. The total volume exhaled is the forced vital capacity (FVC), and the volume exhaled in the first second of the test is termed the **forced expiratory volume in one second** (FEV$_1$). In normal subjects, the FEV$_1$ is usually between 80 and 90% of the FVC (Figure 8.9a). If the test is repeated on a subject with obstructive lung disease such as bronchitis or asthma, the pattern of changes in lung volume is different (Figure 8.9b). Here, there is a much slower timecourse of forced expiration, since there is an increased resistance to flow of air through the airways. The FVC is reduced and the FEV$_1$ as a percentage of the FVC is considerably reduced. In restrictive diseases such as pulmonary fibrosis, the FVC is reduced due to a reduction in the inspiratory reserve volume as a result of the disease condition (Figure 8.9c). There is no increase in resistance to flow through the airways with this condition however, and the FEV$_1$ as a percentage of the (reduced) FVC (%FVC) is normal (in some cases the %FEV$_1$ is actually increased since

the fibrotic changes in the lung tissue prevent airway collapse during forced expiration).

Lung function tests such as these also allow other important parameters to be measured, e.g. peak expiratory flow rate (maximum change in volume per unit time), maximal mid-expiratory flow rate (maximum flow rate during the middle 50% of expiration) and flow–volume patterns (changes in flow at different lung volumes as the lungs empty). A detailed account of lung function tests and their importance is given by Wanger (1992).

Other Respiratory Manoeuvres

Deep-breathing exercises are used to increase functional lung volume, re-opening alveoli. Slow breathing reduces airway turbulence, encouraging ventilation to dependent areas. It is thought that alveoli, once inflated, will remain open for approximately one hour. End-inspiratory holds, or 'sniff' manoeuvres, may be added at maximum inspiration to promote airflow to poorly ventilated lung areas by increasing collateral ventilation.

A **cough** is a release of air from the lungs at high speed. High positive pressure develops in the thorax, causing segments of bronchi to collapse,

Figure 8.9   Spirometer traces obtained from forced expiration tests. (a) Normal subject. (b) Subject with obstructive lung disease. (c) Subject with restrictive lung disease. The pattern and time course of the volume changes shown are clinically useful in the identification of different lung disorders.

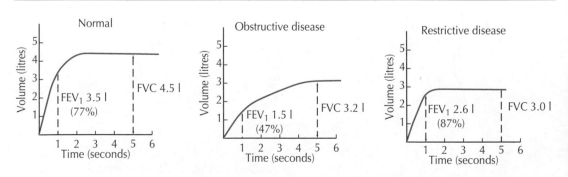

trapping air. Deep breathing is required to re-open these airways, but this may be difficult for some patients with respiratory disease.

Forced expiratory technique (FET) is a combination of forced expiration and relaxed deep breathing. Transpulmonary pressure developed during the forced expiration is less than that developed during a cough, and so the degree of airway collapse is reduced. FET may also be more effective than a cough at clearing secretions from the airways, as the forced expiration causes oscillation of airway walls which may loosen secretions.

Gas Exchange and Transport

Gas Exchange

Air entering the lungs has a higher concentration of oxygen than the blood. The partial pressure of oxygen in the atmosphere is about 158 mmHg. This is calculated by knowing the atmospheric pressure (the pressure exerted by all the gases present in the atmosphere) and the percentage volume of the atmosphere which consists of oxygen. The average atmospheric pressure is 760 mmHg and the percentage oxygen in the atmosphere is 20.9%, i.e. 20.9% of 760 mmHg equals 158 mmHg — the partial pressure of oxygen.

When this atmospheric air enters the respiratory passages, it becomes saturated with water vapour, due to the moist linings of the airways. At body temperature, the water vapour pressure is 47 mmHg. The pressure of the *gases* in the air therefore falls to 760 − 47 = 713 mmHg. The partial pressure of oxygen in the inspired air will therefore also fall to 20.9% × 713 mmHg = 150 mmHg.

Upon reaching the alveoli, the inspired oxygen mixes with the carbon dioxide already present in the alveoli as a result of diffusion from the blood. The partial pressure of carbon dioxide (PCO_2) in the alveoli is 40 mmHg. Knowing these values, the **alveolar gas equation** allows the alveolar PO_2 to be calculated:

$$\text{Alveolar } PO_2 = \text{Inspired } PO_2 - \frac{\text{Alveolar } PCO_2}{RQ}$$

where RQ is the respiratory quotient (volume of CO_2 produced by the tissues divided by the volume of O_2 consumed by the tissues). With an alveolar PCO_2 of 40 mmHg, and a normal RQ of 0.8, this gives an alveolar PO_2 of 100 mmHg.

The PO_2 in the alveoli is therefore about 100 mmHg, whilst that of the venous blood entering the alveolar capillaries is about 40 mmHg. A concentration gradient therefore exists for oxygen which allows diffusion of oxygen from the alveoli, crossing the alveolar wall, the interstitial space and the capillary endothelium into the blood in the capillaries. The blood is constantly flowing through the alveolar capillaries and this concentration gradient is therefore maintained as the oxygenated blood leaves the pulmonary circulation and is replaced by deoxygenated blood entering from the heart.

Diffusion of oxygen continues until an equilibrium has been achieved and the blood leaving the lungs to return to the heart and the arterial system has a PO_2 of 100 mmHg.

The PCO_2 of the venous blood entering the alveolar capillaries is about 46 mmHg. A diffusion gradient therefore exists between the capillaries and the alveoli, allowing carbon dioxide to diffuse from the blood and enter the alveoli where it will then be removed from the lungs during expiration. Since the carbon dioxide in the blood

Figure 8.10   Summary of gas compositions in the atmosphere, alveoli, venous blood and arterial blood.

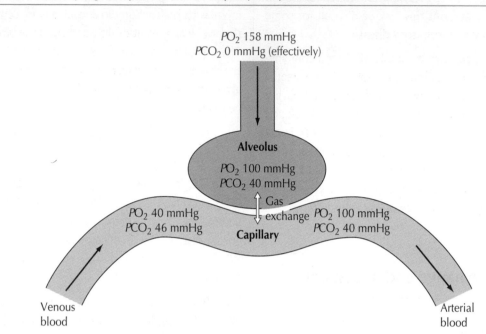

equilibrates with that in the alveoli, the PCO_2 of the blood leaving the pulmonary circulation and returning to the heart and arterial system is 40 mmHg, the same as alveolar air.

Figure 8.10 summarizes the relationships between alveolar and blood gas compositions.

Gas Transport in the Blood

OXYGEN TRANSPORT

Arterial blood contains about 200 ml of oxygen. Of this, approximately 3 ml is in the form of dissolved oxygen and about 197 ml as oxygen chemically bound to haemoglobin in the red blood cells.

Haemoglobin consists of a protein component (globin) and an iron-containing pigment molecule (haem) (Figure 8.11). Each haemoglobin molecule has four haem groups associated with the

Figure 8.11   Structure of haemoglobin. The molecule consists of four polypeptide chains, two alpha-chains and two beta-chains, each of which is associated with a haem group. Each haem group contains an atom of iron which has the ability to combine with one molecule of oxygen.

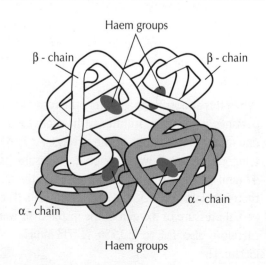

globin component and each haem group has the ability to combine with one molecule of oxygen. Each molecule of haemoglobin can therefore bind four molecules of oxygen. Since each red blood cell contains approximately 280 million molecules of haemoglobin, each red blood cell is therefore capable of carrying over one billion molecules of oxygen.

The average content of haemoglobin in the blood is 150 g l^{-1} (or 15%). Since there is a finite number of oxygen binding sites on the haemoglobin molecule, there is a maximum amount of oxygen which can combine with haemoglobin. The main factor which determines the amount of oxygen bound to haemoglobin – the haemoglobin saturation – is the PO_2 of the blood. The relationship between PO_2 and haemoglobin saturation is shown in Figure 8.12. This graph shows the oxygen–haemoglobin dissociation curve, which is sigmoid in shape with a steep slope between the PO_2 values of 10 and 60 mmHg, and a flatter portion between 60 and 100 mmHg. The shape of this curve represents the affinity of haemoglobin for oxygen and is very important with respect

to the uptake of oxygen by the blood at the alveoli and the release of oxygen from the blood to the tissues.

At sites in the body where the PO_2 is high (e.g. at the alveoli), the affinity of haemoglobin for oxygen is high and so the percentage saturation of haemoglobin with oxygen is increased. Therefore at the lungs, oxygen will readily combine with haemoglobin. However, at sites where PO_2 is low (e.g. at the cells of metabolizing tissues), the affinity of haemoglobin for oxygen is decreased and oxygen will be given up by the haemoglobin molecules to the tissue cells.

The plateau portion of the dissociation curve is also important in providing a safety factor in situations where alveolar ventilation is reduced or atmospheric pressure is less than normal (e.g. at altitude). In these situations, alveolar PO_2 can be reduced to about 60 mmHg, but haemoglobin saturation still remains relatively high – about 90%.

The shape of the oxygen–haemoglobin dissocia-

Figure 8.12   Oxygen–haemoglobin dissociation curve.

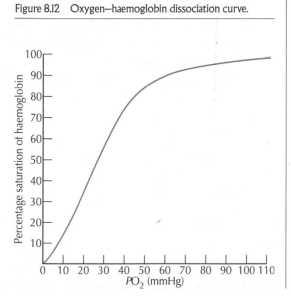

Figure 8.13   The Bohr effect of pH changes on the oxygen–haemoglobin dissociation curve.

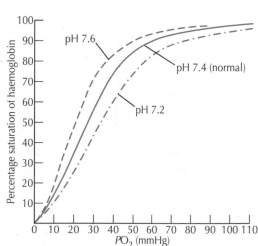

tion curve is not fixed however. Alterations in blood pH can shift the curve to the left and upwards, or to the right and downwards (Figure 8.13). This shift in the position of the curve is known as the **Bohr effect** and has implications for the uptake and delivery of oxygen. A decrease in blood pH results in a lower haemoglobin affinity for oxygen. The excess hydrogen ions in the plasma bind to the protein component of the haemoglobin molecule, producing a conformational change in its structure. This reduces the oxygen binding capability of the molecule, thereby shifting the dissociation curve to the right.

The more metabolically active a tissue is, the more acidic the environment surrounding the tissue cells will become:

$$CO_2 + H_2O \rightarrow HCO_3^- + H^+$$
(from cell
metabolism)

Highly active tissues will therefore reduce the pH of the interstitial fluid, thereby increasing the delivery of oxygen to the tissues due to the Bohr effect. In addition, metabolizing tissues also produce 2,3-diphosphoglycerate, a byproduct of metabolism. This is present in red blood cells and as the concentration rises further, the affinity of haemoglobin for oxygen is decreased. This again means that oxygen will be more readily given up to active tissues.

The concentration of hydrogen ions at the pulmonary capillaries is reduced, thereby increasing the pH at the lungs. This will cause a shift in the dissociation curve to the left and upwards, enhancing the ability of haemoglobin to pick up oxygen at the lungs.

Inhalation of noxious fumes, either in isolation, or associated with burns (smoke inhalation) affects the oxygen-carrying capacity of the blood. The most commonly inhaled noxious gas is carbon monoxide (CO) which has a greater affinity for haemoglobin than oxygen. Carbon monoxide combines with haemoglobin to form **carboxyhaemoglobin**. This reduces the amount of oxygen bound to haemoglobin. The overall effect is to shift the dissociation curve to the left. This has the effect that oxygen already bound to haemoglobin is difficult to release from the haemoglobin at the level of the tissues, even when tissue PO_2 is low. In such cases, increasing the inspired PO_2 by oxygen therapy improves the oxygenation of the blood by displacing carbon monoxide from haemoglobin. Other effects of smoke inhalation include loss of surfactant (see p. 159) and reduced action of the cilia lining the respiratory tract.

CARBON DIOXIDE TRANSPORT

Carbon dioxide is generated as a product of cellular metabolism. It is about 20 times more soluble in water than oxygen, and so more can be transported dissolved in the plasma. Between 8 and 10% of the total carbon dioxide is transported in this way.

Dissolved carbon dioxide can also react with free amino groups of proteins, particularly those of haemoglobin, to form **carbamino** compounds. The **carbaminohaemoglobin** formed in this way accounts for about 25% of the total carbon dioxide transported in the blood. The remaining 65% of carbon dioxide is transported as carbonic acid and bicarbonate ions in the plasma. This is formed from the reaction of carbon dioxide with the water of the plasma and that inside the red blood cells:

$$CO_2 + H_2O \rightarrow H_2CO_3 \rightarrow H^+ + HCO_3^-$$

This reaction proceeds only very slowly in the plasma. However, inside the red blood cell the reaction proceeds at a much faster rate (about

10 000 times faster) due to the presence of the enzyme **carbonic anhydrase**. This enzyme catalyses the formation of carbonic acid.

These reactions are reversible, but they are pushed to the right due to the Law of Mass Action; when the PCO_2 increases, the formation of hydrogencarbonate is favoured. The hydrogen ions formed by this reaction are buffered by combining with haemoglobin in the red blood cell. The hydrogencarbonate ions, however, are free to diffuse out of the red blood cell and into the plasma. This movement of negatively-charged ions out of the red blood cell is balanced by the movement of chloride ions into the cell. This is the **chloride shift**.

In the pulmonary capillaries, this sequence of events is reversed, with the dissolved carbon dioxide diffusing from the plasma to the alveoli. This diffusion of the dissolved carbon dioxide reduces the PCO_2 of the plasma, thereby inducing carbon dioxide to dissociate from haemoglobin and diffuse into the plasma and from there to the alveoli. Simultaneously, hydrogencarbonate in the red blood cells combines with hydrogen ions to form carbonic acid which readily dissociates to form carbon dioxide and water. The carbon dioxide diffuses out of the red blood cell and into the alveoli.

Figure 8.14 summarizes the transport of oxygen and carbon dioxide in the blood and allows the

Figure 8.14 Integration of oxygen and carbon dioxide transport in the blood. Reactions move from left to right at the level of the tissues, where PO_2 is low, and from right to left at the lungs where PO_2 is high. (Hb, haemoglobin)

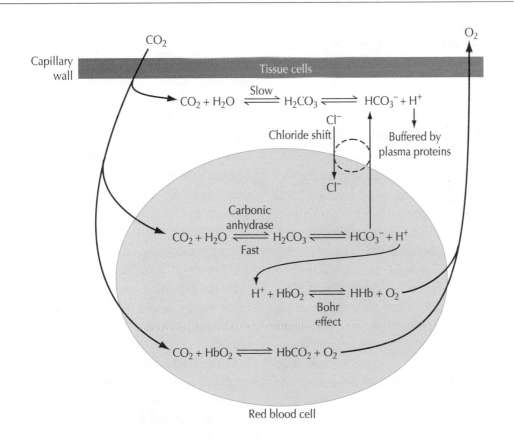

Control of Respiration

Normal breathing depends upon the rhythmic contraction and relaxation of the respiratory muscles. Inspiration is initiated by a burst of nerve impulses from the respiratory centres in the brainstem being sent via the spinal cord to the motoneurones of the respiratory muscles.

The respiratory control system can basically be divided into three main elements (West, 1992):

- **Sensors,** which receive information about the general state of the respiratory system.
- **Central controller,** which integrates and coordinates this information and which alters respiratory behaviour in response to this.
- **Effectors,** which are the respiratory muscles, producing changes in ventilation.

The sensors in this system are **chemoreceptors** which monitor changes in blood gas composition. There are two main types of chemoreceptor — **central** and **peripheral.**

Central chemoreceptors are located on the ventral surface of the medulla in the brainstem. These chemoreceptors respond indirectly to changes in the PCO_2 of the plasma by detecting changes in the pH of the cerebrospinal fluid (remember that increasing the PCO_2 will also increase the concentration of hydrogen ions). Increased plasma PCO_2 will result in diffusion of carbon dioxide from the plasma to the cerebrospinal fluid across the blood–brain barrier, thereby affecting the hydrogen ion concentration. The cerebrospinal fluid contains much less protein than the plasma, and so has a smaller buffering capacity than plasma for hydrogen ions.

Peripheral chemoreceptors are located at the bifurcation of the common carotid arteries in the **carotid bodies,** and also at the aortic arch in the **aortic bodies.** The peripheral chemoreceptors respond to changes in PCO_2, PO_2 and pH of the plasma. These chemoreceptors have an input to the central controller and can alter the rate and depth of breathing.

Other receptors which have an input to the central controller are lung **stretch receptors** which are stimulated by inflation of the lung, **irritant receptors** and **juxtacapillary** (or **J**) **receptors.** These are mechanoreceptors located in the alveolar walls close to the alveolar capillaries which are only weakly stimulated by lung inflation but are more sensitive to stimuli such as pulmonary oedema, pulmonary congestion and pulmonary embolism. These all produce an increase in the alveolar interstitial fluid and this suggests that the J receptors may be sensitive to the interstitial fluid composition.

The central controller is comprised of groups of cells located in the pons and medulla of the brainstem, referred to as the **respiratory centres.** These make up the medullary respiratory centre which has cells responsible for the control of inspiration and expiration. These two groups of cells interact with each other so that, for example, inspiration is switched off when expiration is occurring and vice versa. This interaction produces the background rhythmicity of the breathing pattern at rest. Normally the cells which promote expiration are not active (expiration being mostly passive recoil of the lung tissue and thorax); however, they increase their activity during demand for increased ventilation, allowing forced expiration to occur. Cells in the medullary respiratory centre have an inherent rhythmicity — they are spontaneously active and excite themselves in a cyclical fashion. This rhythmicity is subject to control from other brain areas allowing voluntary alterations to the breathing pattern.

Another component of the respiratory centres is the **pneumotaxic centre,** located in the upper pons. This area influences the inspiratory neurones of the medulla by inhibiting them when lung inflation reaches a certain level. This, therefore, limits the length of inspiration and stimulates the switchover from inspiration to expiration. In this way the pneumotaxic centre regulates the respiratory frequency.

A further element of the respiratory centres is the **apneustic centre** which is located in the lower pons. This coordinates the switchover between inspiration and expiration, but is usually dominated by activity in the pneumotaxic centre.

The respiratory centres are subject to reflex effects arising from the sensors. Increases in plasma PCO_2, or decreases in plasma PO_2 and pH are detected by the chemoreceptors which influence the respiratory centres to produce an increase in the rate and depth of breathing. This therefore improves the delivery of oxygen to the blood and the removal of carbon dioxide from the blood. Similarly, sensory input from stretch receptors in the lung tissue inhibits activity of the inspiratory neurones of the respiratory centres. This reflex inhibition of inspiration by lung stretch is known as the **Hering–Breuer reflex.** The inhibitory effect of this reflex is thought to be relatively weak, with a role in protecting against overstretching of the lungs rather than in controlling respiration.

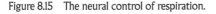

Figure 8.15   The neural control of respiration.

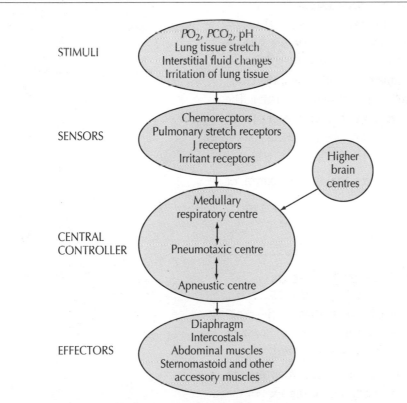

Considering all of the above factors which can influence the control of respiratory function, it is the response to arterial PCO_2 which exerts the most powerful effects. For every 1 mmHg increase in arterial PCO_2 there is an increase in alveolar ventilation of about 2 litres per minute. This ventilatory response to increased PCO_2 is exaggerated if PO_2 is also reduced below normal levels. This increase in alveolar ventilation is not limitless, however. A maximum level of about 100 litres per minute is achieved at a PCO_2 of about 115 mmHg.

Reduced PO_2 on its own can also exert an influence on ventilation. With a constant PCO_2 at normal levels, if PO_2 is lowered there is no real increase in ventilation until the PO_2 is reduced to about 50 mmHg. If PCO_2 is also increased above normal, the response to lowered PO_2 is increased. This **hypoxic drive** to ventilation does not normally play an important part in the control of ventilation, since PO_2 never usually falls this low. However, at high altitudes both PO_2 and PCO_2 are reduced due to lower atmospheric pressure. In this situation, PCO_2 cannot increase sufficiently to stimulate adequate ventilation and, therefore, the low PO_2 is relied upon to drive ventilation. The hypoxic drive is also important in cases of chronic carbon dioxide retention (see the discussion on oxygen therapy on p. 178–179).

Figure 8.15 summarizes the neural control of respiration.

Ventilation:Perfusion Ratios

The amount of blood flowing through the capillaries in the lungs — **perfusion** — is not constant from one region of the lung to the next.

The effects of gravity mean that in an upright subject there is less perfusion to the apex of the

lungs than at the base. This is also due to the balance of hydrostatic pressures inside the capillaries and the atmospheric pressures in the alveoli. Since the alveoli are separated from the capillaries by only a thin layer of tissue, the balance of the forces across this layer — the transmural pressure — is important in determining whether the capillaries are open or closed. At the top of the lung,

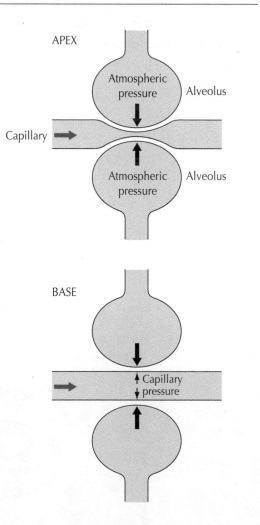

Figure 8.16   Balance of alveolar atmospheric pressure and capillary hydrostatic pressure at the apex and base of the lungs. Atmospheric pressure is greater than capillary hydrostatic pressure at the apex, leading to capillary collapse. At the base, capillary hydrostatic pressure is sufficient to keep the capillaries open against atmospheric pressure.

APEX

Atmospheric pressure

Alveolus

Capillary

Atmospheric pressure

Alveolus

BASE

Capillary pressure

the capillary pressure is relatively low, and therefore the atmospheric pressure inside the alveoli can compress the capillaries, thereby reducing the blood flow. At the base of the lung the capillary pressure is greater than the atmospheric pressure in the alveoli, and so the capillaries can remain open and continuous flow of blood is possible (Figure 8.16).

Similarly, the amount of ventilation to the alveoli is greater at the base of the lungs than at the apex. Again, this is due to gravity, where the weight of the lungs tends to pull on the alveoli of the apex, distending them and making it difficult for them to be inflated further. At the base of the lungs, the alveoli are more compressed, and so are more capable of further inflation.

There is, therefore, a regional distribution of ventilation and perfusion throughout the lungs and the ratio of ventilation (V) to perfusion (Q) (the $V{:}Q$ ratio) will also vary from the apex to the base of the lungs (Figure 8.17). This variation in $V{:}Q$ ratios is very important in determining the

final blood gas composition. To look at how $V{:}Q$ ratios affect the oxygen and carbon dioxide content of arterial blood, it is firstly useful to consider a perfect ventilation–perfusion match ($V{:}Q = 1$), together with two extremes of ventilation perfusion ratios, $V{:}Q = 0$ and $V{:}Q = \infty$ (Figure 8.18)

- $V{:}Q = 1$. Figure 8.18(a) shows a lung unit (alveolus + capillary) where the ventilation is exactly matched by perfusion. The partial pressures of oxygen and carbon dioxide are shown for inspired air, alveolar air, venous blood and arterial blood.
- $V{:}Q = 0$. A reduction in the $V{:}Q$ ratio would occur in any situation where ventilation is reduced or impaired. If this is taken to the extreme of complete airway blockage (no ventilation), then the ratio will be zero. In this case, it is clear that the PO_2 of the alveolus will fall, while the PCO_2 will rise until it is in equilibrium with venous blood. After this, no gas exchange will occur and the blood leaving this lung unit to join the rest of the arterial blood will have an elevated PCO_2 and reduced PO_2 (Figure 8.18b).
- $V{:}Q = \infty$. If the flow of blood to the lung unit is gradually reduced, the $V{:}Q$ ratio will rise. If this is taken to the extreme of complete occlusion of the capillary, the ratio will be infinite. In this case, no gas exchange will occur with the pulmonary venous blood and there will be a decreased contribution of oxygenated blood to the final arterial blood (Figure 8.18c).

These $V{:}Q$ ratios represent extreme situations. In the normal, upright lung, however, the value of the ratio in different lung regions varies as shown in Figure 8.17. Since there is a variety of such ratios throughout the lung, they will contribute differently to the overall arterial blood oxygen and carbon dioxide content.

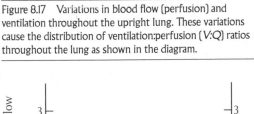

Figure 8.17 Variations in blood flow (perfusion) and ventilation throughout the upright lung. These variations cause the distribution of ventilation:perfusion ($V{:}Q$) ratios throughout the lung as shown in the diagram.

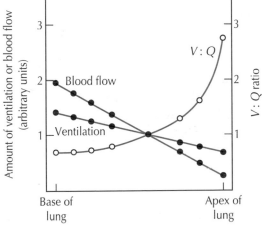

Figure 8.18 Ventilation:perfusion ratios in different situations, and their effects on alveolar and blood gas compositions (see text for details). (Adapted from West, 1995)

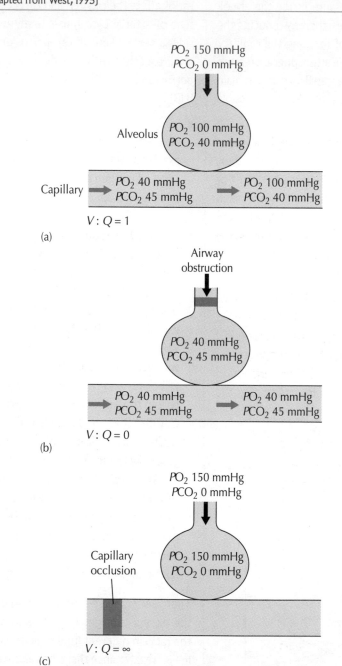

Figure 8.19   Effect of *V:Q* variations on alveolar PO_2 and PCO_2. As the *V:Q* ratio increases, alveolar PO_2 also increases, and PCO_2 decreases. As the *V:Q* ratio decreases, alveolar PO_2 decreases and PCO_2 increases. The numbers on the O_2–CO_2 curve relate to the numbered segments of the upright lung shown at the top of the figure, showing how *V:Q* ratios throughout the upright lung affect alveolar gas composition. [Adapted from West, 1995]

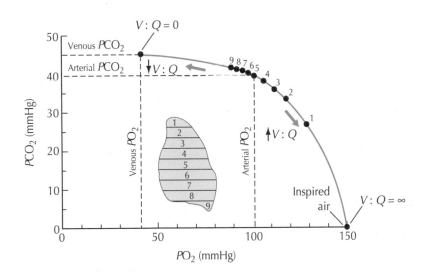

Figure 8.19 shows the variation in alveolar PO_2 and PCO_2 in lung units with different *V:Q* ratios. This graph represents *all* of the possible alveolar gas compositions which are obtained with different amounts of ventilation and perfusion throughout the lung. Figure 8.19 also shows how these ratios are distributed in different areas of the upright lung.

With the subject in a supine position, the regional variation in *V:Q* ratios is more or less abolished. Apical blood flow increases from that seen in the upright posture, while basal blood flow is not much altered. Perfusion therefore becomes almost uniform from the apex to the base, although there will now be a slightly higher blood flow in the posterior portions of the lungs.

With the subject lying on her or his side, the diaphragm on the lower side is pushed slightly higher into the thoracic cavity, thereby giving it a greater capacity to move further during inspiration. This allows for greater volume changes dur-

ing inspiration and, consequently, the lower lung is relatively better ventilated in this position [Figure 8.20].

In subjects with pulmonary disease, positioning may be important in redistributing *V:Q* ratios throughout the lung in order to optimize plasma PO_2 and PCO_2.

Figure 8.20   Increased capacity for expansion of the lower lung by lying on the side. The lung on the lower side is pushed higher into the thoracic cavity by the diaphragm, allowing it a greater relative volume change during inflation [arrows] than the upper lung.

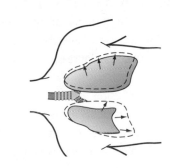

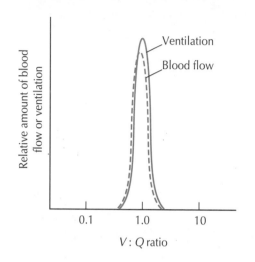

Figure 8.21 Distribution of ventilation and blood flow to lung units with different $V:Q$ ratios in the normal lung. Most blood flow and ventilation goes to lung units with $V:Q$ ratios of about 1. (Adapted from West, 1992)

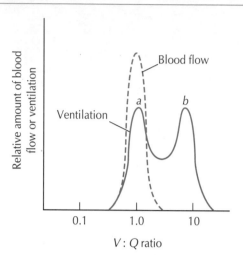

Figure 8.22 Distribution of ventilation and blood flow to lung units with different $V:Q$ ratios in a subject with emphysematous disease (see text for details). (Adapted from West, 1992)

Effects of Obstructive Disease on $V:Q$ Ratios

The distribution of ventilation and blood flow to lung units with different $V:Q$ ratios in the normal lung is shown in Figure 8.21. This demonstrates that most blood flow goes to lung units which are well ventilated ($V:Q$ ratios around 1.0), and that most ventilation goes to lung units which have a good blood supply ($V:Q$ ratios around 1.0).

In *type A (emphysematous) chronic obstructive airway disease*, there is a general enlargement of the airways after the terminal bronchioles, with wall destruction and loss of alveolar capillaries. In essence, this results in an increase in the anatomical deadspace. In such cases, the distribution of ventilation and perfusion to lung units with different $V:Q$ ratios is radically altered (Figure 8.22). Although there is a general reduction in the blood flow to the alveoli, the blood which *does* get

through generally goes to lung units which are well ventilated (Figure 8.22, dashed line, $V:Q$ ratios are about 1.0). The distribution of ventilation (solid line), however, shows that some ventilation goes to lung units which have an adequate blood flow (at point *a* $V:Q$ ratios are about 1.0) whereas large amounts of ventilation also goes to lung units which have poor or no blood supply (at point *b* $V:Q$ ratios are about 10.0). These high $V:Q$ ratios are effectively alveolar deadspace. Patients with this type of disease would show a mild degree of hypoxaemia (low blood PO_2), with a PO_2 approximately 60–70 mmHg. This is because there is not much blood flow to lung units with low $V:Q$ ratios (i.e. areas of low ventilation).

In *type B (bronchitic) chronic obstructive airway disease*, airway narrowing (or sometimes complete blockage in the smaller bronchi) occurs due to excess mucus production, and again can substantially alter the pattern of ventilation and blood flow to lung units with different $V:Q$ ratios (Figure 8.23). Here, the distribution of ventilation

Figure 8.23 Distribution of ventilation and blood flow to lung units with different $V:Q$ ratios in a subject with bronchitic disease (see text for details). (Adapted from West, 1992)

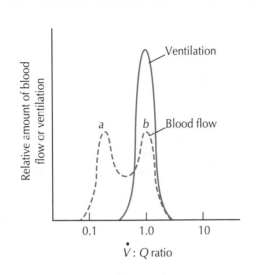

and perfusion to lung units with different $V:Q$ ratios shows that, although alveolar ventilation is poor, the alveoli which *are* ventilated generally have a good blood supply (Figure 8.23, solid line, $V:Q$ ratios are about 1.0). Of blood supply to the lungs in this condition (dashed line), some blood flow supplies regions which are adequately ventilated (at point *a* $V:Q$ ratios are about 1.0), whilst a large proportion of the blood flow goes to regions which are poorly ventilated due to the bronchitic changes (at point *b* $V:Q$ ratios are about 0.1). This blood flow to low $V:Q$ lung units can produce a severe hypoxaemia, with an arterial PO_2 in the region of 40–50 mmHg.

The effects of airway obstruction can be reduced to a certain extent by **collateral ventilation**. The existence of small communicating channels between adjacent alveoli and small airways means that air flow can sometimes be directed into better-ventilated areas. This redirection of ventilation may be induced by a decrease in PCO_2 in the affected alveoli. **Hypoxic vasoconstriction** (constriction of blood vessels due to low PO_2) also allows blood flow to be diverted from areas of poor ventilation to better-ventilated regions of the lung. Both of these compensatory mechanisms produce 'silent' lung units which make no contribution to the distribution of $V:Q$ ratios throughout the lung, since they are effectively unused (no ventilation and no perfusion). In doing so, these mechanisms may help to reduce the effects of ventilation–perfusion mismatching in disease.

Effects of Restrictive Disease on Lung Function

We have already looked at the effects of obstructive lung disease on the ventilation–perfusion relationships in the lungs. We should also consider the effects of restrictive disease such as *pulmonary fibrosis* where there are changes in the supporting structures of the lung tissue, with a general thickening of the interstitium of the alveolar walls. This occurs as a result of deposition of collagen fibres in the interstitial space, restricting the amount of inflation which can occur, thereby reducing the total lung capacity, functional residual capacity and the residual volume. Elastic recoil is increased and hence compliance is reduced. The consequence of this is that unusually high pressures are required in order to inflate the lungs. In addition, the fibrotic changes increase the amount of radial traction acting on the airways, increasing their diameter. This reduces the resistance to flow through these airways, accounting for the increased FEV_1 often seen in lung function tests on these subjects (see Figure 8.9).

As a result of these changes, inequalities in ventilation and perfusion can arise, causing hypoxaemia. This is more noticeable on exercise, and the degree of hypoxaemia cannot be accounted for by altered $\dot{V}:\dot{Q}$ ratios alone. The greater level of hypoxaemia on exercise is accounted for by the fact that fibrosis of the lung tissue increases the diffusion distances for transfer of oxygen between the alveoli and the capillaries. The increased blood flow through the lungs on exercise means that there is a reduction in the time available for diffusion to take place. This is exacerbated by the increased diffusion distance due to the fibrosis.

Subjects with fibrotic lung disease often breathe in a rapid, shallow pattern. This may be a reflex breathing pattern brought about by the activation of J receptors which are stimulated by the increased traction on the airway walls.

Another restrictive disease, which does not affect the lung tissue directly, is *ankylosing spondylitis*. In this condition, reduced mobility of the vertebral joints and the ribs greatly restricts the movements of the chest wall, resulting in a reduced vital capacity and total lung capacity.

Oxygen Therapy and Mechanical Ventilation

In many cases, the effects of pulmonary disease necessitate the use of artificial means to improve the oxygen supply to the blood and relieve possible hypoxaemia. This is used either to improve short-term function, or may be used longer term in cases where voluntary ventilatory drive is diminished or absent.

OXYGEN THERAPY

This therapy relies on alterations in the composition of inspired gas to change alveolar gas concentrations. Increasing the alveolar PO_2 increases the concentration gradient for diffusion of oxy-

gen from the alveoli to the capillary blood. This is useful in situations where the diffusion distance has been increased, e.g. in pulmonary fibrosis. In cases where ventilation is impaired (e.g. by obstructive disease), increasing inspired PO_2 will help to increase alveolar PO_2. The effects of altering inspired PO_2 can be calculated using the alveolar gas equation (Equation 1) where the respiratory quotient has a value at rest of 0.8. Using 100% oxygen as the inspired gas, and assuming an atmospheric pressure of 760 mmHg and an alveolar PCO_2 of 40 mmHg, therefore gives an alveolar PO_2 of

$$760 \text{ mmHg} - \frac{40 \text{ mmHg}}{0.8} = 710 \text{ mmHg}.$$

100% oxygen is rarely used for any great length of time. It is useful in providing a rapid and massive rise in alveolar PO_2 in acute situations. However, 100% PO_2 used for extended periods is toxic, causing damage to both the alveolar / capillary membrane and the central nervous system. This damage can appear in as little as 24 hours exposure to 100% oxygen. The use of 100% oxygen is therefore recommended only for relatively short durations, and the balance of relief from hypoxaemia and the possible resultant pulmonary damage has to be considered. The cause of oxygen toxicity is thought to involve oxygen free radicals (a highly reactive ionic form of oxygen).

It is not always essential, however, to use oxygen contents as high as 100%. Even small increases in inspired oxygen can substantially improve the oxygen diffusion gradient. For example, the normal diffusion gradient from alveoli to capillaries is 60 mmHg (100 mmHg alveolar − 40 mmHg capillary). If the inspired oxygen is increased from the normal 20% to 30%, the alveolar PO_2 will increase to 178 mmHg (from the alveolar gas equation). The diffusion gradient for oxygen is now 138 mmHg (178 − 40 mmHg), more than double the normal diffusion gradient. This can produce a substantial improvement in arterial PO_2 in cases of hypoxaemia.

In practice, use of inspired PO_2 values of <60% are regarded as being relatively free from the effects of toxicity.

Care has to be taken in administering oxygen therapy in cases where ventilation has been depressed for a considerable period of time. In these cases, there may be a considerable retention of carbon dioxide in the blood − **hypercapnia**. With elevated plasma PCO_2, bicarbonate ions may be transported across the blood–brain barrier to enter the cerebrospinal fluid (CSF). This increase in CSF bicarbonate concentration increases the buffering of hydrogen ions in the CSF and will therefore reduce the stimulus to ventilation acting on the central chemoreceptors. In such circumstances, the subject can therefore no longer rely on a high plasma PCO_2 as the stimulus to breathe and instead must rely on a low PO_2 − the hypoxic drive − in order to maintain a reasonable level of ventilation. If oxygen therapy is administered to such a patient in an attempt to improve plasma PO_2, then this hypoxic drive will be removed and the patient's ventilation will be depressed even further.

This, therefore, appears to be a catch-22 situation, where the attempted treatment for low arterial PO_2 will exacerbate the problem by further reducing the level of ventilation. In such cases, an alternative approach must be taken − if the patient cannot breathe automatically, then breathing must be assisted.

MECHANICAL VENTILATION

Mechanical ventilation is used to provide adequate ventilation in patients where normal respiration is depressed or absent. There are several different types of mechanical ventilation which can be used in different clinical circumstances. One common method of mechanical ventilation is **intermittent positive pressure ventilation (IPPV)**. As the name suggests, positive pressure (greater than atmospheric pressure) is applied to the airways for a period of time to inflate the lungs, before being switched off to allow the lungs to deflate passively by elastic recoil. Positive pressure is then re-applied and removed to maintain and control a constant respiratory frequency. The positive pressure which is applied must be of a sufficient level to overcome airway resistance to flow as well as the elastic recoil forces of the lungs and chest wall.

IPPV can be used to manipulate many ventilatory parameters such as tidal volume, inspiratory flow rate, inspiratory duration, respiratory frequency and minute ventilation. In doing so, these parameters can be adjusted for individual patients in order to provide the optimum respiratory pattern for their condition. For example, prolonging inspiratory duration may allow normally unventilated alveoli to become ventilated, possibly improving $V:Q$ ratios in that area of the lung.

Some IPPV machines monitor the patient's own respiratory attempts and allow these to occur when they happen. This allows some degree of voluntary ventilation to be superimposed on the mechanical ventilation.

Normal ventilation arises from negative pressure created within the thorax, drawing air into the lungs. In contrast, during IPPV, air is forced into the lungs under positive pressure. Positive pressure ventilation reverses the ventilation distribution in the lungs, with most ventilation going to the non-dependent areas where the alveoli are open, thus providing the route of least resistance to incoming air. A reduction of ventilation to dependent parts of the lungs leaves these areas at risk of atelectasis (alveolar collapse).

The raised alveolar pressure may, in nondependent areas, cause compression and collapse of the pulmonary blood vessels, diverting blood away from the ventilated areas and increasing the perfusion gradient from the bottom to the top of the lung as more blood flows to the dependent areas.

The reversal of the normal ventilation distribution and an increase in the normal perfusion gradient lead to a ventilation–perfusion mismatch. Supplementary oxygen is therefore required in patients on IPPV to counteract the resultant hypoxaemia.

Other adverse effects of IPPV include an increase in deadspace as the positive pressure increases the radial traction in the airways, enlarging their diameter. The positive pressure which develops in the thoracic cavity causes a reduction in venous return, with a consequent reduction in cardiac output.

Positive end expiratory pressure (PEEP) is the application of a small positive pressure to the airways at the end of expiration. In this case, the patient breathes unassisted, but deflation of the lungs is prevented from going beyond the functional residual capacity by the application of positive pressure. This technique is useful in situations where elastic recoil of the lung is increased, e.g. in respiratory distress syndrome. This prevents collapse of the lungs and airway closure at low lung volumes.

Manual hyperinflation (or bagging) is a form of positive pressure ventilation which may be used by the clinician to re-inflate areas of atelectasis or to assist the clearance of secretions.

The patient's breathing circuit is attached to a 2-litre rebreathing bag. The clinician squeezes the bag, delivering a slow inspiration and inflating the patient's lungs. A short inspiratory pause may be held at maximum inspiration, and the bag is then released quickly, encouraging a high expiratory flow rate to mobilize secretions. A PEEP valve may be added to the rebreathing bag if required.

As with other forms of positive pressure ventilation, incoming gas will preferentially ventilate non-dependent areas. Thus, patients with atelectasis should be positioned in side lying with affected lung uppermost.

Exercise – Acute Responses

The respiratory responses to exercise are aimed at improving the delivery of oxygen to tissues which have increased their metabolism and removing the increased output of carbon dioxide from these same tissues to the outside atmosphere.

During exercise, tidal volume and respiratory frequency increase to produce an increase in overall ventilation. From a resting level of about 5 litres per minute, minute ventilation can increase

---

Figure 8.24   General ventilatory responses to exercise. Actual values for increases in minute ventilation are dependent on the severity of the exercise.

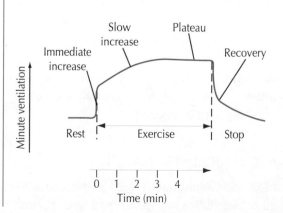

during heavy exercise to over 100 litres per minute. This is brought about initially by an increase in tidal volume, with increasing frequency becoming more predominant with progressive exercise. This increase in ventilation is matched by an increase in oxygen consumption from a resting level of about 200–250 ml O_2 per minute to $\geqslant$ 5 litres O_2 per minute in highly trained athletes.

At the start of exercise, ventilation increases immediately or just before exercise begins. This is followed by a slower increase in ventilation to reach a steady level which is maintained for the duration of the exercise period (Figure 8.24).

There are several mechanisms which may be responsible for producing these ventilatory responses to exercise. Arterial gas composition remains relatively constant during exercise, and in some cases PCO_2 may actually be reduced below normal levels. This suggests that changes in PO_2 and PCO_2 alone cannot be responsible for inducing the ventilatory changes in exercise.

Furthermore, since ventilation increases immediately at the start of (or even before) exercise, changes in arterial gas composition cannot be responsible. It is suggested that nervous stimuli from limb proprioceptors and/or from higher brain centres are responsible for generating this initial ventilatory response.

Other factors which have been postulated as contributing to the increased ventilatory drive during exercise include increased body temperature and decreased plasma pH.

Aging

Age-related changes in the respiratory system affect both the lung tissue itself and also the thorax, respiratory muscles, blood vessels and other tissues. All can have important consequences for altered respiratory function.

It is important to distinguish between true changes associated with age and those that are associated with other diseases which may be present in aged subjects. Age-related factors which affect the lung tissue include enlargement of the alveolar ducts, together with a separation of the alveolar epithelium from the capillary endothelium. There is therefore no longer close contact between these membranes resulting in an effective increase in deadspace.

A loss of some of the capillary blood supply to the alveoli again increases the amount of deadspace, and will affect $V:Q$ ratios.

Some capillaries also exhibit an increase in the amount of fibrous material in the capillary wall. This increases the distance for diffusion of gases and therefore reduces the effectiveness of gas exchange.

A decrease in the number and thickness of elastic fibres in the connective tissue in the lung reduces the elastic recoil of the lungs. This results in a reduction in passive deflation of the lung during breathing, although the work of breathing may also be reduced as less effort is required to inflate the lungs.

Airway resistance may be increased in some cases due to decreased distensibility of the smaller airway walls. This will affect the distribution of ventilation to different regions of the lung.

In the thorax, there may be an increase in the amount of calcification of the cartilage of the bronchial airways and of the ribs. This increases the resistance of the chest wall to expansion and increases the work of breathing.

Joint disease can afflict the costovertebral joints,

Table 8.1

Changes in Lung Function Parameters with Age: Comparison of Representative Values for 20- and 60-year-old Men and Women, Standardized for Height and Weight

Parameter	Age, men		Age, women	
	20 years	60 years	20 years	60 years
Total lung capacity (litres)	7.2	6.9	5.1	4.7
Vital capacity (litres)	5.2	4.0	4.17	3.29
Functional residual capacity (litres)	2.2	3.5	2.4	2.5
FEV_1	81%	71%	80%	70%
	(4.45 l)	(3.17 l)	(3.26 l)	(2.26 l)
Maximum voluntary ventilation (litres min^{-1})	150	99	110	77

Adapted from Reddan, WG (1980). Respiratory system and aging. In: *Exercise and Aging — The Scientific Basis*. Edited by Smith, EL and Serfass, RC. Enslow Publishers.

as well as other joints in the body, which leads to an increased stiffness of these joints. This results in an increased use of the diaphragm in ventilation.

Wasting of the respiratory muscles reduces the capacity of these muscles to do work, thereby reducing the maximum amount of voluntary ventilation that can be achieved. This becomes especially important if any degree of exercise is undertaken.

Table 8.1 shows a comparison of respiratory parameters in 20- and 60-year-old individuals, demonstrating the changes in respiratory function which can accompany aging.

Role of Respiratory System in Regulation of Blood pH

The normal pH of plasma is around 7.4, and the pH is very carefully regulated within very tight limits around this value. This is an important homeostatic mechanism in the body, requiring the integrated functions of both the respiratory and renal systems. If the plasma pH deviates from this normal to any great degree there are effects on the functioning of many enzyme and metabolic systems throughout the body.

Before commencing an explanation of how the respiratory and renal systems are involved in plasma pH regulation it is useful to study some of the factors that determine pH in the blood.

Plasma pH can be calculated by knowing the plasma PCO_2 and the plasma concentration of hydrogencarbonate ions (HCO_3^-). The reaction of carbon dioxide with water in the blood can be summarized as:

$$CO_2 + H_2O \rightleftharpoons H_2CO_3 \rightleftharpoons H^+ + HCO_3^-$$
$$\text{Carbonic acid}$$

From this equation, the relationship between carbon dioxide, hydrogencarbonate ions and pH (hydrogen ions) can be seen. In fact, pH can be calculated using the following equation:

$$pH = 6.1 + \log \frac{[HCO_3^-]}{(PCO_2 \times 0.03)}$$

This is the **Henderson-Hasselbalch equation,** which allows pH to be calculated knowing plasma hydrogencarbonate concentrations, and plasma PCO_2. (The derivation of this equation can be found in West, 1995.)

The normal values for the parameters in the equation are:

plasma $[HCO_3^-] =$ 24 mM and arterial $PCO_2 = 40$ mmHg.

Therefore, substituting these values into the equation we can calculate normal plasma pH:

$$pH = 6.1 + \log \frac{24}{40 \times 0.03}$$

$$= 6.1 + \log \frac{24}{1.2}$$

$$= 6.1 + \log 20$$

$$= 6.1 + 1.3$$

$$= \underline{7.4}$$

A simpler way of looking at the Henderson–Hasselbalch equation is to state that plasma pH is proportional to the ratio of plasma hydrogencarbonate divided by plasma $PCO_2 \times 0.03$. To maintain a normal plasma pH, this ratio must equal 20 (as shown above). As a consequence of this, if either of these two factors are altered by changes in normal function, then the pH will also be altered.

An example of this is when a patient is experiencing some degree of respiratory distress (due to some pathological condition perhaps) and, as a result, plasma PCO_2 goes above the normal level of 40 mmHg. This reduces the hydrogencarbonate:carbon dioxide ratio, thereby reducing plasma pH below the normal level of 7.4. This is a condition known as **respiratory acidosis,** since the blood has now become more acidic than normal and the change is respiratory in origin. If this situation persists, the body must attempt to return plasma pH towards normal by restoring the bicarbonate:carbon dioxide ratio to 20. This is achieved by the cells of the **kidneys** increasing the reabsorption of hydrogencarbonate ions back into the blood, also increasing the reabsorption of hydrogencarbonate ions back into the blood

and also increasing the secretion of hydrogen ions into the kidney tubule fluid to be excreted in the urine.

The resulting increase in the plasma concentration of hydrogencarbonate ions will take the ratio of hydrogencarbonate:carbon dioxide towards 20, and thus restoring plasma pH towards 7.4.

Although plasma pH can now be said to be near normal, the same cannot be said of the patient's acid–base status. This still remains abnormal since both plasma carbon dioxide and hydrogencarbonate are elevated. In this condition the patient's acid–base status would be described as **compensated respiratory acidosis.** Since the compensatory mechanisms involved the kidneys, this mechanism is referred to as **renal compensation.**

An alternative scenario that would cause acidosis is a reduction in plasma hydrogencarbonate levels. In a metabolic disorder such as diabetes mellitus, the subject has a lack of the hormone **insulin** (type I diabetes) or a lack of insulin receptors on the cell membranes (type II diabetes). If the condition is not remedied, for example by injecting insulin for type I diabetes, the subject does not have access to glucose as a fuel molecule for cellular metabolism. In order to obtain energy, the cells must therefore switch to fat metabolism. A byproduct of fat metabolism is the build up of keto-acids such as aceto-acetic acid and hydroxybutyric acid in the blood. Essentially, hydrogen ions are being added to the plasma as a result of fatty acid metabolism. These extra hydrogen ions are buffered by plasma proteins, haemoglobin and also by plasma hydrogencarbonate. Therefore the concentration of free plasma hydrogencarbonate decreases below the normal level of 24 mM. As a result, the ratio of plasma hydrogencarbonate:carbon dioxide is again decreased, leading to a reduced plasma pH. This condition is known as **metabolic acidosis.**

In order to compensate for this condition, the ratio of plasma hydrogencarbonate:carbon dioxide must be restored. One way of doing this is to reduce the level of plasma carbon dioxide, this is achieved by hyperventilation. By blowing off more carbon dioxide from the lungs, plasma carbon dioxide will be lowered, and so will restore the hydrogencarbonate:carbon dioxide ratio to 20, taking plasma pH towards the normal value of 7.4. As before, while pH might be near to normal, the patient's acid–base status is still abnormal, this time with reduced plasma hydrogencarbonate and carbon dioxide. The patient's acid–base status in this condition is therefore described as **compensated metabolic acidosis**. Since the compensation is achieved through hyperventilation, it is said to be **respiratory compensation**.

Changes in blood pH *above* the normal level of 7.4 can also occur. In **respiratory alkalosis**, there is a reduction in plasma PCO_2 caused, for example, by voluntary hyperventilation or high altitude. The compensation for this condition is renal, by increasing hydrogencarbonate ion excretion. Similarly, excess alkali ingestion or loss of acid from the body (i.e. by vomiting) leads to an effective increase in plasma hydrogencarbonate concentration – **metabolic alkalosis**. The compensation for this condition is respiratory, reducing ventilation so that plasma PCO_2 levels increase.

Acid–base balance is an extremely complex subject which has only briefly been dealt with here. However, the principles involved allow the integrated roles of the respiratory and renal systems in homeostasis to be seen. It is important, especially when dealing with patients with respiratory problems, that physiotherapists bear in mind the possible consequences of treatments such as oxygen therapy and mechanical ventilation on the acid–base status of a patient.

Bibliography

Bouhuys, A (1977) *The Physiology of Breathing – A Textbook for Medical Students.* New York, Grune and Stratton.

Harper, RW (1981) *A Guide to Respiratory Care – Physiology and Clinical Applications.* JB Lippincott, Philadelphia.

Levitzky, MG (1986) *Pulmonary Physiology.* McGraw-Hill, New York.

Nunn, JF (1987) *Applied Respiratory Physiology.* Butterworth, London.

Shapiro, BA, Harrison, RA, Trout, CA (1991) *Clinical application of respiratory care.* Year Book, Chicago.

Wanger, J (1992) *Pulmonary Function Testing – A Practical Approach.* Williams and Wilkins, Baltimore.

West, JB (1990) *Ventilation/Blood Flow and Gas Exchange.* Blackwell Scientific Publications, Oxford.

West, JB (1992) *Pulmonary Pathophysiology – The Essentials.* Williams and Wilkins, Baltimore.

West, JB (1995) *Respiratory Physiology – The Essentials.* Williams and Wilkins, Baltimore.

Widdicombe, J, Davies, A (1991) *Respiratory Physiology.* Edward Arnold, London.

9

Exercise

Exercise and a Healthy Lifestyle

Since the turn of this century there has been a transformation of a society who were predominantly physically active into one which is predominantly sedentary. In industrialized countries and particularly within the cities, statistics would indicate that 90–95% of total activity is very light. Three times per week for twenty minutes is known to be the minimal level of activity in order to promote physiological change. However, in a survey conducted in the UK (Sports Council, 1992) only 14% of men and 4% of women achieved this target. These data are against a backdrop where the health benefits to be gained from a physically active health style are real and well documented.

It is possible to look at the benefits of exercise by looking at the possible outcomes of inactivity. Physical inactivity, either as a result of illness or because of a prolonged period of a sedentary lifestyle, leads to a progressive decline in the ability to perform relatively simple tasks. This can occur to the point where individuals find that walking at a 'normal' pace may place them in a stressful state and that they will be required to utilize the anaerobic energy systems which are limited and cause early fatigue. This population is therefore working at near maximum levels for routine activities.

Fortunately, it would appear that, at any age,

physiological and biochemical changes of inactivity can be reversed, by an exercise programme. The programme need not be extensive and changes can occur within 8–10 weeks.

Training for a healthy lifestyle is predominantly concerned with training which enhances the aerobic capacity of the individual and with training which offsets the muscle fibre atrophy noted with age in Chapter 6.

Exercise Prescription for a Healthy Lifestyle

A comprehensive exercise programme should focus on more than one area of development, although the most fundamental of these is aerobic endurance exercise. Exercise prescription varies depending on the initial physiological status of the individual. In general, two sets of guidelines are available and are complementary. They represent a staged approach to increasing population activity and fitness levels.

The first set was devised by the American College of Sports Medicine, together with the Center for Disease Control (1993), and was aimed at the essentially inactive population in order to reduce mortality from coronary heart disease. This guideline suggests an accumulation of 30 minutes of moderate intensity physical activity on most days per week. The emphasis is on increasing habitual activity of moderate intensity, such as walking and stair climbing.

The second set is aimed at those who are already moderately active, or fit, but who wish to improve their fitness or performance. These guidelines follow those published by the American College of Sports Medicine (1990).

The activity, although aerobic, must be relatively vigorous and for a sufficient period of time otherwise no training effect will take place. In order to stimulate the cardiovascular system it is necessary to increase the heart rate during exercise to >70% of the theoretical maximum heart rate. For 20-year-old subjects, this corresponds to an exercising heart rate of about 130–140 beats per minute. The percentage will vary with age; the maximum heart rate decreases with age and therefore the 70% value also decreases. It is important also, however, that the heart rate should not exceed 90% of the maximum as this would take the individual almost certainly into an anaerobic activity. The effective training zones for each age group are depicted in Figure 9.1.

With respect to the frequency of participation, it would appear that 3–4 days per week represents an optimal frequency; in this case 'optimal' is used to indicate the greatest return relative to the amount of time invested. For people who are already in relatively good condition, two days a week may suffice; however one day of aerobic exercise per week does very little to increase one's aerobic capacity. It is generally agreed that

Figure 9.1 Training zone for exercising heart rate for people of various ages. (Available as a commercial package from Bodycare Products Ltd, Princes Drive Industrial Estate, Kenilworth, Warks, UK.)

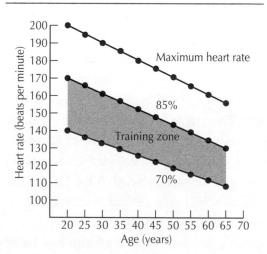

each of these sessions should last 20–40 minutes per day. It must be understood that the 20–40 minutes represents the time invested in cardio-respiratory endurance conditioning activities and does not include the initial warming-up phase or the final cool-down phase.

An appropriate warm-up and stretching period must be included to enable the muscles to stretch before the impending exercise and also to maintain proper flexibility of the major joints. The warm-up and stretching period can last for several minutes to 10 or 15 minutes depending on the needs of the individual. A warm-down period is also important to facilitate the removal of waste products from the muscle and to return heart rate and respiration to resting levels.

Relative to the duration of the total training programme the greatest improvement normally occurs during the first six months. Beyond the initial six months progress will be seen but the rate of progress will tend to diminish, although this is necessarily dependent on the initial fitness level, i.e. the lower the fitness level the greater the potential improvement.

Compliance in Exercise Programmes

Adult exercise programmes have reported considerable variability and drop-out rates of 9–87% are common, indicating substantial non-compliance among those individuals who voluntarily enter physical conditioning programmes. Numerous variables, such as inconvenience, excessive cost, lack of variety, exercising alone, lack of positive feedback, medical problems and lack of spouse support are related to, and predictive of, exercise drop-out. In addition, a deterrent to both short- and long-term adherence to an exercise programme is excessive duration (longer than one hour) and a high proportion of high-intensity exercise. Increasingly, evidence would suggest, however, that the exercise leader is the single most important variable affecting exercise compliance. Knowledgeable and trained exercise leaders therefore play a critical role in the development and implementation of adult fitness programmes.

Exercise programmes for adults should include an educational component and selected motivational strategies. These would include caloric expenditure, appropriate exercise intensity, frequency, duration, modes of training, concepts of perceived exertion, importance of warm-up and cool-down, exercise myths and misconceptions, suitable exercise clothing and shoes, and nutrition. Group meetings for participants and partner also allow for discussion of the topics. Motivation to exercise must be high therefore there should be an emphasis on variety and enjoyment. Personal goal-setting (established by the exerciser) provides the greatest potential for long-term exercise success. This can be arranged alongside periodic testing to assess the participant's response to the training programme.

Physical Fitness and Habitual Physical Activity in Children

The literature surrounding the effect of exercise on fitness levels of children is confusing, principally because it is difficult to differentiate those changes which are occurring with natural growth of the child from the effects of exercise. It is also not ethically acceptable to operate controlled trials where the physical activity of a child is limited in order to act as a control group. In spite of this, evidence suggests that the natural activity found in the young child decreases significantly by the early teens and is predominantly associated with a lack of regular vigorous exercise outside school hours. Provision for exercise in schools cannot compensate for this out of school inactivity. It is important, therefore, to ensure that a child adopts a lifestyle which incorporates physical activity.

The aerobic fitness of children and adolescents seems to respond to training in a manner similar to that of adults although there is some evidence to suggest that a maturational threshold exists below which prepubescent children do not respond. The evidence in the literature, however, is conflicting and probably depends on the initial level of fitness of the child and the corresponding intensity of exercise. The limited data available investigating the metabolic response of children to exercise would suggest that more of the energy needs of the child are met through the tricarboxylic acid (TCA) cycle after a training period. In general, the lactate levels of children and adolescents after the same relative workload will be lower than those of an adult.

The evidence documenting the effect of exercise on anaerobic capacity of the young is even more sparse. It is clear that prepubescent children are known to have a low anaerobic capacity and power but little or nothing is known about the trainability in this dimension.

Weight-bearing activities are necessary for normal growth and development. The most efficient and safe way of developing that strength is through exercise. Due to the possible damage which could occur to the growth zones of the skeleton (epiphyses), it is best to be cautious about maximal resistance training until the growth spurt is virtually over. However, there are advantages in submaximal loading in that the bone mineral content will increase with physical activity and will give the bone a greater mechanical strength. Prepubescent children are capable of increasing muscular strength in response to resistance training although they experience more difficulty in increasing muscle mass, probably due to the immature nervous system and the low levels of male sex hormones (androgens). Any exercise, however, designed to improve a child's strength, should incorporate a large percentage of the body's muscle mass and be varied to ensure that no particular joint is overloaded. This type of exercise not only enhances the strength of the bone but increases the muscle strength. If an endurance factor can be added to the strength training programme, it is possible simultaneously to develop local muscular endurance. The best types of exercise to increase muscle strength therefore are probably those which use the child's own body weight on a large muscle mass and involve many repetitions. Alongside the training programme, it is important to maintain flexibility to avoid any overuses or imbalances of muscle strength.

The case for ensuring that a child and young adult adopt habitual exercise patterns is strengthened through the evidence which is accumulating that the course of events leading to heart disease begins in childhood and adolescence, in spite of symptoms not appearing for many years. It is also known that former athletes have a reduced risk of heart disease but this is only true if a habitual pattern of exercise is continued into later life. Inactive children are likely to become inactive adults.

Physical Activity and the Elderly

With aging, there is a progressive decline in aerobic capacity and strength. The extent of the decline is, however, variable and very much depends on the activity of the individual. Many older people are having to apply maximum effort to achieve simple tasks. The National Fitness Survey (Sports Council, 1992) which was conducted on an English population indicated that 30% of men aged between 65 and 74 years had quadriceps strength below that required to stand up from a chair unaided. The equivalent percentage in women was 56%. Within the same population, 45% of men and 79% of women were not fit enough to sustain continuous normal-paced walking. These figures were in contrast to the self-assessment of fitness levels of men and women where the individuals believed themselves to be very fit.

There is clearly a loss in muscle strength with age, which is accelerated from the age of 60 years onwards. As a consequence of this loss of strength, subjects aged over 70 years show at least 20% lower strength values than those of young adults (average on all muscle groups). This differential between the young adult and the elderly person of 70 years can be reduced if activity is maintained. The ability to generate power is also an important index to measure as it determines how quickly strength can be generated and is important in activities such as going up stairs, or responding to a reaction. The decline in that extensive power of the quadriceps is about 3.5% per annum. The decline in power is greater than that noted in pure strength, i.e. the speed with which movement can be made also decreases. Connective tissue also undergoes structural change which makes it stiffer, thereby affecting joints, tendons, ligaments and muscles. This, together with a reduction in blood supply to the soft tissues, lengthens the time for recovery from minor sprains and strains.

Endurance activity too reduces greatly with age. A 10% decrease of endurance capacity per decade is normal over middle life. At the level of the muscle, this may be due to the reduced muscle mass or to a decreased ability to utilize oxygen because of a change in the cellular enzymes. Centrally, aging affects the structure and function of the heart, the major vessels and lungs. The general decline in aerobic capacity and the subsequent necessity for some older people to utilize anaerobic systems to achieve normal daily activities does not make it surprising that many elderly people will fall and stumble just as athletes finishing a maximal effort race will tend to fall over and stumble under parallel fatigue situations.

Maintaining the integrity of the central nervous system is essential to avoid falls and accidents. Diminution of proprioceptive function affects the coordination of body movements, particularly the correction of externally exposed forces. There is an increase in movement and reaction time and a slowing of the central processing of information. All of these aging processes contribute to a decrease in skill with the older person.

Regular exercise can offset all of these aging processes, aging itself and the deterioration of the physiological mechanisms will occur, but it is clear that these occur at a slower rate. Exercise prescription for older individuals requires development. Much of the prescriptive data available is based on evidence which refers to healthy younger people.

As the number of elderly people in the community increases and the morbidity rate decreases then it is essential that the quality of life and the independence of these older people is enhanced through exercise.

Exercise and Mental Health

It is clear that physical fitness and mental health are related in a positive manner. There is no evidence, however, which demonstrates that the relationship of physical fitness to mental health reflects more than a mere association, i.e. there is no consistent evidence to suggest that the relationship is causal. There are few longitudinal studies dealing with the psychological consequences of exercise interventions. It is not possible, therefore, to accept or refute the hypothesis that vigorous exercise leads to an alteration in mental health. This absence of general agreement motivated the National Institute of Mental Health (NIMH, 1987) to release a consensus statement which identified the following:

- Physical fitness is positively associated with mental health and wellbeing.
- Exercise is associated with the reduction of stress emotions such as states of anxiety.
- Anxiety and depression are common symptoms of failure to cope with mental stress and exercise has been associated with a decreased level of mild-to-moderate depression and anxiety.
- Long-term exercise is usually associated with reduction in traits such as neuroticism and anxiety.
- Severe depression usually requires professional treatment which may include medication, electroconvulsive therapy, and/or psychotherapy, with exercise as an adjunct.
- Appropriate exercise results in reductions in various stress indices such as neuromuscular tension, resting heart rate and some stress hormones.
- Current clinical opinion holds that exercise has beneficial effects across all ages and in both sexes.
- Physically healthy people who require psychotropic medication may safely exercise when exercise medications are titrated under close medical supervision.

It has also been noted that regular exercisers, such as joggers, can become dependent on the running experience. Groups of runners defined as being dependent on running have been described as compulsive exercisers, they have a bizarre occupation with food, and they place an unusual emphasis on lean body mass.

Exercise and Disease Prevention

CARDIOVASCULAR DISEASE

The literature relating to cardiovascular disease has identified a number of risk factors which predict coronary heart disease. Some of these factors cannot be altered such as heredity, gender, race and age. Other factors can be altered and these fall into two categories – primary and secondary. Primary factors include cigarette smoking, hypertension and elevated serum cholesterol, triglycerides or low-density lipoproteins, and fibrin. The secondary factors of this group include diet, obesity, physical inactivity, diabetes, emotional stress and anxiety, and electrocardiogram abnormalities.

Since the classical work of Morris in 1953, which identified that the conductors of London's double-decker buses had about 30% less heart disease than their coworkers who drove the buses, it has been accepted that physical activity has a potential role in both the prevention and treatment of cardiovascular disease. Inactivity increases the risk of coronary disease by about a factor of two and activity is linearly related to the degree of protection against coronary disease. The minimal amount of physical activity which is required to produce a protective effect has been quoted to be equivalent of approximately 5 hours of very brisk walking (7 km per hour) or 3.5 hours of running (9 km per hour) per week. It is clear that the protective effect against coronary disease can only be demonstrated in those taking relatively vigorous aerobic exercise. Recreational work such as heavy gardening or DIY activities as opposed to sport, do not appear to give protection, although this may also be due to their irregularity. If regular exercise is not continued then the protection is lost, i.e. a past history of taking regular exercise does not appear to offer protection.

Cholesterol, an identified risk factor, is an essential component of cell membranes and is transported in the blood in combination with protein. The combination is referred to as a **lipoprotein**. The two most important lipoproteins for cholesterol transport are **low-density lipoprotein (LDL)** and **high-density lipoprotein (HDL)**. LDL is the main source of cholesterol for the membranes whereas HDL accepts cholesterol from the tissues. Due to this function of HDL, it has been suggested that increased levels of HDL-cholesterol may protect against **atherosclerosis** and thus **coronary heart disease**. Sustained exercise has been reported to increase the level of HDL-cholesterol and lower LDL-cholesterol and therefore potentially has a role directly in the prevention of coronary heart disease. However, more recent evidence would suggest that the results are confounded by an associated weight loss and dietary change.

Exercise has been shown to have a beneficial effect in mild-to-moderate hypertension. However, in established severe hypertension, exercise does not lower the blood pressure.

CONTROL OF OBESITY

It has been reported that of adults older than 30 years of age in the UK, 40% are obese, that is, they are 10% above the generally accepted desirable weight for their height. This degree of obesity is associated with increased morbidity from cardiovascular disease and diabetes. Considerable controversy surrounds both the cause and management of obesity. Undoubtedly the most effective therapy for the treatment of obesity is dietary but there is probably a place for regular exercise. During caloric restriction it is possible that the resting metabolic rate of obese subjects falls and that a programme of aerobic physical activity can offset this decrease, not only during the period of exercise but for several hours afterwards.

JOINTS, LIGAMENTS AND TENDONS

With age, joint mobility generally decreases. Moving and exercising the joints through their full range of movement can maintain or improve their mobility and thus prevent strains and potential rupturing around the joint.

DIABETES

Physical activity reduces blood glucose levels, increases the number of insulin receptors and increases the effect of insulin hence supporting the insulin-dependent diabetic.

PREVENTION OF INFECTIOUS DISEASES

Vigorous physical activity produces a stimulus to increase the concentration of white blood cells in the circulation and thus, potentially, has the effect of reducing the incidence or severity of infectious diseases.

Nutrition

In man, all movements are related to muscular activity. The amount of movement, described as energy expenditure, is of the range of 20 000 kilojoules (kJ) or 4760 kilocalories (kcal) every 24 hours (1 kcal = 4.2 kJ).

Energy expenditure is a combination of basal metabolism and voluntary muscular work. The basal metabolic rate provides energy for the work done by the heart, respiratory movement, digestive movement, maintenance of body temperature and all chemical reactions that require energy. The adult rate varies, predominantly because of differences in body mass. In women the range is approximately 5490–6940 kJ and in men about 6850–8110 kJ. This represents at most 50% of the normal work done in a 24-hour period. Basal metabolism is little affected by age although it can be altered during prolonged fasting, after a bout of high-intensity muscular effort or psychological tension.

The greatest variation, however, in energy expenditure comes from the energy cost of muscular work. The energy cost of muscular activity must be measured both in its intensity and its duration. It is clear that the higher the intensity of any work, the shorter will be the duration. Table 9.1 gives a sample of a number of activities with the appropriate energy expenditure. It should be noted, however, that they are all expressed per minute in order to make them comparable. It is unlikely, however, that the intensity of effort in sprinting could be maintained for that one-minute period.

Table 9.1
Energy Expenditure of Various Activities

Activity	Duration	kJ min^{-1}
Vigorous isolated movement (pure strength)	1 s	269
Sprint	20 s	134
1500 metres or comparable effort	5 min	67
Marathon or similar performance	2 h	21
A day of manual labour	8 h	8

Source: Nutrition and Sport (1980) Nestlé Products Technical Assistance.

There is not only considerable variability in energy expenditure between individuals but also within individuals on different days and if body weight is to be maintained then the energy input must match the energy output.

Body weight = [energy input] − [energy output]

Obviously any increase in energy input over energy output will cause a weight gain and the converse will cause a weight loss with a concomitant lack of ability to exercise.

The total amount of energy supplied to the muscles is critical but also the type of energy is important.

There are three principal nutrients which supply energy: carbohydrates, lipids (fats) and, to a lesser extent, protein. It is generally agreed that the amount of protein in the diet of a healthy person should be in the region of 12% (of requirements), i.e. the lipids and carbohydrates supply at least 88% of our energy.

Carbohydrates

Carbohydrate is the nutrient most important to exercise performance. The energy from carbohydrate can be released within exercising muscles up to three times as fast as energy from fats. However, the stores in the body are limited and when depleted, athletes cannot exercise intensely and may experience fatigue. Carbohydrates are composed of carbon, hydrogen and oxygen. The basic unit of a carbohydrate is the monosaccharide, the most common of which is glucose. Glucose and other monosaccharides, such as fructose and galactose, are usually combined together in foods as larger compounds. When two monosaccharides are joined together they are termed 'disaccharides' and the most common disaccharide in the diet is sucrose or table sugar.

The best high carbohydrate foods are those such as wholemeal bread, flour and crispbreads, wholemeal pastas, brown rice, pulses, potatoes, cereals, nuts, fresh fruit, dried fruit and tinned fruit. The carbohydrate in these foods is mainly found in the form of polysaccharide (multiple monosaccharides).

The other carbohydrate foods are sweet-tasting foods. These would be things such as sugar, syrups, jams, confectionery, sugary drinks such as lemonade, drinking chocolate, sugar-coated cereals, etc. These tend to be highly processed foods and the carbohydrate is mainly in the form of disaccharides and monosaccharides which can be rapidly absorbed following relatively little digestion.

Ingested carbohydrate is transported by the bloodstream to the liver where it can be converted to fat, stored as glycogen or released into the bloodstream for transport to other tissues such as muscle, where it can be utilized or stored as glycogen. When glycogen is broken down within muscle, energy can be released at rates which can power sprinting at 150% of maximal oxygen uptake. (It should be noted that unlike liver glycogen, muscle glycogen when broken down does not release glucose into the bloodstream; muscle glycogen is solely for muscle use.) By comparison the energy in fat cannot be released rapidly enough to allow a person to exercise more intensely than about 50% of maximal oxygen uptake. When muscle glycogen concentration is normal, it is sufficient to fuel most athletes' workouts and other activities completed within 90–120 minutes. At 1–3 hours of continuous running, cycling or swimming at 65–80% of maximal oxygen uptake or after repeated bouts of intense exercise, muscle glycogen stores will be depleted and this is when it is necessary to provide additional sources of energy and carbohydrate

feedings. Ideally, in an athlete's diet, at least 60–70% of the calories should come from carbohydrate. Although it is recognized that this is the amount of carbohydrate required, many athletes' diets contain <40% of carbohydrates and therefore they are presenting themselves for training or competition already in a potentially fatigued state.

After exhaustive exercise, it takes approximately 20 hours to totally restore the glycogen stores in the muscle. This is provided that approximately 600 g of carbohydrate are consumed. It is almost impossible to achieve this through eating complex carbohydrate because of the sheer volume and it is almost certainly necessary to supplement the complex carbohydrate with the simple sugars. This, of course, has to be balanced against the concerns relating to dental caries. When successive days or successive bouts of exercise are required, approximately 100 g of carbohydrate should be taken 15–30 minutes after exercise followed by additional 100 g feeding every 2–4 hours thereafter. There appears to be no differentiation in the replenishment rates whether the carbohydrate is in the form of simple sugar or complex carbohydrate. The feedings seem to be equally effective.

It is possible to manipulate one's diet in order to create additional muscle glycogen deposits prior to exercise. The higher-level glycogen stores will allow the onset of fatigue to be delayed, thus improving performance by allowing the athlete to be active for longer periods. The most practical method of glycogen loading for a given sport involves training intensely 5 or 6 days prior to competition. During the remaining days before competition athletes gradually reduce the amount of training and eat high carbohydrate meals on each of the three days before competing. The regimen will increase muscle glycogen stores 20–40% or more above normal.

As exercise progresses, the carbohydrate source, however, changes from predominantly muscle glycogen to the source of carbohydrate being blood glucose derived from the breakdown of glycogen in the liver. After 2–3 hours of exercise this blood glucose level will fall and the individual can become hypoglycaemic (low blood glucose). By taking carbohydrate throughout the exercise this fatigue can be delayed. In exercise, therefore, which is longer than 2 hours or in games such as rugby or soccer, it my be beneficial to consume carbohydrate supplements during competition as the glycogen levels can become particularly low. Further discussion of supplementation during exercise is given on p. 195.

Fats

In contrast to the limited carbohydrate stores the lipid stores in the human body are, for all practical purposes, unlimited. A jog at about two-thirds of maximal aerobic power uses one kilogram of fat to supply energy for approximately 10–20 hours. Similarly, a marathon run of 4–5 hours duration would require less than one kilogram of body fat, provided only fat was utilized for combustion. Élite endurance athletes usually have several kilograms of body fat, whereas an average, middle-aged man would have approximately 10 kg. Therefore, there is sufficient reserve to run multiple marathon races, and there is no parallel in terms of food supplementation for supplementing any athlete with fat.

Lipid for utilization during exercise is in three forms: triglycerides in adipose tissue (the main store), triglyceride within the muscle and circulating triglycerides primarily in the form of very low density lipoproteins produced by the liver. It is the triglyceride stores in muscle which are utilized during work and it is these which have to be replenished from the circulating free fatty acids. Immediately upon the start of exercise, muscle capillaries dilate facilitating free fatty acid uptake. This process is reversed at the end of the exercise.

The fat depot decreases with physical training to facilitate body movements; however, there is no reliable evidence to suggest a local effect of training to deplete selectively regional adipose tissue stores.

Protein

Due to, in part, the complexity of measuring protein metabolism, the question of how much dietary protein is necessary for optimal athletic performance is still unclear. The recommended protein intake, based on a number of expert committees on nutrition throughout the world ranges from 0.8 to 1.2 $g\,kg^{-1}\,day^{-1}$. These figures are derived from individuals who are essentially sedentary although there is a general consensus that exercise, particularly where attempts are made to increase muscle mass or in ultramarathon-type events, that the protein should be increased to around 1.2–1.7 $g\,kg^{-1}\,day$.

Although many proteins exist, each is made up of amino acids. There are two types of amino acids: those which the body can produce and those which are essential from the diet. Very high protein intakes can be harmful; however, intakes at the levels quoted above do not cause any problems. It may not be necessary to supplement athletes' diets as they will already contain sufficient quantities of proteins because of the large volume of food that an athlete eats. Therefore a complete dietary evaluation should be performed to determine if additional protein is necessary.

Vitamins

Vitamins are chemical compounds needed in minute amounts but they are, in the main, not made by the body or, if they are, they are not made in sufficient amounts. The most important vitamins, concerned with energy needs for exercise, are vitamins B, C and E. Although most of the recent well-controlled experiments have demonstrated that for individuals eating a well-balanced diet, supplementation with one or more vitamins does not result in increased physical performance, there are continued claims that vitamin supplements, especially the B-complex vitamins and vitamin C, are beneficial. This may be because, although vitamin supplementation has no effect when the diet is adequate, it remains possible that it may be important when an athlete is consuming relatively low energy intakes. The B-complex vitamins have been reported to enhance endurance capacity by improving mitochondrial transport, enhancing glycogen utilization by decreasing plasma free fatty acids, improving sensory motor control (and thus firing accuracy in shooting performers) and to be of value when high sweating rates are encountered. Vitamin C supplementation may enhance heat acclimatization. Vitamin E has also been recommended at high altitudes as it may have a beneficial effect on physical performance under these conditions and a partially protective effect of cell membranes.

The general consensus, however, is that these effects are only attained if the diet itself is deficient.

Fluid and Electrolyte Loss and Replacement in Exercise

The primary cause of fatigue in exercise lasting more than one hour, but not more than four to five hours, is usually the depletion of the body's carbohydrate reserves. The ambient temperature and the humidity can also, however, significantly affect performance. Prolonged exercise can be reduced to as much as half through the effect of dehydration and thermal regulatory problems. In order to maintain body temperature during exercise, it is necessary to increase water loss (sweat). Sweat is associated, not only with water, but with a loss of electrolytes. Fluid ingestion during long-term exercise, therefore, not only has to replace carbohydrate but it also needs to supplement the body stores of water and in some cases electrolytes. Replacement of carbohydrate and water are not necessarily compatible, in that, when the carbohydrate content of drinks increases, there will be a tendency to decrease the rate at which water is absorbed from the stomach. Low levels of glucose, however, will aid water uptake from the small intestine and where fluid replacement is a priority, it is recommended that approximately 2.5% glucose solutions are appropriate.

Evidence would suggest that the only electrolyte that needs to be added to drinks during exercise is sodium and this is normally done in the form of sodium chloride. Sodium will stimulate sugar and water uptake while in the small intestine and is therefore helpful when the rate of water uptake is of concern. Most soft drinks contain virtually no sodium whereas sports drinks will commonly contain $10-25^{-1}$mmol l^{-1}. Those solutions, which are used to rehydrate subjects with diarrhoea, will have $30-90^{-1}$mmol l^{-1} of sodium.

In general it would appear therefore, that low levels of sodium and low levels of glucose would help restore fluid loss during exercise. The balance of these components in various sports drinks varies considerably and the carbohydrate and electrolyte content of some commonly used sports drinks is given in Table 9.2.

Table 9.2
Composition of a Variety of Commercially Available Sports Drinks

Sports drink	Carbohydrate	Na$^+$	K$^+$	Cl$^-$	Osmolality
Isostar	73	24	4	12	296
Gatorade	62	23	3	14	349
Lucozade Sport	69	23	4	1	280
Pripps Energy	75	13	2	7	260
Coca-Cola	105	3	0	1	650
WHO-ORS	20	90	20	80	331
Dioralyte	16	60	20	60	240

Source: Maughan, RJ (1991) Fluid and Electrolyte Loss and Replacement in Exercise. In Williams, C, Devlin, JT (eds) *Foods, Nutrition and Sports Performance*. London: E & FN Spon.

It is difficult to predict the volume of water required because of the effect of the environment, the wind conditions and indeed the individual's sweating rate on any particular day. A variety of figures have been suggested which range somewhere between about 300 ml every 10–15 minutes during exercise to 100–200 ml every 2–3 km. In practice, however, it would appear that the maximum fluid intake of élite marathon runners never exceeds about 600 ml per hour.

Principles of Sports Training

The purpose of training is to improve performance. Therefore, training methods must relate to that performance and be specific to the performance. The principle of specificity requires that the training regimen overloads the metabolic system that supports the activity. That overload can be accommodated by manipulating two basic factors; the training intensity and/or the training volume. In general, the greater the overload the greater the resulting adaptation and increase in functional capacity. Because it takes time for physiological responses to occur following the application of a training stimulus, it must

be applied progressively. A rapid and continuous increase in training will possibly result in breakdown of the athlete. This concept of heightened training dispersed with recovery periods is illustrated in Figure 9.2. Ideally, loadings should be

Figure 9.2 The relationship between training load frequency and recovery time. (Dick FW, 1991)

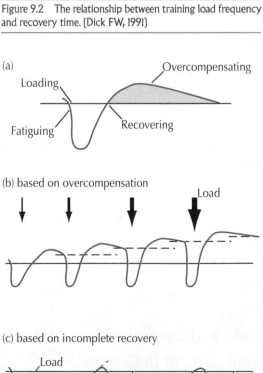

introduced at the peak of the overcompensating period allowing progression. However, if the loading is continually placed on the recovery phase, then progress is not seen.

Most athletes when planning their year will divide it into different phases. Each phase will carry objectives which allow a sense of achievement. In a single periodized year the competition phase will be restricted to essentially one block. Double periodizing of the year plans for an initial short competition period followed later in the year by a major competition period. This latter format has been shown to improve maximal performance at the time of the major competition.

The basic training model is built upon strength, speed and endurance. It is unlikely, however, that any sporting event requires only one of these components and the art of coaching necessitates that the correct proportions of each of these are matched to the athlete's event. Further refinement of the model can identify such things as strength endurance, elastic strength and speed endurance (Figure 9.3).

Training for Strength

There exists many methods of training to develop strength and increasingly there are a number of strength training devices to support the activity.

Figure 9.3 The principal components of a training model.

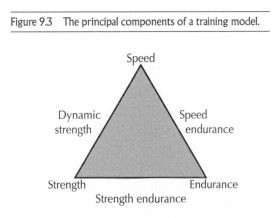

By far the most common method of strength training is with **free weights**. The loading for the free-weight movements is determined before training by establishing the **one-repetition maximum** (1 RM). This is carried out by lifting a maximum weight, recovering and trying to lift a heavier one. Once established, the 1 RM is used as a measure of the maximal force of the muscle and repetitions and training regimens are worked out on a percentage of that 1 RM. In general, it has been shown that to increase strength, three sets of six repetitions at a frequency of three times per week would appear to be optimal. More on this subject is given on p. 212.

A variant of this method of weight training is **pyramid training** which consists of training sets with an increase in load for example 6, 4, 2, 1 RM. In practice this would mean that the weight would be the maximum that could be lifted on 6, 4, 2, 1 consecutive repetitions. Physiological benefits of using the pyramid system are stated to be that activation of all motor units is ensured, whereas this is not necessarily the case with using constant percentages. This evidence, however, tends to be subjective. Physiologically, increased motor unit recruitment would only increase with increased speed of movement.

A disadvantage of free weights is that the load which can be lifted is limited by the weakest point during the movement and therefore not all muscle fibres are fully activated. This is in addition to the general safety problems in using free weights.

These observations have led to the development of strength training apparatus such as **isokinetic training** where the muscle fibres are fully activated throughout the range of movement. (The physiology of isokinetic work is discussed more fully on p. 212.) Isokinetic training is particularly advantageous for competitive swimmers because movement of the leg and arms in the water is very similar to the isokinetic movement on the machine. Isokinetic exercise is limited, however, where movement involves acceleration, which is the case in most other sports.

Training eccentrically does not appear to have any great advantages over concentric training. However, eccentric training is a component in any free-weight system, i.e. during a weight lift, a concentric contraction is always followed by an eccentric contraction when the weight is lowered again. Increased damage to the skeletal muscle caused by eccentric training would tend not to advocate this form of training for sports people.

Plyometrics is a technique used to bridge the gap between speed and strength training and is used particularly by those sports involving jumping. It uses the stretch reflex to facilitate recruitment of additional motor units and also loads both the contractile and elastic components (fascia and tendons) of the muscle. When stretched, the elasticity of the contractile and elastic components are stored as energy. During subsequent muscle activity, this stored energy is released, increasing the amount of force. Plyometric training is almost exclusively applied to extensor muscles of the legs and consists of a vigorous lengthening of the active extensor muscles, immediately followed by a maximal concentric contraction. This sequence of muscle activity is usually accomplished by having a person jump from a vaulting horse or a box down onto the floor and immediately leaping out of that position to touch a basketball net. Optimum heights, for the initial jump down, have been determined experimentally and plyometric training has been shown to improve jumping height. However, the improvement is no greater than that found with isokinetic training. Again the disadvantage of plyometric training is the risk of injury during touch down and take off from the floor, where

the tension in the muscle will reach supramaximal values.

The subject's own body weight can be used for strength development in an infinite number of ways and in a sport such as gymnastics it is the common way of strength training. Such exercises as push-ups, pull-ups, turn-ups, back-lifts, etc. can be enhanced by wearing vests with extra loadings.

Strength endurance is the expression of force in a climate of endurance factors. In order to develop this characteristic, then it is necessary to introduce an endurance component into the strength programme. The most effective way of doing this is to introduce circuit training. The loading suggested for the development of strength endurance are four to six repetitions at 25–50%. In order to achieve a circuit, a number of whole-body exercises are utilized and the athlete does one set of all the exercises and then undertakes a recovery and then does a further set to make up the appropriate number of repetitions. A modification of circuit training which involves more of a local muscular endurance, is **stage training**. This type of training ensures that all the repetitions of one exercise are done before proceeding to the next exercise, i.e. the athlete undertakes all three repetitions of one exercise prior to progressing on to the next exercise. The repetitions are normally less in stage training.

Training for Endurance

Aerobic endurance is developed through continuous training methods and by interval training methods. Both continuous exercise and interval training would appear to produce similar improvements in aerobic potential but it is generally agreed that interval training provokes endurance adaptations more rapidly than continuous training. Differentiation has been claimed, based on the case that interval training may be superior in bringing about the adaptations to replenish the energy systems whereas continuous training increases the capacity to sustain exercise for prolonged periods at a high percentage of the maximal oxygen consumption $V_{O_2\,max}$. Normally, athletes will use both types of exercise if for no other reason than to prevent boredom.

As with any other training, the training must be specific to the event and the duration of the event must be covered in the training programme. The onset of **blood lactate accumulation,** OBLA (the assessment method is discussed on p. 209) appears to be one of the best ways of improving aerobic performance by steady-state running. This involves running for 25 minutes at a steady pace which maximally works the aerobic system. When using interval training, it is important to achieve maximal or near maximal uptakes during the exercise period. Therefore the intensity of the intervals tends to be higher than the OBLA steady-state pace. The length of the interval is variable and there is little evidence to identify whether short or long intervals cause any differential effect on performance. It is probably best to involve both long and short intervals within any athlete's programme. The emphasis should be placed on equal work and recovery periods, i.e. if short work intervals are used, then rest intervals should also be shortened.

Training for Speed

It is generally accepted that improvements in speed progress minimally with training. Out of all the components which contribute to performance this aspect is influenced most by genetics. However, training does have a role in trying to teach the body how to recruit all the muscular

resources available without consideration of energy cost or economy. Motor units are not normally 100% activated and would only be recruited in 'fright-or-flight' situations. This is normally mediated through the hormone adrenaline which is released from the adrenal medulla in response to stimulation from the sympathetic nervous system. The nervous part of the competition is an essential part of any speed performance if maximal recruitment is to be achieved. One effect of adrenaline may be to alter the balance between fructose 6-phosphate and fructose biphosphate by affecting the enzyme phosphofructokinase. This could cause high rates of glycolysis. Another effect may be to lower the threshold for the firing of some of the large type IIB fibres (see Chapter 6). There is evidence that some of these IIB motor units are recruited when speed demands are high and that repeated recruitment in this way tends to reduce the level of inhibition and make such motor units more 'available' to the sprinter. This effect is likely to be very specific, only working on those motor units in the motoneurone pool which are utilized and are part of a rehearsed motor programme. This process has been labelled 'discipline disinhibition'. Sprinters include starting and forms of very fast sprinting in their training and precompetition warm-ups, in order to try to trigger this response.

The inability of sprinters to run in training as quickly as they can in competition poses problems if the assumptions about motor recruitment noted above are true in that they are not recruiting a similar pattern to that which they will require in the competition event itself. To compensate for this, many athletes employ a variety of speed drills. Also speed-assisted techniques have ranged from sprinting down slight gradients to running on high speed-treadmills and being pulled on a rope behind cars and motorcycles.

Obviously the latter has inherent problems of danger but the intention is that sprinters are given the sensation of speed that forces them to recruit muscle fibres that otherwise they would be incapable of doing. These training techniques have been taken to their extreme where electrical stimulation of muscle has been used to provoke the neuromuscular changes.

Speed Endurance

Speed endurance can be defined as high quality speed of movement (purely speed) no endurance factors. To develop this aspect of performance, repetition training methods are used where sets and repetitions are organized in such a way that the required intensity of each repetition is maintained throughout the unit. The intensity is normally in excess of 85% of maximum sprinting speed. By necessity, then, the numbers of sets

are high and the repetition within the sets are low in number. Distances run vary from 60 to 120% of racing distance. Relaxation is suggested as one of the most important factors involved and practices such as speed ball work have been introduced to develop relaxation at a high speed of arm movement.

The Performance

Although theoretically and in training we can separate the different components of an event, how these are integrated into a single maximal performance is left to the planning and management of the coach. The coach requires to quantify each of the sessions by their nature (e.g. contributing to speed, speed endurance, strength, strength endurance or endurance of the athlete). The balance of each of these depends on their relative priority in the event. Figure 9.4

Figure 9.4   The type of data which could be collected by a coach for evaluation. (Nimmo MA, 1994)

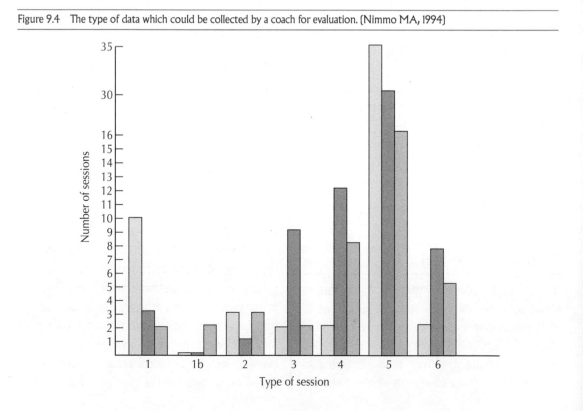

illustrates the type of information which can be gathered by a coach.

The Effect of Chronic Training on Physiological Systems

Cardiovascular Adaptations to Endurance Training

Blood volume increases with endurance training as a consequence of an increased plasma volume. It is believed that two mechanisms are involved in increasing the plasma volume. Firstly, exercise causes the release of the antidiuretic hormone (ADH) and aldosterone. These hormones cause the kidneys to retain water, which increases blood plasma. Secondly, exercise increases the amount of plasma proteins which will increase the potential to retain fluid in the blood.

Although resting heart rate is influenced by genetic components, endurance exercise can reduce heart rates to as low as 30–40 beats per minute in some cases. Heart rates recorded at standardized submaximal workloads will also be reduced although maximal heart rates vary only very slightly, if at all. Because maximal heart rate is relatively stable throughout the training cycle, it can be used as a reference point for judging the relative intensity of a workload. After exercise, the time it takes for an individual's heart rate to return to resting levels is termed 'heart rate recovery period'. After a period of endurance training, heart rate returns to its resting level much more quickly than prior to training. This factor, heart rate recovery period, can also therefore be used to monitor cardiorespiratory fitness.

The reduction in heart rate does not reflect a reduction in cardiac output as there is a concomitant rise in stroke volume. The maximum increase is reported to be around 20%. Reports of very high values in some élite athletes is thought to be genetically determined rather than a response to training directly. The increase in stroke volume arises because the lowered heart rate and increased plasma volume cause the left ventricle to fill more completely during diastole. This in turn activates the Frank–Starling mechanism (see Chapter 7), which enhances the ejection.

In response to these changes in the ventricular filling, the cardiac muscle and that of the left ventricle, in particular, undergoes hypertrophy. This concept of 'athlete's heart' caused initial concern as it was thought to be pathological. However, it is now accepted to be a normal adaptation to chronic training.

The heart works relatively less to meet the needs of any given workload after training. This reduces its oxygen consumption and a slight decrease in coronary blood flow is evident at rest and during standardized submaximal exercise. There is an increase in coronary flow at maximal exercise, however, reflecting the increased cardiac output. Coronary blood flow therefore reflects the metabolic load on the heart.

Increased capillaries around the muscle fibres of the heart does not appear to take place as a consequence of training; however, it does occur in the skeletal muscles that have been adapted by training as will be noted on p. 204. Blood flow to the skeletal muscle is further enhanced by a more effective redistribution of the cardiac output. This ability to redistribute blood to active muscle sites has, at least in animal studies, been shown to be enhanced by training.

Endurance training causes little or no change in blood pressure at standardized or maximal workloads although a lowering of blood pressure can be noted at rest, particularly in hypertensive individuals.

As a consequence of the increased plasma volume, relative measures of red blood cells such as haematocrit tend to be lowered. This reduces the viscosity of the blood facilitating blood movement through the capillary beds. Overall absolute values of red blood cells are typically unchanged in the highly trained athlete.

Functionally, the most significant change for the athlete is possibly the enhanced blood volume because this allows maximal cardiac output to increase. Increasing maximal cardiac output makes more oxygen available to the muscles thus improving the maximal oxygen consumption ($V_{O_2 max}$). Increases in $V_{O_2 max}$ with endurance training can be around 20%.

Cardiovascular Adaptations to Strength and Sprint Training

Ventricular hypertrophy has been noted with strength and sprint training programmes although the effect in endurance trained individuals is greater.

Reductions in resting and standardized submaximal heart rates are not so evident with strength and sprint training programmes and the result clearly depends on the specific nature of the programme, i.e. the volume, the recovery between sets, the muscle mass involved and the intensity (i.e. the size of the endurance component). Any reductions with maximal strength or speed programmes which have full recoveries are likely to be due to the changes in heart size.

Strength training, although constantly elevating the blood pressure during acute exercise bouts, does not result in elevations of resting blood pressure. There are reports of the converse, i.e. resistance training causing reductions in hypertensive patients which quantitatively were greater than those reductions with endurance training although conclusive evidence for this is not available.

Respiratory Adaptations with Exercise

Respiratory factors are seldom limiting in exercise performance and thus the adaptations with chronic training are relatively small. Lung volume measures and respiratory rate alter little with training and the maximum diffusion capacity and pulmonary capillary blood volume are similar in athletes and non-athletes.

Pulmonary ventilation, however, can increase two-fold with highly trained endurance athletes such as rowers, who are reported to have maximal pulmonary ventilation rates in excess of $120 \, l \, min^{-1}$.

The oxygen content of the arterial blood does not alter with training but the arteriovenous oxygen difference does increase with training, particularly at maximal levels of exercise. The increase results from a lower mixed venous oxygen content. This reflects a greater extraction of oxygen at the tissues and a more efficient distribution of the blood to the active tissues.

Athletes would appear to be able to adapt their respiratory muscles. Maximum pressure development against an occluded airway (MVV test) shows that the endurance athlete can achieve and sustain a higher percentage of their MVV (75%) than non-athletic populations (68%). This would imply a training effect on respiratory muscles with endurance training. No similar work has been conducted on strength trained individuals.

Skeletal Muscle Adaptation to Strength and Speed Training

An increase in size of skeletal muscle after strength training has only been identified in a few longitudinal studies; the majority of information arises from cross-sectional studies where muscles from so-called normal subjects are compared with muscles from groups of subjects engaged one way or another in strength training. Values ranging from 8 to 23% improvements in the cross-sectional area of muscle have been found. It is unclear whether the increased cross-sectional area is caused by hypertrophy or hyperplasia. In animal studies, both possibilities have been put forward; however, in humans it is more likely to be due to fibre hypertrophy rather than to hyperplasia.

The nature of the weight-lifting programme can also affect the degree of increase of cross-sectional area of the muscle. Weightlifters have a similar percentage of the main fibre types as normal subjects but, with training, show preferential hypertrophy of the type II fibres, whereas body-builders do not show this preferential hypertrophy. These differences are probably related to the fact that, while the aim of training for the body-builder is only hypertrophy, the weightlifter is interested in the development of power as well as muscle strength. The hypertrophy training programme consists of many sets with loads usually not exceeding 8 RM. Some muscle groups are trained with loads as small as 20–30 RM but all muscles are exercised to complete exhaustion. In contrast, weightlifters exercise using heavier loads, 2–6 RM, and fewer sets, and a high speed of contraction is constantly emphasized. Apart from this very broad differentiation in the type of adaptation of skeletal muscle to resistance training, there is little further evidence to differentiate between, for instance, pyramid-type sessions and repetition maximums.

In explosive-speed and sprint events for which strength training is important, much of the energy is derived from the glycolytic system together with adenosine triphosphate (ATP) and creatine phosphate systems. The evidence currently would suggest that training bouts require to be about 30 seconds before they will enhance the enzymes of these pathways. Shorter activity bouts tend to develop strength and neuromuscular components rather than the enzyme systems.

Anaerobic training also improves the capacity of muscles to tolerate lactic acid. The production of lactic acid and the consequent increase in hydrogen ions is thought to contribute to fatigue in sprinting events. Buffers (such as bicarbonate) combine with hydrogen ions to reduce the acidity of fibres; thus, they can delay fatigue. Anaerobic training has been shown to improve the buffering capacity of muscles.

Skeletal Muscle Adaptation to Endurance Training

The major effects of endurance training on skeletal muscle are on its metabolic capacity and its capillary supply.

Many studies have shown that endurance training increases the mitochondrial content and oxidative capacity of skeletal muscle. The major effect of the enzymatic changes is to increase the contribution of fat and correspondingly decrease the contribution of carbohydrate to the oxidative energy supply during submaximal exercise. The increased oxidation of fat is probably a consequence of an increase in the potential for oxidation of substrates as the glycolytic capacity shows little adaptive response to endurance training. The trained runner not only uses more fat and less carbohydrate at the same running speed but also at the same relative exercise intensity when it is expressed as a percentage of $V_{O_2 max}$. At an intensity, therefore, within the normal range of endurance exercise, the trained individual has a lower blood lactate concentration than the untrained individual. These two effects of decreased carbohydrate oxidation and decreased lactate production result in a sparing of the body's limited carbohydrate stores, which is a major factor in improving endurance performance.

Studies of endurance-trained muscles show an increase in the capillary density expressed as capillaries per fibre and as capillaries per unit area. This provides an increased surface for exchange between blood and muscle. Capillary density increases, resulting from growth of new capillaries, occur within the first few weeks of training.

The diffusion distance is also enhanced by a decrease in the muscle fibre size with endurance training. In addition, myoglobin, which is responsible for shuttling the oxygen molecules from the cell membrane to the mitochondria within the cell, increases by 75–80% with endurance training.

Adaptations to Heterogeneous Training Programmes

It is clear that the adaptations to strength training are different from those induced by endurance training. This is true particularly with the skeletal muscle adaptations. Studies have therefore investigated whether simultaneous training for strength and endurance compromises single-discipline training. Evidence would suggest that gains in strength are compromised by endurance training. The effects on endurance performance of a strength training programme are more variable and probably depend on the endurance component of the strength programme.

Specific Issues Relating to Females

Increased participation of women in sport and the continuous improvement in the quality of their performances has led to an increasing number of investigations looking at the differences in physiological response of males and females to an exercise stimulus. These differences have been discussed in relation to skeletal muscle in Chapter 6. In summary, the data available suggest that women are predisposed to low-intensity, long-duration work because of a predominance of type I fibre tissue and a greater preference than males to utilize fat as a fuel.

Non-athletic females have a higher body fat content than do non-athletic males (25–30% and 15–20%, respectively). Body fat, however, in excess of 10% is reported to hamper endurance performance. It is, therefore, relatively common to see athletic women with body fat contents of < 10% and ths can have secondary physiological consequences which are discussed below.

The onset of puberty can sometimes be a traumatic time for a young athlete. The young female beginning intense exercise before puberty may have a delayed menarche and will develop a long, lithe figure ideally suited for endurance work. At the onset of puberty, however, she is likely to experience an increase in body weight and her performance is likely to deteriorate.

It is also common to experience irregularities in the menstrual cycle in young athletes. This is often referred to as 'athletic amenorrhoea' and is not peculiar to the élite. The young are particularly vulnerable to these irregularities which may lead to anovulation (menstrual bleeding without ovulation), amenorrhoea (no menstrual bleeding), as well as transient infertility.

There are classes within distance running which are particularly susceptible to menstrual cycle irregularities. These are:

- Females under 18 years of age.
- Females who initially weigh under 50 kg and drop their weight by more than 4.5 kg.
- Females whose average training is greater than 35 miles per week.
- Females who have trained for a number of years.
- Females who experience late menarche.

It is clear, therefore, that menstrual cycle irregularities are not peculiar to the élite. Prevalence rates have been estimated from 1 to 44% in athletes and from 1.8 to 5% in the general population. Although it is evident that those disturbances are caused by hormonal disturbances, the reason for the hormonal disturbances is not clear. Several mechanisms have been proposed explaining the menstrual changes in athletes. One theory identifies that it is the intensity of physical training which is the cause and there is support for this theory through a study showing normalization of menstrual function when exercise diminishes due to injury or an off-season. It certainly seems clear that a sudden increase in intensity will cause irregularity in the menstrual cycle. The critical fat hypothesis maintains that a specific percentage of body fat is needed to initiate menarche (17%) and to sustain fertility thereafter (22%). Other groups of researchers believe that regional fat distribution is the important factor in triggering amenorrhoea whereas the most recent evidence would now suggest that it is not so much the total calorific intake but the composition of the intake. All of these theories, however, have been criticized and it is likely that there is no one cause but a combination of many.

The irregularities in the reproductive cycle are believed to be reversible and fertility in later life is not affected. However, the associated lower level of oestrogen which may accompany amenorrhoea can have secondary effects. Lower bone densities have been found in amenorrhoeic runners and rowers when compared with a similarly active control group. The bone densities of these young athletic women are comparable to 55-year-old menopausal women. The low bone densities can make the athlete, however, susceptible to bony disorders including stress fractures. However, exercise in part compensates for the bone loss. This is evidenced when a group of inactive amenorrhoeic women were compared to an exercised amenorrhoeic group and were found to have higher bone densities.

Treatment can partially reverse the bone loss if given within the first three years (see below). Also, the bone loss can be offset if calcium intake is not allowed to fall lower than 1500 mg per day. Excessive dosages of calcium above requirement, however, are ineffectual.

Female athletes with menstrual irregularities (dysmenorrhoea) may benefit from taking low-dose oral contraceptives. The effects of these low-dose oral contraceptives on aerobic and anaerobic athletic performance, however, must be further studied.

In general, it is clearly advantageous to manage an athlete's training in such a way that excessive stress is avoided. This is true whether the athlete is male or female. It is merely fortunate in some ways that the effect of stress, in the form of a lack of menstrual bleeding is easily detectable in females. The effect of exercise stress on the male hormonal system may be just as problematic.

Fitness Assessment

Measurement of Aerobic Performance

The classical method of estimating aerobic capacity is by measuring the maximum oxygen consumption ($VO_{2\ max}$). Measurement of $VO_{2\ max}$ is intended to evaluate cardiovascular performance since it is a function of cardiac output and arterial mixed venous oxygen difference.

The laboratory protocol consists of 9–15 minutes of continuous incremental exercise. The actual intensities at which the increments are accelerated vary greatly, depending on the population. The important factor is that volitional exhaustion should occur between 9 and 15 minutes. A number of prescribed protocols exist in the literature, the most common of which are outlined in Figure 9.5. Recently, a new treadmill protocol,

---

Figure 9.5   A sample of published treadmill protocols. (Hayward VH, 1991)

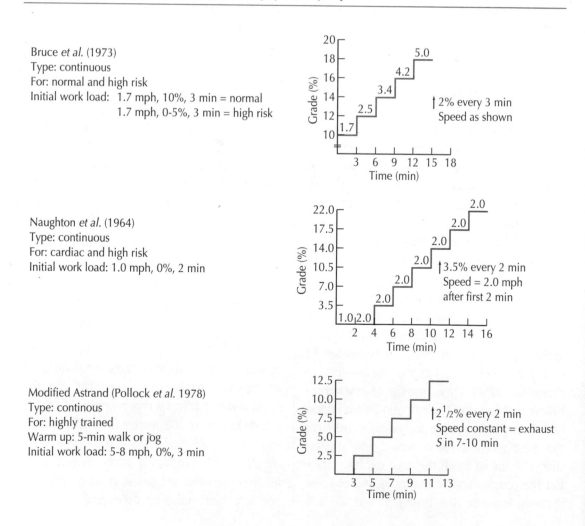

Bruce *et al.* (1973)
Type: continuous
For: normal and high risk
Initial work load: 1.7 mph, 10%, 3 min = normal
                     1.7 mph, 0-5%, 3 min = high risk

Naughton *et al.* (1964)
Type: continuous
For: cardiac and high risk
Initial work load: 1.0 mph, 0%, 2 min

Modified Astrand (Pollock *et al.* 1978)
Type: continous
For: highly trained
Warm up: 5-min walk or jog
Initial work load: 5-8 mph, 0%, 3 min

standardized exponential exercise protocol (STEEP), has been introduced which appears to be more sensitive to functional performance of limited subjects such as cardiac patients. Measurements of $VO_{2\ max}$ may be carried out. Symptoms of ECG changes may terminate the protocol. Throughout the test period, expired air is collected either continuously or at the end of each workload. Generally, four criteria need to be met in order to justify that it is a true maximum oxygen consumption. These are:

1. That an increase in workload does not increase the oxygen consumption >2 ml kg^{-1} min^{-1} or 5%.
2. The highest respiratory exchange ratio is >1.15.
3. The final value for heart rate should be within 10 beats per minute of the age-related maximum.

4. A post-exercise blood lactate level consistent with considerable reliance on anaerobic metabolism (e.g. $\geqslant 8.0$ mmol l^{-1}).

Some $VO_{2\ max}$ values taken from a number of sources are presented in Table 9.3.

It is not always advantageous to exercise an individual to maximum and an estimate can be made from the oxygen consumption measured at submaximal work intensites. This method is based on the fact that there is a linear increase in oxygen consumption with heart rate. Therefore, it is possible to extrapolate from the submaximal heart rate (Figure 9.6) to the predicted maximum heart rate. Maximum heart rate is closely related to age and is estimated from the simple formula $(220 - age)$. Two estimates are made in this prediction method of $VO_{2\ max}$. Firstly, the continued

Table 9.3a
Cardiorespiratory Fitness Classification

Women maximal oxygen uptake (ml kg^{-1} min^{-1})

Age (years)	Low	Fair	Average	Good	High
20–29	<24	24–30	31–37	38–48	49+
30–39	<20	20–27	28–33	34–44	45+
40–49	<17	17–23	24–30	31–41	42+
50–59	<15	15–20	21–27	28–37	38+
60–69	<13	13–17	18–23	24–34	35+

Men maximal oxygen uptake (ml kg^{-1} min^{-1})

Age (years)	Low	Fair	Average	Good	High
20–29	<25	25–33	34–42	45–52	53+
30–39	<23	23–30	31–38	39–48	49+
40–49	<20	20–26	27–35	36–44	45+
50–59	<18	18–24	25–33	34–42	43+
60–69	<16	16–22	23–30	31–40	41+

Source: From Preventative Medicine Centre, Palo Alto, CA, and from a survey of published sources. Table modified from *Exercise Testing and Training in Apparently Healthy Individuals: A Handbook for Physicians.*

Table 9.3b
Range of $VO_{2\ max}$. Reported for International Athletes in a Variety of Sports. Units are ml kg^{-1} min^{-1}

Sport	Range	
	Males	Females
Nordic skiing	65–95	56–74
Middle distance running	70–86	
Distance running	65–80	55–72
Rowing	58–74	48–68
Cycling	56–72	
Swimming	54–70	48–68
Soccer	50–70	
Figure skating		42–54
Wrestling	50–70	
Gymnastics	48–74	38–48
Hockey	45–65	
Field hockey	39–49	
Basketball	45–65	42–54
American football	40–60	
Baseball	40–60	
Untrained	38–52	30–46

Source: From MacDougall, JD, Wenger, HA, Green, H (eds) *Physiological Testing of the Elite Athlete.* New York: Movement Publications.

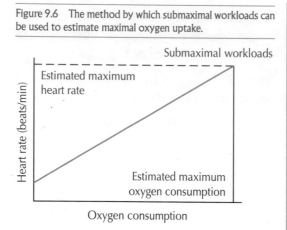

Figure 9.6 The method by which submaximal workloads can be used to estimate maximal oxygen uptake.

linear relationship of heart rate and $VO_{2\ max}$ and secondly, the maximum heart rate. It is not surprising therefore an error of $\geqslant 10\%$ can be introduced. A number of submaximal exercise test protocols are available. References, giving the details of these tests, are presented in the bibliography.

Estimates of aerobic capacity can also be achieved through merely making an estimate from work done where neither heart rate nor oxygen consumption is measured. An example of this is with a number of standardized exercise protocols such as the Bruce protocol or the Ellestad protocol. Further details of these protocols are presented in a paper by Pollock *et. al.*

Whether estimating $VO_{2\ max}$ or measuring it directly, a decision has to be taken on which ergometer should be used. In general, it is always best to measure an individual on an ergometer which is closest to the individual's activity. If not dealing with sports people, then the chosen ergometer is most usefully a treadmill. **Treadmill ergometry** involves a larger active muscle mass than **bicycle ergometry,** therefore there is less risk of elevated blood pressure and this is always a risk in older or sedentary patients. It is also easier to devise a protocol that ensures that fatigue is at the

level of the heart and lungs and not at the local muscular level which is common in bicycle ergometer tests.

Treadmill and bicycle work tests, whether maximal or submaximal, are too impractical to use with large numbers and therefore tests are available which predict maximal oxygen uptake from walking/running performance have been devised. All that is required is a non-slippery surface at least 20 metres in length and a cassette player. The concept for a progressive shuttle run test for the prediction of maximal oxygen update was first introduced by researchers from the University of Montreal in Canada and it was first published by Leger and Lambert. Hence, the test is often called the Leger test. During this test, the individual shuttle runs between two cones 20 metres apart, at a pace dictated by a timer on a cassette tape. Each subject runs for as long as possible until he/she can no longer keep up with the speed set by the tape at which point he/she voluntarily withdraws from the test. The predicted $VO_{2\ max}$ is then worked out depending on the level that the individual achieved. Errors noted in this type of test, is the assumption that the work capacity/oxygen consumption is common in all subjects. The test, however, is maximal and does not introduce the estimation of heart rate.

Other assessments of 'aerobic' performance include norms for walking/running set distances, although many of these are not designed to give a prediction of $VO_{2\ max}$, nor on many occasions is it the cardiorespiratory system which is the limiting factor.

In recent years it has been identified that improvements in endurance performance can be achieved without improving the $VO_{2\ max}$ and hence tests have now been devised which look at the aerobic capacity of the skeletal muscle in addition to looking at the cardioarterial level. This is routinely carried out by using one of two procedures: blood lactate and respiratory parameters.

BLOOD LACTATE

Blood lactate values have been shown to reflect the muscle lactate fairly closely up to 4 mmol l^{-1}. It is, therefore, possible to estimate the muscle lactate by measuring blood lactate. Blood lactate concentration is the result of production by the muscle and removal by the liver. When the production matches removal, blood lactate levels are constant. When production exceeds removal, blood lactate levels will increase. When this happens it is thought to be reflective of the body's systems working anaerobically although this has been questioned. It is this principle which was used to develop a method for measuring the aerobic capacity of skeletal muscle in the mid-1970s. The protocol involves individuals walking or running for a 25-minute period at a steady state on a treadmill. Blood lactate is measured every 5 minutes. On subsequent visits to the laboratory the intensity (i.e. the speed of the treadmill) is increased until the blood lactate levels increase more than 1 mmol l^{-1} over the last four measurements. The results of such a protocol are shown in Figure 9.7. When this test was applied to a large number of individuals it became clear that the average lactate level at which most people were able to maintain their steady state lactates was at 4 mmol l^{-1}. Subsequently, therefore, it has been possible to use an incremental test to identify the intensity which will elicit 4 mmol l^{-1} of lactate (Figure 9.8). This assessment is referred to as the 'onset of blood lactate accumulation' or **OBLA test**. However, it must be stressed that the figure of 4 mmol l^{-1} is an average value and that the range of values can be anything between 3 and 5.6 mmol l^{-1}. The incremental test can only be used, therefore, when applying to a general population and would not be appropriate to be used with élite or specific sports performers.

Because there is this possible error with the OBLA test, an alternative which still allows the maximum aerobic capacity of skeletal muscle to be identified from one visit is the identification of the **lactate

Figure 9.7   Determination of training pace using OBLA (units refer to training pace in minutes per mile). (Nimmo, 1992)

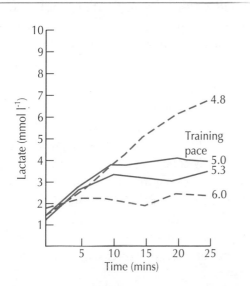

Figure 9.8   Identification of the intensity which elicits 4 mmol l^{-1} lactate and the identification of the lactate inflection point.

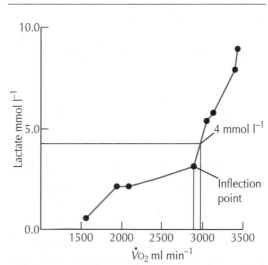

inflection point (Figure 9.7). An argument against the use of this latter test is that it necessitates a large number of blood samples for a meaningful result. Investigators therefore need to decide on the most appropriate assessment for the population that they are studying.

RESPIRATION

When lactic acid is transferred to the venous system, it dissociates to lactate and hydrogen ions. The hydrogen ions are buffered by the plasma bicarbonate resulting in an increase in carbon dioxide production and an accompanying increase in pulmonary ventilation. This increase in ventilation offers a method of identifying increases in blood lactate by a non-invasive method. The anaerobic threshold, as it is referred to, is identified during an incremental test as the point at which ventilation increases in a non-linear fashion. The use of this method has become widespread and there are many reports which identify a close relationship between lactate inflection and ventilatory inflection. However, studies on McArdle's syndrome patients, who lack the enzyme myophosphorylase and thus are incapable of producing lactate, identified an 'anaerobic threshold' at 81% of $VO_{2\ max}$. The conclusion therefore is that the close relationship is fortuitous rather than causal and the use of this assessment procedure is now questionable.

Training at the identified work intensity, which represents the maximum steady state, (however it is determined) has been shown to be one of the most effective ways of raising aerobic performance. Levels below that intensity may maintain the aerobic capacity but are less efficient in improving it. Intensities above that would take the individual into an anaerobic metabolism and thus would be detrimental to the aerobic profile of that individual. This concept of measuring OBLA and its transfer into training practice has made 'OBLA training runs' a common practice in athletic training.

Measurement of Anaerobic Performance

The Wingate test has been used more than any other to assess the characteristics of anaerobic performance. It was described initially in 1974 as a leg performance test and since then it has been adapted to test anaerobic performance of the arm. The test itself takes 30 seconds. The subject is instructed to pedal as fast as possible for 30 seconds against a resistance which is calculated from his or her age and weight. The results from this test allow the calculation of mean power, which is the work output over the 30 seconds period, peak power which is the highest power output in a 5-second period and the fatigue index which is the difference between the peak power and the lowest 5-second power output divided by peak power. Power decline can also be assessed. A characteristic trace of the output from the Wingate test is given in Figure 9.9. The reliability of the Wingate test, particularly with reference to peak power and to mean power, is very high. The power decline component however is more variable.

More recently, maximal isokinetic tests have been used to determine aerobic performance. The individual is asked to perform as many flexions and extension movements as possible. The tests are normally conducted on the leg in the seated position, measuring the quadriceps. The power output per kilogram of body weight can be calculated and also the total work output over a given period. The validity of these tests as true measures of anaerobic capacity, however, is questionable.

Figure 9.9   Characteristic output from a 30-second leg Wingate test

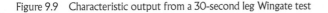

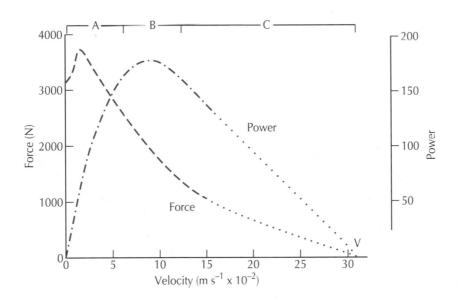

For sport activities, specific anaerobic performance tests can be developed. For example 60–120-second maximal tests can be designed for running, ice skating, speed skating, cycling as well as others.

Although the Wingate test has been the most commonly used assessment of anaerobic capacity, in the 1980s it was criticized over reports that up to 20% of the energy source during the 30-second period is derived from the aerobic system. Therefore, the validity of the test as a true anaerobic capacity test is being questioned. Considered now to be the most acceptable anaerobic capacity test is one which was developed by Medbo and colleagues. This test involves two pretest assessments involving running on a treadmill at a 10.5% incline at intensities between 85 and 95% $VO_{2\ max}$. The actual test is carried out on a separate day and involves running to volitional exhaustion on a 10.5% gradient for a 2–3-minute period. Oxygen consumption is measured throughout the test. The two submaximal values

along with the resting oxygen consumption, assumed to be 5 ml kg^{-1} min^{-1}, is plotted on a graph as illustrated in Figure 9.10(a). The oxygen consumption is extrapolated to a theoretical point for oxygen consumption at the running speed of the maximal test. That theoretical oxygen consumption, established via these procedures in Figure 9.10(a) is then used to calculate the anaerobic contribution as shown in Figure 9.10(b) where the actual oxygen consumption is measured throughout the 2–3-minute maximal test then subtracted from the theoretical oxygen consumption required for that intensity of work. The difference reflects the anaerobic capacity. Because this test requires perhaps four or five visits to the laboratory, it is not routinely used when assessing athletes and many investigators are now looking to adapt this test in a way which can be routinely applied.

None of these anaerobic tests clearly differentiates between the alactic acid component and the lactic acid component. The alactic component

Figure 9.10   (a) Relationship between exercise intensity (treadmill speed) and O_2 demand. (b) Accumulated O_2 deficit is calculated as the difference between accumulated O_2 demand and accumulated O_2 uptake of exercise.

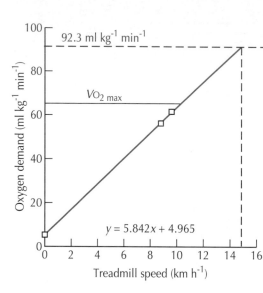

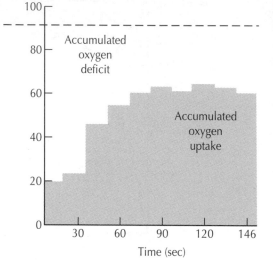

concerns the utilization of ATP and creatine phosphate which are virtually impossible to measure by non-invasive methods. The only valuable method is to estimate the content by muscle biopsy or more recently through the use of magnetic resonance imaging (MRI). This was discussed in some detail in Chapter 6.

Measurement of Muscle Strength

A common method of estimating strength in a particular muscle group is by measuring the heaviest weight that can be lifted once (one repetition maximum or 1 RM; see p. 197) through a specified range of movement. This is a measure of concentric contraction strength. Classically, weight-training strength is measured in kilograms although correctly it should be measured in newtons which accounts for gravity. A simple conversion can be made by multiplying the kilogram value by 9.8.

Isotonic testing is sometimes related incorrectly

to weight-lifting exercise but a truly isotonic system does not allow a preset force to be exceeded. The comparison is therefore incorrect. An isotonic system allows the measurement of acceleration, peak velocity, work and power at a specific force.

An alternative to weight-lifting and isotonic measurement, is a model which measures isometric strength. This measures the strength of a muscle at a certain length and it may be necessary to measure at a number of set angles of the joint and this can become tedious. However, because of the simplicity of the measurement, there is a great deal of normative data available using this model, particularly with relevance to the quadriceps muscle. A classical isometric model for measuring quadriceps strength is presented in Figure 9.11. Some normative data are given in Table 9.4.

Isokinetic testing involves testing the muscle through a range at a constant velocity. It is possible using this method to measure both concentric

Figure 9.11   Measurement of quadriceps isometric force using a Tornvall chair.

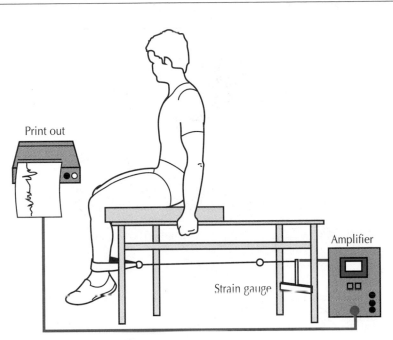

and eccentric contractions. The isokinetic dynamometers allow strength to be measured at preset velocities. The principle of such measurements is that the body part being measured is not allowed to exceed the velocity of the dynamometer. If it is faster than the preset velocity, then it creates a force or torque against the dynamometer and is measured in newtons per second. Although the test measures isokinetic movement, much of the movement through the range is not isokinetic. It is only when the body part engages with the resistance arm of the dynamometer that the movement is isokinetic. When the dynamometer is set at the higher velocities (e.g. 400° per second) then only 15% of the movement is isokinetic. The rest of the movment is the body part accelerating to engage with the resistance arm.

Limitations of this type of assessment are often due to the limitations of commercially available dynamometers. Many will only preset to velocity values well below functional requirements and also many will only measure one joint angle where most functional movements involve multiple joints. A sample result produced from measuring the quadriceps muscle of a healthy male at 30° per second can be seen in Figure 9.12.

Rating of Perceived Exertion (RPE)

It is helpful to be able to evaluate ratings of perceived exertion to assess whether or not a test is truly maximal and to assess when maximum exercise is being approached. This is particularly important if patients are taking medications that restrict heart rate responses to exercise. Perceived exertion skills provide methods to quantify subjective exercise intensity. RPE from the category scale correlates closely with several exercise variables including percentage

Figure 9.12   Mechanical properties measured on the Cybex. (Top) Knee extension is performed at a velocity of $30°\ s^{-1}$ through a range of approximately 90°. (Bottom) A recording of a concentric contraction shows a peak torque of 300 Nm. (MacDougall, Wenger and Green, 1991)

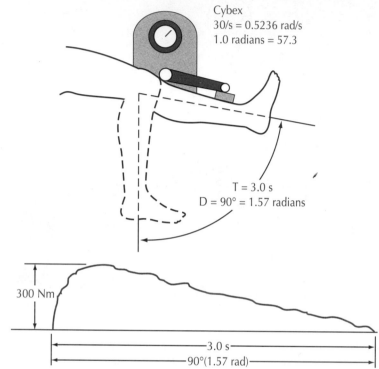

Cybex
30/s = 0.5236 rad/s
1.0 radians = 57.3

T = 3.0 s
D = 90° = 1.57 radians

300 Nm

—3.0 s—
—90°(1.57 rad)—

$VO_{2\ max}$ percentage heart rate reserve, minute ventilation and blood lactate levels. RPE scales are given in Table 9.4a. Numerous clinical studies have illustrated that the category RPE scale is a reproducible measure of exertion within a wide variety of individuals, regardless of age, gender or race. The validity is also unaffected by beta-blocking agents. Most individuals rate the lactate inflection to RPEs of about 13–16 and reach exhaustion at an RPE of 18–19. There is a small proportion of individuals who tend to underestimate RPE at submaximal levels and it is useful to have some practice, i.e. learning trials, before actual testing.

Although the category ratings work well for exercise-tested procedures, Borg has developed a new scale which has ratio properties. True psychophysical responses to intensity stimuli appear to increase as a power function rather than a linear or logarithmic response. Thus, at both low and high intensities of exertion, subjects may need an opportunity to pick scale numbers that provide a more finely tuned subjective response to small increases in objective exercise intensity. The new category ratio RPE scale is preferred when testing angina patients and it should better approximate changes in blood lactate response. When using the ratio scale it is important to understand that a rating of 10 is not maximal. If the subjective intensity rises above 10 then the person is free to choose any larger number in proportion to 10 that describes the proportionate growth of the sensation. For example, if an increase in exercise intensity feels 20% harder than it did at a rating of 10 the RPE would be 12. If it feels 50% harder then

Table 9.4

Normative Data for the Force Production from the Quadriceps Muscle of Different Populations.

Subject Group	Isometric Strength (mean +/−SD)
Normal males*	675 +/− 120
Normal females*	485 +/− 89
Male international rugby players	718 +/− 9
Female international squash players	548 +/− 96

Source: Reproduced from Nimmo, M (1987) How science can help sport. *Analytical Proceedings*, **24**: 68.
*Harman, M, Leiper, JB, Litchfield, PE, Maughan, RJ (1984) *Journal of Physiology*, **357**: 103.

Table 9.4a

RPE scales. Original Scale (6 to 20) on Left and Revised Scale (1 to 10) on Right

Category RPE scale		Category-Ratio RPE Scale	
6		0	Nothing at all
7	Very, very light	0.5	Very, very weak
8		1	Very weak
9	Very light	2	Weak
10		3	Moderate
11	Fairly light	4	Somewhat strong
12		5	Strong
13	Somewhat hard	6	
14		7	Very strong
15	Hard	8	
16		9	
17	Very hard	10	Very, very strong
18			Maximal
19	Very, very hard		
20			

Source: From Borg, GA (1982) *Medicine and Science in Sports and Exercise*, **14**: 377–387.

the RPE would be 15. Using the ratio scale therefore requires some very clear and explicit instructions from the operator. It is also misinterpreted at times for sports persons. Use of the scale describes the exercise as 'strong'. This can be interpreted by an athlete in a different way, i.e. the word 'strong' in terms of an athlete is some-

times used when the athlete feels good, i.e. they feel strong in spite of the intensity being particularly hard. Meaning of words in this context is very important and the athlete must understand what is being required if the ratio scale is to be used.

Body Composition

Most body composition methods are based upon the model in which the body consists of two chemically distinct compartments, **fat** and **fat-free compartments**.

Because water is not stored in fat and it occupies approximately 72–74% of the fat-free mass, total body water has been used as an index of human body composition. The total body water of an individual is estimated from ingestion of a radioisotope or tracer, normally deuterium. The protocol requires the individual to ingest or have injected a specified quantity of the tracer, which is followed by an equilibrium period before sampling. The calculation of the total body water volume is based upon the simple relationship $C_1 V_1 = C_2 V_2$ where C_1 is the concentration of tracer given, V_1 is the volume of the tracer, C_2 is the final concentration of tracer in a biological fluid and V_2 is the volume of total body water. Although this is a fairly reproducible method of estimating body fat it involves radioisotopes and therefore cannot be used routinely.

Similarly, because fat contains no potassium and the fat-free mass contains 60–70 mmol l^{-1} in men and 50–60 mmol l^{-1} in women, the quantification of the total body potassium allows an estimation of body fat to be made. Quantification of total body potassium requires specially constructed counters that consist of a large shielded room containing a gamma-ray detection system connected to a suitable recording device. Therefore, again this makes this method of estimating total body fat relatively inaccessible for most people.

Human body composition can probably be most accurately estimated from body density measurements. The relationship, as defined by Siri (1961), between body density (BD) and body fat is:

$$Fat\% = (4.95/BD - 4.50) \times 100$$

Body density is estimated by weighing individuals in air and then in water. Because the density of the fat-free body is 1 g cm^{-3} and fat has a density of 0.9 g cm^{-3} the difference between the two weighings will be less in an individual with a high lean-body mass (LBM). The claim for validity of densitometry as a means of predicting fat, however, depends on the assumption that each component of the two-compartment model, i.e. fat and fat-free, has a constant density. It is well known that exercise will influence bone mineralization and variation in bone density can influence lean body mass figures by around 2%. Densitometry methods are therefore perhaps not the best measure to use on athletic populations where the bone is obviously in a dynamic state. This is similarly true in patients who have forced inactivity or osteoporosis.

Skinfold measurements are based upon the assumption that the thickness of the subcutaneous adipose tissue reflects a constant proportion of the total body fat and the site selected for measurement represents the average thickness of subcutaneous tissue. These are obviously very general rules. The validity of using skinfold equations to predict body composition is therefore restricted to populations from whom these equations were derived. A variety of equations have now been derived and the appropriate one should always be sought. The measurement of skinfold thickness is made by grasping the skin and adjacent subcutaneous tissue between the thumb and

forefinger and pulling it gently away from the underlying muscle. Various sites of estimating the skinfold thickness have been developed.

The precision of a measurement of skinfold thickness is dependent upon the skill of the anthropologist and the site measured. In general, a precision of within 5% can be attained easily by properly trained experienced individuals.

Body impedance measures have become popular in recent years and are based upon the fact that fat-free mass contains virtually all the water and conducting electrolytes in the body. Conductivity is far greater therefore in the fat-free mass than in the fat mass of the body. Aluminium foil spot-electrodes are positioned in the middle of the dorsal surfaces of the hands and feet. The exact positioning of the electrodes is critical in order to ensure reproducibility. The precision of the method determined in 14 men has been shown to be < 2%. The 2% variability is thought to be due to true changes in the body-water compartments. Preparation of the subject prior to assessment is variable depending upon the manufacturer. As a general procedure measurements should be made approximately 2 h after eating and within 30 min of voiding. It should be noted that the equations transferring impedance to body fat are different between commercial products and therefore the instructions for each individual product should be followed. The validity of this method's use in populations at the extremes of the body fat range are yet to be proven.

A variety of other methods of estimating body fat including total body electrical conductivity (TOBEC), ultrasound, infrared interactance, neutron activation analysis, photon absorptiometry, computed tomography and MRI have all been used to a limited extent in the estimation of body fat. Table 9.5 presents a summary of the

Table 9.5
Limitations of Methods of Determining Human Body Composition*

Method	Cost	Technical difficulty	Precision	
			Fat-free mass	% Fat
Water				
Deuterium	2	3	3	3
Oxygen-18	5	5	4	4
Tritium	3	3	3	3
Potassium	4	4	4	3
Creatinine	2	3	2	1
Densitometry				
Immersion	3	4	5	5
Plethysmography	4	3	5	5
Skinfold thickness	1	2	2	2
Arm circumference	1	3	2	2
Neutron activation	5	5	5	5
Photon absorptiometry	4	4	4	4
3-Methylhistidine	2	3	3	?+
Electrical				
Conductivity	5	1	4	4
Impedance	2	1	4	4
Computed tomography	5	5	?	?
Ultrasound	3	3	3	3
Infrared interactance	4	3	3	3
Magnetic resonance	5	5	?	?

Source: Taken from Lukaski, HC (1987) *American Journal of Clinical Nutrition*, **46**: 537–556.
*Ranking system: ascending scale, 1 = least and 5 – greatest
+ Unknown at this time.

cost, the technical activity and precision of estimating the compartments.

Pulmonary Rehabilitation

Whereas the overall mortality rate from heart disease is generally on the decline, in contrast, the prevalence of chronic lung disease in the Western world is increasing – most notably in females.

The majority of research evaluating the effectiveness of pulmonary rehabilitation programmes for those with chronic lung disease has focused on patients suffering from chronic obstructive airway disease. This encompasses a number of pathologies including chronic bronchitis, emphysema and asthma.

Chronic obstructive airway disease not only results in early mortality, but it also leads to a significant morbidity, disability, absenteeism from work and early retirement. It has been estimated that 10% of all hospital beds in the UK are occupied by patients suffering from chronic obstructive airway disease. It therefore has obvious economic, medical and social implications for the individual sufferer and for society in general. It should be noted that, due to the slow, insiduous onset of 20–30 years, patients presenting with noticeable symptoms are usually middle-aged or elderly.

Various definitions exist for pulmonary rehabilitation, but overall the aim is to minimize the symptoms of pulmonary disease and optimize the functional capacity of the sufferer. Before interest developed in pulmonary rehabilitation, the preferred treatment for those suffering from chronic lung disease was inactivity and rest, which led increasingly to physical deconditioning. Pulmonary rehabilitation encourages physical reconditioning, and an improvement in exercise capacity.

Prior to undertaking a pulmonary rehabilitation programme, all patients must be fully assessed. If possible, an exercise test should be performed. This is generally an incremental, symptom-limited test using an ergometer. Patients are closely monitored throughout the test, particularly for oxygen saturation, VO_2, VCO_2, minute ventilation and by electrocardiography, if necessary. VO_2 is an indicator of metabolic work and anaerobic threshold. However, due to the ventilatory limitations of a lot of these patients, many never attain anaerobic threshold.

If ergometer tests are not available, simple walking tests such as the 6- or 12-minute walking test also give a good, though basic, indication of exercise tolerance.

Throughout the assessment, patients grade their shortness of breath using the Borg scale.

In addition to physical assessment, psychosocial evaluation is necessary, as many patients suffering chronic respiratory disease also have symptoms of anxiety, depression, fear and apprehension which may affect their exercise capabilities and their activities of daily living (ADL).

The only reported contraindications for inclusion in pulmonary rehabilitation programmes are psychotic disorders, severe weight loss, cor pulmonale or other serious cardiac disorders.

The programme is tailored to the individual and consists in education of both the patient and their family, patient training and exercise. The education component consists in advice on drug management, anatomy and physiology of the lungs, preventing infection and exacerbation, sexuality, smoking cessation and nutrition information. Undernourishment, a problem for many chronic obstructive airway disease patients, adversely affects respiratory function due to reduced lung surfactant metabolism and lung defence mechanisms, as well as weakening of respiratory muscles due to loss of muscle protein.

The patient-training component may include methods of breathing control, positioning, relaxation and methods of chest clearance.

No agreement exists for the best form of exercise. Studies have examined upper limb exercise, lower limb exercise, walking, stair climbing, modified aerobics, exercise in water and respiratory muscle training. Upper limb exercise has been reported to require higher ventilatory demand for a given workload than lower limb exercise or respiratory muscle training. Although respiratory muscle training has been found to reduce respiratory rate, increase tidal volume and overall exercise tolerance, it must be avoided in patients with existing fatigue of the diaphragm, as further loading may lead to respiratory failure and the need for mechanical ventilation. Patients prone to exercise-induced hypoxaemia will require supplementary oxygen throughout the exercise sessions. Patients are monitored during the sessions by respiratory rate, heart rate, oxygen saturation or the Borg scale. Researchers agree that submaximal exercise sessions should be undertaken a minimum of three times per week. The length of each session has been variable (20–90 minutes), perhaps reflecting the disability of the participants. The rehabilitation programmes studied have lasted 6–12 weeks, with patients being advised to continue at home.

Regardless of the exercise programme, reconditioning has been found to increase exercise capacity with reduced heart rate, reduced minute ventilation and reduced carbon dioxide production. The exact mechanism responsible for these changes is uncertain, but is thought to be increased efficiency of movement and enhanced uptake of oxygen in exercising muscles. Other proposed improvements following pulmonary rehabilitation are shown in Table 9.6. Although the subjective improvements in respiratory symptoms have been found, no significant changes in pulmonary function tests, specifically FEV_1 and the FVC measures of airway obstruction, have been reported. It has been suggested that the main benefit of pulmonary rehabilitation is an improvement in psychosocial wellbeing, and that any increase in exercise capacity is as a result of this.

No significant changes in cardiac function have been seen following pulmonary rehabilitation, due to respiratory symptoms limiting the intensity of the exercise before reaching a level appropriate for cardiac training. Similarly, no change in mortality has been found.

Overall, the outcome of pulmonary rehabilitation may depend on the severity of signs and symptoms, previous levels of fitness, ventricular function, reactivity of bronchi and social circumstances.

Ultimately, more research is required into pulmonary rehabilitation to understand how improvements can be obtained. In addition, expansion of programmes to include those suffering from restrictive lung disease, postoperative pulmonary surgery and children with asthma and cystic fibrosis must be considered. The exercise prescription also requires further assessment — general exercise or specific respiratory muscle training? New developments such as passive mobilization of the joints and soft tissues of the thorax and shoulder girdle should also be considered. The availability of objective data in many areas would supplement the subjective clinical judgements often relied upon in the current practice of pulmonary rehabilitation.

Table 9.6
Proposed Improvements following Pulmonary Rehabilitation

- Reduced anxiety and depression
- Increased $VO_{2\ max}$
- Reduced blood lactate
- Increased endurance
- Reduced smoking
- Reduced respiratory symptoms
- Reduced hospitalization
- Improved quality of life
- Increased knowledge
- Increased early return to work

Cardiac Rehabilitation

Since the 1970s, there has been a radical change in the care of patients with cardiac conditions, with a much more active approach being adopted. Prior to 1970, patients who had suffered a myocardial infarction (MI) were almost completely immobilized for six weeks or more. It was thought that the damaged myocardium required time to form scar tissue. Studies in the early 1980s found that no adverse effects were obtained with early mobilization. On the contrary, there were detrimental physiological and psychological effects with prolonged bed rest, such as reduced physical work capacity, reduced $VO_{2\ max}$, increased resting heart rate, wasting of skeletal muscle, demineralization of bone, loss of postural vasomotor reflexes, reduced pulmonary function and an increase in the number of red blood cells relative to plasma volume, contributing to the risk of thromboembolism. Bed rest can also contribute to a deterioration in psychological health.

The promising results of the more active approach to rehabilitation during hospitalization immediately after MI have led to a similarly more active approach to rehabilitation post-MI after discharge from hospital. The value of this active approach has been confirmed by the Royal College of Physicians (1992) which recommended that every major district hospital treating patients with heart disease should provide a multidisciplinary cardiac rehabilitation programme, with exercise forming the basis of that programme, to be supplemented by education and counselling if available.

The potential benefits of exercise for post-MI patients and for coronary artery bypass graft surgery (CABGS) patients are well established. Patients with other groups of cardiac conditions can also benefit from exercise, including those with valve surgery, cardiac transplantation, angina pectoris, mild cardiac failure, percutaneous transluminal coronary angioplasty and congenital heart lesions in young patients.

More specifically, the goals for cardiac rehabilitation are as follows:

- Counteract the deleterious effects of inactivity.
- Improve cardiovascular efficiency.
- Reduce atherogenic risk factors in the development of coronary heart disease.
- Reduce future coronary events.
- Reduce and manage limiting symptoms.

- Maintain and enhance mental wellbeing and quality of life.

There are two phases of cardiac rehabilitation: in hospital where early mobilization reduces the effects of bed rest and after hospital, where programmes can start as early as four weeks' post-MI and six weeks for CABGS. Cardiac rehabilitation can take the form of organized classes or can be home-based. Long-term maintenance programmes are often continued in the community.

Exercise prescription should ensure that physical activity is delivered in a systematic, individualized and safe manner. The prescription will also encompass the patient's own needs, current level of activity and other aspects of health status (e.g. presence of arthritis). The prescription will include variables of mode, intensity, duration and frequency of exercise. If the prescription is satisfactory, the patient will be exposed to their training sensitivity, or zone, for long enough and often enough to experience physiological and psychological benefits.

The structure of an exercise class is similar to that described above on exercise and lifestyle. Warm-up and warm-down are incorporated, and the training overload period will primarily be aerobic/endurance in nature. The mode of activity may be walking, aerobic dance, swimming, etc. requiring large muscle mass and movements which are rhythmic in nature. High-intensity isometric activity or high resistance weight-lifting are not recommended since they also tend to raise arterial blood pressure. The intensity of the exercise need not be of a high level (e.g. between 40% and 80% of functional capacity). As heart rate correlates closely with myocardial oxygen uptake, it is often used as the basis of appropriate exercise intensity prescription.

Exercise tolerance testing, usually on a treadmill,

may be carried out at approximately six weeks. During the test, onset of symptoms or electrocardiographic changes can determine the percentage of the patient's maximum heart rate used for training. Many protocols may not always achieve the patient's true maximum.

More recently, the STEEP treadmill protocol has been more widely used, as it also appears to be more sensitive to the abilities of the patient. Not all programmes are able to have exercise tolerance testing for all cardiac rehabilitation patients. Other, less accurate, methods may be required (e.g. the age-adjusted maximum heart rate using the formula [220 − subject's age] to determine the percentage of maximum heart rate). The Borg scale for the rating of perceived exercise is extensively being incorporated, with the addition of other verbal or visual cues to determine the patient's perceived level of activity. Approximately 12–16 on the Borg scale is recommended for cardiac rehabilitation. This scale is very useful for patients on beta-blocker medication or transplant patients, where the use of heart rate to determine appropriate exercise intensity is difficult or impossible.

The standard duration and frequency of aerobic activity in this context are three sessions of 15–30 minutes' aerobic exercise per week. In addition, there are warm-up and warm-down periods in each session. It is thought that if the intensity of the session is light to moderate, the duration and frequency can be increased (e.g. five sessions of 20 minutes). The rate of progression depends on the individual.

Improvements in cardiovascular efficiency with cardiac rehabilitation are *not* concerned with improvements in *peak* performance, i.e. ability to work at near maximum levels of $VO_{2\ max}$. Instead, the ability to maintain activity at lower percentages of $VO_{2\ max}$ is the desired outcome of cardiac rehabilitation. An augmented $VO_{2\ max}$ has the advantage that the patient can now accomplish ordinary tasks (e.g. stair climbing) at a lower percentage of their $VO_{2\ max}$. This is primarily achieved by enhanced peripheral circulation in skeletal muscle and improved ability to utilize oxygen. In turn, the ability of the patient to perform normal activities at decreased levels of perceived effort will enhance the quality of life.

The lowering of heart rate both at rest and during submaximal activity results from improvements in left ventricular contractile function, increasing stroke volume and cardiac output. Contributing to this decreased heart rate is the reduced sympathetic and increased parasympathetic influence on the heart.

A slowing of the heart rate prolongs the diastolic phase of the cardiac cycle, during which the coronary artery blood supply is at its peak. This decreases demand from the myocardium at these submaximal levels. Both the improved contractile performance of the myocardium and the reduced heart rate contribute to the increased level of activity before exertional angina occurs, and to the possibility of reducing anti-anginal and beta-blocker medication. An alternative mechanism for lowering anginal threshold is increased myocardial collateral vasculature, although the evidence for this at this time is not conclusive.

The effects of cardiac rehabilitation include improvements in the following modifiable cardiovascular risk factors: hypertension, elevated serum cholesterol, cigarette smoking, levels of triglycerides, low-density lipoproteins and fibrinogen, obesity, diabetes, physical inactivity, emotional stress and ECG abnormalities, as discussed on p. 191.

There is evidence that cardiac rehabiliation not only has a beneficial effect on future cardiac events, but also on rate of re-admission, reduction of medication and return to work.

Bibliography

EXERCISE AND A HEALTHY LIFESTYLE

American Academy of Physical Education Papers (1988) *Physical Activity and Ageing 22.* Champaign, IL: Human Kinetics Books.

Armstrong, N, Welsman, J (1993) Training young athletes. In Lee (ed) *Coaching Children in Sport.* London: E. & F.N. Spon.

Dishman, RD (1988) *Exercise Adherence: Its Impact on Public Health.* Champaign, Il: Human Kinetics Books.

Golanty, E (1992) *Health and Wellness,* 4th edn. London: Jones and Bartlett.

Grimley Evans, J, Goldacre, MJ, Hodkinson, M, Lamb, S, Savoy, M (1992) *Health: Abilities and Well Being in the Third Age.* Carnegie Trust Research Paper No. 9 Fife, Scotland: Carnegie Trust.

Rollands, TW (1990) *Exercise and Children's Health.* Champaign, IL: Human Kinetics Books.

Royal College of Physicians (1991) *Medical Aspects of Exercise: Benefits and Risks.* London: Royal College of Physicians.

Sports Council, Allied Dunbar, Health Education Authority (1992) *Fitness Survey.* London: The Sports Council.

Wilmore, JH (1986) *Sensible Fitness.* IL: Leisure Press.

NUTRITION

Katch, FI (ed.) (1986) *Sport Health and Nutrition 2.* Champaign, IL: Human Kinetics Publishers Inc.

Williams, C, Develin, JT (eds) (1992) *Foods, Nutrition and Sports Performance.* An International Scientific Consenus Organised by Macro, Incorporated with International Olympic Committee Patronage. London, Chapman and Hall.

Woofton, S (1989) *Nutrition for Sport.* New York: Simon and Schuster.

PRINCIPLES OF SPORTS TRAINING

Brooks, GA, Fahey, T (1984) *Exercise Physiology: Human Bioenergetics and its Application.* New York: Collier.

Dick, FW (1991) *Training Theory,* 3rd edn. London: British Amateur Athletic Board.

Fox, EL, Bowers, RW, Fosse, ML (1989) *The Physiological Basis of Physical Education and Athletics,* 4th edn. Dubuque, Iowa: WC Brown Publishers.

Reilly, T, Secler, N, Swell, P, Williams, C (eds) (1990) *Physiology of Sports.* London: E and F.N. Spon.

Shakey, BJ (1990) *Physiology of Fitness.* Champaign, IL: Human Kinetics.

THE EFFECT OF CHRONIC TRAINING ON PHYSIOLOGICAL SYSTEMS

Dudley, GA, Djanil, R (1985) Incompatibility of endurance- and strength-training modes of exercise. *Journal of Applied Physiology* 59(5): 146–151.

Hortobagyi, T, Katch, FI, Lachance, PF (1991) Effects of simultaneous training for strength and endurance on upper and lower body strength and running performance. *Journal of Sports Medicine and Physical Fitness,* 31: 20–30.

Lamb, DR, Murray, R (eds) (1988) *Perspectives in Exercise Science and Sports Medicine: Prolonged Exercise.* Benchmark Press, Inc.

Reilly, T, Secler, N, Swell, P, Williams, C (eds) (1990) *Physiology of Sports.* London: E and F.N. Spon.

Wilmore, JH, Costill, DL (1994) *Physiology of Sport and Exercise.* Champaign, IL: Human Kinetics.

SPECIFIC ISSUES RELATING TO FEMALES

American Orthopaedic Society for Sports Medicine (1993) *The Athletic Female* Pearl, AJ (ed). Champaign, IL: Human Kinetics Publishers.

Brownel, KD, Nelsonstein, S, Wilmorn, JNH (1987) Weight Regulation Practices in Athletes: An Analysis of Metabolic and Health Effects, *Med Sci Sports Exercise,* 19(6): 546–556.

Drinkwater, B (1984) Woman and Exercise; Physiological Aspects. *Exercise and Sport Science Reviews,* 12: 21–25.

Loucks, A (1987) Skeletal demineralisation in the amenorrheic athlete. In McLeod, D, Maughan, R, Nimmo, N, Reilly, T, Williams, C (eds) *Exercise Benefits Limits and Adaptation.* London: E. & F.N. Spon.

Shangold, M, Rebarr, RW, Wentz, AC, Schiff, I (1990) Evaluation and management of menstrual dysfunction in athletes. *Journal of the American Medical Society,* 23(12): 1665–1669.

FITNESS ASSESSMENT

American College of Sports Medicine (1991) *Guidelines for Exercise Testing and Prescription.* London: Lea and Febiger.

Astrand, I (1960) Aerobic work capacity in men and women with special reference to age. *Acta Physiologica Scandinavica,* 49(Suppl.): 169.

Barr-Orr, O, Dotan, R, Inbar, O (1977) A thirty second all-out ergometric test: its reliability and validity for anaerobic capacity. *Israel Journal of Medical Sciences,* 13: 126.

Durnin, JVGA, Womersley, J (1974) Body fat assessed from total body density and its estimation for skinfold thickness measurement on 481 men and women aged 16 to 72 years. *British Journal of Nutrition,* 32: 77-97.

Jackson, AS, Pollock, ML (1978) Generalised equations predicting body density of men. *British Journal of Nutrition,* 40: 497–504.

MacDougall, DD, Wenger, HA, Green, HJ (1991) *Physiological Testing of the High Performance Athlete,* 2nd edn. Champaign, Illinois: Canadian Association of Sports Scientists and Human Kinetics.

PULMONARY REHABILITATION

Shephard, RJ (1994) *Aerobic Fitness and Health.* Leeds: Human Kinetics.

Webber, BA, Pryor, JA (1993) *Physiotherapy for Respiratory and Cardiac Problems.* Edinburgh: Churchill Livingstone.

CARDIAC REHABILITATION

Bouchard, C, Shephard, RJ, Stephens, T (1994) *Physical Activity, Fitness and Health — International Proceedings and Consensus Statement.* Leeds: Human Kinetics.

Connors, G, Hilling, L (eds) (1993) *Guidelines for Pulmonary Rehabilitation Programmes.* Champaign, Illinois: Human Kinetics.

Horgan, J, Bethel, C, Carson, P *et al.* (1992) Working Party Report on Cardiac Rehabilitation. *British Heart Journal,* **67**: 462–468.

Meade, TW, Mellows, S, Brozovic, M *et al.* (1986) Haemostatic function and ischaemic heart disease — principal results of the Northwick Park Heart Study. *Lancet,* **2**: 553–557.

Royal College of Physicians (1992) Working Party Report on Cardiac Rehabilitation. *British Heart Journal,* **67**: 412–418.

Shephard, RJ (1968) Exercise and lifestyle change. *British Journal of Sports Medicine,* **23**: 11–22.

Todd, IC, Ballantyne, D (1990) Antianginal efficacy of exercise training: a comparison with beta-blockade. *British Heart Journal,* **64**: 14–19.

Webber, BA, Pryor, JA (1993) *Physiotherapy for Respiratory and Cardiac Problems.* Edinburgh: Churchill Livingstone.

Glossary

Acinar Gland Gland with sac-shaped secretory portion(s).

Acne A skin disorder characterized by the inflammation of sebaceous glands.

Actin Thin filamentous protein involved in muscle contraction.

Active transport Energy-dependent movement of a substance, via a carrier molecule, across a membrane against its concentration gradient.

Adenosine triphosphate (ATP) Energy storage molecule containing adenine and three phosphate groups. The bonds between the adenine and the phosphate groups store energy which can be released for use inside the cell when a phosphate is cleaved from the molecule.

Adipocyctes Connective tissue cells which store neutral fats.

Adipose tissue Fatty tissue made up of accumulations of adipocytes.

Adrenal gland Endocrine gland found at the apex of each kidney, comprising a clearly distinguishable cortex and a medulla.

Adrenal medulla The middle portion of the adrenal gland, which synthesizes and releases the hormones noradrenaline and adrenaline.

Aerobic Uses oxygen.

Agglutination The process of clumping of red blood cells which occurs upon contact of cells of one blood group with those of a different group due to the reaction of agglutinogens on the cell surfaces with agglutinins in the plasma.

Agglutinin Plasma antibodies which react with agglutinogens such as red blood cells of a different blood group or bacteria.

Agglutinogen Antigens present on the surface of red blood cells. Used to group specific blood types.

Agonist muscle A muscle which works with another muscle to develop the same movement pattern by contracting as the original muscle contracts.

Akinesia Absence of normal movement and muscle tone.

Alpha motoneurone Motor nerve fibres located in the anterior horn of the spinal cord grey matter. Supply extrafusal fibres of the skeletal muscles.

Alveolar duct A branch of the respiratory bronchiole leading to the alveolar sacs.

Alveolar sac A group of alveoli leading from the alveolar duct.

Alveolus Small air sac in the lungs, forming part of the respiratory portion of the lung tissue.

Amenorrhoea The absence of a menstrual cycle.

Anaerobic Does not use oxygen.

Anaerobic threshold The point during exercise at which it is believed the body requires to involve the anaerobic energy pathways. It is evidenced by an increase in blood lactate.

Anatomic dead space The proportion of the tidal volume which does not take part in respiratory gas exchange, comprising the nasal passages, pharynx, larynx, trachea, bronchi and conducting bronchioles. Normally about 150 ml of the tidal volume is dead space.

Angina pectoris Chest pain, usually induced by exercise, which accompanies an inadequate blood supply to the heart muscle.

Angle of pennation This refers to the angle of the muscle fibres relative to the shaft of the bone over which the muscle fibres lie.

Ankylosing spondylitis Rheumatic condition affecting the joints of the spine, among others. In severe cases, rib cage movement may be affected.

Antagonist A muscle which works with another muscle to develop the same movement but contracts if the original muscle is relaxing or vice versa.

Anterolateral system Spinal cord pathway responsible for the transmission of sensory information concerning pain, temperature and crude touch to higher centres of the nervous system.

Antiporter A carrier molecule which, as it transports one substance across a membrane, it simultaneously transports another molecule in the opposite direction.

Aortic body Peripheral chemoreceptor responding to changes in blood levels of oxygen, carbon dioxide and pH. Located near the aortic arch.

Apneustic centre Portion of the respiratory centre in the medulla which coordinates inspiratory activity.

Apocrine A method of secretion in exocrine glands whereby a large portion of the apical membrane of a cell, full of secretion, buds off, releasing the secretion into the glandular duct.

Areolar Loosely arranged fibrous connective tissue.

Arrector pili The smooth muscle attached between hair follicles and the dermis, which upon contraction elevates the hair shaft.

Arteriole A small branch of the arterial blood supply which gives rise to the capillary blood vessels. Smooth muscle in the walls of the arterioles allows constriction and dilation of these vessels thereby regulating blood flow and arterial blood pressure.

Artery A blood vessel which transports blood away from the heart.

Astrocytes Nervous system supporting cells particularly at the blood–brain barrier.

Ataxia Impaired voluntary muscle coordination, displayed as unsteady gait and shaky movements.

Atherosclerosis Deposition of fatty plaques in the walls of arterial blood vessels, narrowing their diameter and therefore reducing flow.

Atrophy The process by which tissue loses mass.

Atrium One of the upper chambers of the heart.

Auscultation Procedure for listening for sounds within the heart or blood vessels using a stethoscope.

Avascular No blood supply.

Axon The long process extending from the cell body of a neurone which conducts impulses away from the cell body.

Baroreceptor Sensory nerve endings located in the walls of the carotid sinuses and aortic arch which respond to changes in blood pressure.

Basal ganglia Collection of deep subcortical nuclei of the cerebral hemispheres involved in motor control. *See also* Caudate nucleus, Globus pallidus, Substantia nigra, Corpus striatum.

Basal metabolic rate Metabolic rate when one is resting but not sleeping; requires a 24-hour fast preceding measurement.

Basement membrane The specialized membrane on which epithelial cells lie, separating them from the connective tissue.

Basket cells Inhibitory interneurones located in the cerebellar cortex

Bipolar neurone A type of neurone which has two processes, one axon and one dendrite, beginning from opposite poles of the cell body.

Bohr effect Displacement of oxygen from haemoglobin as a consequence of increased plasma acidity causing the oxygen–haemoglobin dissociation curve to shift to the right and downwards.

Bradykinesia Slowness of voluntary movement and initiation of movement.

Brainstem The central portion of the brain, consisting of the midbrain, pons and medulla oblongata.

Bronchitis Inflammation of the bronchi causing excess secretion of mucus from the goblet cells, leading to obstructive airway disease.

Bronchus Airways branching from the trachea, supported by cartilagenous rings in the wall.

Brown adipose tissue A tissue made up of adipocytes which are cells that store fat. Brown adipose tissue is involved in the regulation of energy balance and also in cold-induced thermogenesis.

Bundle of His Conducting fibres within the heart muscle. These are modified cardiac muscle fibres which transmit the wave of electrical excitation from the atrium into the ventricles. Also known as the atrioventricular bundle.

Callus An area of tissue repair, particularly in broken bones, where re-unification of the broken ends occurs, initially resulting in a thickened area of that particular tissue.

Calmodulin A protein which can bind calcium ions regulating their free concentration, found, for example, in smooth-muscle cells.

Canaliculi Fine small channels found in bone that link the spaces in which the bone cells are found.

Cancellous bone Spongy bone.

Capillary The smallest of the blood vessels, which form networks of vessels in the tissues – the capillary beds. These vessels are the site of exchange of respiratory gases and nutrients from the blood to the tissues and vice versa.

Carbaminohaemoglobin Haemoglobin bound to carbon dioxide.

Carbonic anhydrase Enzyme present in the red blood cells which catalyses the formation of carbonic acid from water and carbon dioxide.

Carotid body Peripheral chemoreceptor responding to changes in blood levels of oxygen, carbon dioxide and pH. Located in the carotid sinus.

Cardiac cycle The complete series of events from the beginning of one heart beat to the next. The cycle comprises contraction of the atria pushing blood into the ventricles (atrial systole) followed by relaxation of the atria (atrial diastole) and contraction of the ventricles ejecting blood into the pulmonary and systemic circulations (ventricular systole). This is followed by relaxation of the ventricles (ventricular diastole) before the next cycle begins. The duration of the cycle is variable depending on the heart rate.

Cardiac output The volume output of the heart per unit time, given as the product of heart rate and stroke volume.

Cardiovascular centre Medullary controlling centre for cardiovascular function. Output is via the autonomic nervous system.

Carrier-mediated transport Transport processes which rely on a protein molecule to move substances across a membrane.

Cartilage A highly resilient dense connective tissue of which there are three types. It is found, for example, on the ends of long bones in the trachea, intervertebral discs, etc.

Caudate nucleus One of the basal ganglia.

Cell body The portion of a neurone containing the nucleus.

Central sulcus Deep fissure of the surface of the cerebrum forming the boundary between the frontal and parietal lobes of the cerebral hemispheres.

Centrioles Paired cylindrical microtubular structures with a role in cell division.

Centrosome An area of the cytoplasm in which the centrioles are found.

Cerebellum 'Little brain'. Consists of two highly folded hemispheres lying at the base of the brain, over the pons and medulla. Has an important role in motor control.

Cerebral cortex The surface layer of the cerebral hemispheres. Different cortical areas have different functional specialisms.

Cerebrospinal fluid The fluid which surrounds the brain and spinal cord, secreted by cells in the cerebral ventricles.

Cerebrovascular accident A sudden decrease in blood supply to an area of the brain due to a blood clot, or atherosclerosis, leading to a stroke.

Chemoreceptors Specialized receptors responsible for detecting changes in the oxygen, carbon dioxide and pH levels of the blood and cerebrospinal fluid.

Chloride shift Movement of chloride ions from the plasma into the red blood cells in order to balance the diffusion of bicarbonate ions out of the red blood cells.

Cholesterol A lipid molecule found in blood and tissues which is also an important constituent of cell membranes. Excessive cholesterol is associated with atheroma.

Chondrocytes Connective tissue cells which produce cartilage.

Chondroitin sulphate A mucopolysaccharide produced by chondrocytes which is an important component of the extracellular matrix of cartilage.

Chordae tendinae Fibrous cords connecting the heart valves with the papillary muscles in the wall of the ventricles. These prevent eversion of the heart valves during ventricular contraction.

Chromatin The content of the nucleus comprising DNA (the genetic material) and proteins.

Chromosome One of the 46 structures that carry genetic information and which are formed from the chromatin during cell division.

Chylomicron A droplet consisting of protein and lipid which is absorbed into the lacteal of the villus of the small intestine.

Cilia Motile hair-like structures formed from microtubules, that project from the surface of some types of epithelial cells.

Cisternae The interior portions of the endoplasmic retiulum and the Golgi apparatus.

Climbing fibre Excitatory inputs to the Purkinje cells of the cerebellar cortex, arising from the inferior olive.

Coagulation The process of blood clotting.

Collagen A type of connective tissue protein with high resistance to tensile strains.

Collateral circulation An alternative pathway for the flow of blood via a different set of blood vessels when the main pathway becomes blocked or closed.

Colloid osmotic pressure The osmotic pressure produced by the presence of proteins in the plasma.

Compact bone Dense bone.

Compliance Volume change per unit pressure change in the lungs, giving a measure of the distensibility of the lungs – the ease with which the lungs can be expanded.

Compound gland A single gland but made up of numerous secretory portions all leading into one duct.

Compound or **stratified epithelium** Multilayered structure of epithelial cells.

Concentric contractions Contraction of the muscle which results in shortening.

Conductive zone The part of the respiratory passages which are responsible for conducting air to the respiratory portion of the lungs.

Congestive heart failure Impaired cardiac function as a consequence of congestion of blood within the heart chambers.

Connective tissue One of the four main classes of tissues within the body. It consists of varying types of extracellular matrix.

Contraction The ability of a structure to shorten (e.g. in muscle) where the shortening results in the generation of tension and a subsequent movement.

Contralateral Referring to the opposite side of the body.

Cordotomy A pathological condition where the spinal cord is severed.

Coronary arteries The arteries which supply blood to the heart muscle itself.

Corpus callosum 'Hard body'. Connecting bridge of nerve fibres running between the right and left cerebral hemispheres.

Corpus striatum Collective name given to the caudate nucleus and the putamen of the basal ganglia. The name derives from the striped appearance of these nuclei.

Corticospinal tract Spinal cord pathway running from the motor cortex to the motoneurones of anterior horn of the spinal cord. The lateral corticospinal tract carries crossed fibres from the opposite cerebral hemisphere and supplies the motoneurones of distal muscle groups. The ventral corticospinal tract carries uncrossed fibres from the cerebral hemisphere of the same side and supplies motoneurones of proximal muscle groups.

Co-transport Carrier-mediated transport mechanisms which move two or more substances in the same direction across a membrane.

Cristae The foldings of the inner membrane of a mitochondrion which are the sites of chemical reactions producing ATP.

Cuneate fascicle Cuneate = 'wedge-shaped'. Ascending spinal cord pathway making up the lateral portion of the dorsal columns. Carries sensory axons from receptors involved in touch and proprioception in the upper portions of the body to the cuneate nucleus of the medulla.

Cuneate nucleus One of two medullary nuclei which receive input from ascending fibres of the dorsal columns.

Cystic fibrosis A genetically inherited condition which affects the exocrine glands of the body. There is production of a thick mucus which can obstruct the respiratory passages, among others.

Cytoplasm The semi-fluid-like environment within a cell.

Cytoskeleton Protein scaffolding found within a cell.

Dendrite A process of a neurone that receives inputs and which transmits them to the cell body.

Dense bodies Sites of attachment for actin filaments inside smooth cells.

Dentate nucleus A deep nucleus of the cerebellum.

Dermis The loose connective tissue layer of the skin underlying the epithelial layer which contains blood vessels and nerve fibres.

Deoxyribonucleic acid (DNA) Genetic material of a cell.

Diaphragm Dome-shaped muscle separating the thoracic and abdominal cavities. Contraction of the diaphragm flattens the muscle, thereby enlarging the volume of the thoracic cavity and causing the lungs to expand.

Diaphysis The shaft or central portion of a long bone.

Diastole The period of relaxation of the heart during the cardiac cycle.

Dicrotic notch A small deviation in the aortic pressure wave caused by the closure of the aortic valve.

Discipline disinhibition The ability to remove inhibition from some motor units facilitating their recruitment. Believed that it can be accomplished with speed training techniques.

Dorsal column/medial lemniscal pathway Ascending sensory pathway conveying proprioceptive and touch information to higher centres.

Dorsal columns Ascending spinal cord pathway located in the dorsal portion of the spinal cord white matter. Conveys proprioceptive and touch information to higher centres.

Dorsal horn The posterior portion of the spinal cord grey matter.

Dysarthria Disorder affecting the control of muscles responsible for speech.

Dysdiadochokinesia A disorder associated with cerebellar disease demonstrated as an inability to perform rapid, alternating movements such as tapping a surface or rotating the wrists.

Dystrophin A cytoskeletal protein.

Eccentric contraction A muscle contraction where the external forces exceed the tension in the muscle. The muscle therefore lengthens.

Eccrine A mode of secretion where the secretory products pass from the cell through the membrane with no apparent loss of membrane.

Elastic recoil Elastic forces generated by stretching of a tissue (especially the elastic connective tissue elements) which tend to produce collapse (recoil) of the tissue when the stretch is removed. It is of particular importance in the major arteries and in the lungs.

Elastic strength The ability to develop a rebound force from an eccentric contraction.

Elastin A connective tissue protein with the ability to stretch and return to its original size.

Electrolyte A substance which becomes ionized when it is immersed in an aqueous solution.

Electromyography The technique of recording the electrical potentials associated with muscle contraction. Recordings can be made via surface electrodes placed on the skin overlying the muscle, or by needle electrodes placed directly into the muscle itself.

Electron transport chain A series of enzymes and proteins found on the mitochondrial cristae through which electrons are transferred during oxidation–reduction reactions. The electrons are used in the formation of ATP and metabolic water.

Emphysema Disease causing enlargement of the air sacs of the lungs and destruction of alveolar capillaries.

End-diastolic volume The volume left in the ventricles at the end of the relaxation phase of the cardiac cycle, during which the ventricles have filled with blood.

Endochondrial Within cartilage.

Endocrine A ductless gland whose secretion passes directly from the secretory cells into the blood. Secretions are normally hormones.

Endocytosis The uptake of large amounts of material into the cell by membrane-bound vesicles.

Endoneurium The fibrous connective tissue that separates individual nerves within nerve fibres.

Endoplasmic reticulum Membrane-bound series of interconnected channels throughout the cell. When ribosomes are present on the surface, it is classed as 'rough', when no ribosomes present it is regarded as 'smooth'.

Endosteum The membrane that lines the marrow cavity of bone tissue.

End-systolic volume The volume left in the ventricles at the end of the ejection phase of the cardiac cycle.

Endurance The ability to perform for a prolonged period.

Eosinophil Type of white blood cell.

Epidermis The epithelial outer layer of the skin.

Epimysium The fibrous connective tissue that surrounds bone.

Epiphysis The end of a long bone.

Epithelium A tissue that lines or covers all surfaces of the body.

Erythrocytes Red blood cells

Erythropoiesis The process of formation of red blood cells in the bone marrow.

Erythropoietin A hormone produced by cells in the kidney which stimulates the process of red blood cell formation.

Exocrine Glandular tissue where the secretory product is released from the cells into a duct which transmits the secretion on an epithelial surface.

Exocytosis Bulk movement of substances from within a cell to the outside of the cell via membrane-bound vesicles.

Expiratory reserve volume The volume of air which can be expelled from the lungs following a normal tidal expiration.

Extracellular matrix Chemical substances located between cells.

Extrafusal muscle fibres The main muscle fibres of a skeletal muscle (not those within the muscle spindles).

Facilitated diffusion Transport of substances across the cell membrane which requires the presence of a carrier molecule but which does not require the expenditure of energy.

Fasiculus A bundle of muscle fibres.

Fast twitch fatigue-resistant muscle fibre A fibre within skeletal muscle which is fast contracting but fatigues quickly.

Fast twitch fatigueable muscle fibre A fibre within skeletal muscle which is fast contracting and has the biochemical attributes to contract for long periods.

Fibrillation Uncoordinated contraction of cardiac muscle cells, resulting in impaired contractile efficiency of the heart.

Fibrin An insoluble plasma protein formed at the last stage of blood coagulation.

Fibrinogen Soluble precursor of fibrin.

Fibroblast A connective tissue cell that produces connective tissue fibres.

Flagella A microtubular organelle on some cell surfaces, that produces a 'whip-like' action to move the cell along.

Flocculonodular lobe A lobe of the cerebellum formed from the flocculus and the nodulus (smaller lobes of the cerebellum). This lobe receives inputs from the vestibular system.

Forced expiratory volume in 1 second (FEV$_1$) The volume of air which is expired after one second during a maximum forced expiration. In normal circumstances this is about 80% of the forced vital capacity. Obstructive and restrictive lung diseases may alter this figure.

Forced capacity The maximum amount of air which can be expelled from the lungs during a maximum forced expiration.

Frontal lobe The front portion of the cerebral hemispheres.

Functional residual capacity The total amount of air left in the lungs after a normal tidal expiration.

Gamma motoneurone Small motor nerves supplying the muscle fibres of the muscle spindle (*see* Intrafusal fibres).

Genes The hereditary material of the cell. Also known as DNA, chromosome, chromatin.

Globus pallidus One of the basal ganglia. One of the major outputs from the basal ganglia to the thalamus.

Glycolysis The process of enzyme activities which breaks down glucose to two molecules of pyruvate (aerobic) or two molecules of lactate (anaerobic).

Goblet cells Unicellular exocrine glands that produce mucus.

Golgi apparatus A series of membrane-bound sacs within a cell that are involved with the sorting, packaging and processing of manufactured proteins.

Golgi tendon organ A sensory receptor located at the musculotendinous junction responsible for detecting changes in muscle tension. Gives rise to type Ib afferent fibres.

Gracile fascicle Gracile = 'thin'. Ascending spinal cord pathway making up the medial portion of the dorsal columns. Carries sensory information concerning touch and proprioception from the lower body to the gracile nucleus of the medulla.

Gracile nucleus One of two medullary nuclei which receive input from ascending fibres of the dorsal columns.

Granule cells Excitatory cells located in the cerebellar cortex. These cells, in turn, receive excitatory inputs from mossy fibres.

Grey matter The central portion of the central nervous system, consisting of nerve cell bodies.

Haematocrit The proportion of red blood cells in a sample of blood.

Haemoglobin Oxygen-carrying molecule within red blood cells, composed of the protein globin and the pigment haem.

Haversian system The concentric ring structure of compact bone.

Heparin An anticoagulant produced by liver cells.

Hering–Breuer reflex Reflex arising from stretching of pulmonary stretch receptors causing inhibition of lung inflation.

Histochemical profiling Frozen tissue is cut into very thin sections. Serial sections of tissue are then reacted for different enzyme activities. The deposit arising from the enzyme activity is deposited at the site of the reaction. Therefore it is possible, if it is in muscle tissue, to build up a picture of the enzyme activities of any one fibre.

Holocrine Mode of secretion whereby the secretory cell disintegrates releasing its contents.

Homeostasis The maintenance of a relatively constant internal environment within the human body.

Huntington's disease Degenerative disease of the basal ganglia affecting cholinergic and GABA-ergic cells of the corpus striatum.

Hydroxyapatite Calcium phosphate salts in bone tissue.

Hypercapnia Increased levels of carbon dioxide in the blood.

Hyperkalaemia High blood levels of potassium.

Hypernatraemia High blood levels of sodium.

Hyperosmotic Solutions with a greater salt concentration than a reference solution.

Hyperplasia An increase in the size of a tissue due to an increase in the number of cells.

Hypertension High blood pressure.

Hypertonia Increased muscle tone.

Hypertrophy An increase in the size of a tissue due to an increase in the size of the cell.

Hyperventilation Increased rate and / or depth of breathing resulting in an increased total ventilation.

Hypo-osmotic Solutions with a salt concentration less than a reference solution.

Hypothalamus A region of the forebrain which contains several important centres for controlling thirst, satiety, temperature regulation and water balance. The hypothalamus secretes hormones and has both nervous and vascular connections with the endocrine pituitary gland.

Hypoxaemia Low oxygen levels in the blood.

Hypoxia Low oxygen levels in the tissues.

Inspiratory capacity The total amount of air that can be taken into the lungs during a maximum inspiration.

Inspiratory reserve volume The total amount of air that can be taken into the lungs after a normal tidal inspiration.

Integral proteins These are proteins that span the width of the plasma membrane.

Intention tremor Tremor affecting the limbs of subjects with cerebellar disease, manifested only during actual movement.

Intercalated discs These are structures that link the ends of different cardiac muscle cells to one another. The discs anchor the cells to one another and allow electrical connection through gap junctions present in their structure.

Intercostal muscles Muscles lying in the spaces between the ribs. The outer external intercostals elevate the ribs to cause inspiration, while the deeper internal intercostals pull the ribs together during forced expiration.

Intermittent positive pressure ventilation (IPPV) Mechanical ventilation produced by intermittent application of positive pressure to the airways in order to inflate the lungs. When the positive pressure is removed, the lungs are allowed to deflate passively.

Interneurones Small neurones responsible for relaying information from one nerve cell to another — the overall balance of excitatory and inhibitory input to the interneurones is important for integration of information within the nervous system.

Intrafusal fibres The small muscle fibres found inside the muscle spindle. These muscle fibres can alter the sensitivity of the spindle to stretch.

Intramembranous Between membranes.

Ipsilateral Referring to the same side of the body.

Ischaemia Reduced blood supply to a tissue.

Isovolumic contraction The period during the cardiac cycle when the ventricles are contracting, but pressure within the ventricles has not risen to a sufficient level to open the valves. Blood is therefore not ejected from the ventricles during this time.

Isovolumic relaxation The period during the cardiac cycle when the ventricles are relaxing and pressure within the ventricles is falling, but there is no change in ventricular volume.

J-receptors (juxtacapillary receptors) Receptors located in the alveolar walls close to the capillaries which respond to chemical changes in the pulmonary interstitial fluid.

Keratin Tough protein that is produced in the cells of the uppermost layers of the epidermis.

Korotkoff sounds The sounds generated by turbulent blood flow within the brachial artery during the measurement of blood pressure. These sounds are heard using a stethoscope placed over the artery.

Krebs/TCA (tricarboxylic acid) cycle A cyclic set of enzyme-catalysed reactions that occur inside the matrix of the mitochondrion in which electrons, removed from substrates, are utilized in the electron-transport chain to produce ATP.

Lactate A product of the anaerobic metabolism of glucose.

Lacunae Spaces in compact bone occupied by osteocytes.

Larynx The air passage between the pharynx and the trachea, responsible for the generation of vocal sounds.

Lean body mass The body mass which does not include fat.

Leukocytes White blood cells.

Ligament Dense connective tissue made up of collagen fibres bundled together. Ligaments have strength and flexibility but cannot stretch.

Lymphocyte A type of white blood cell involved in immunity. Found in the lymph nodes and spleen.

Lysosomes Intracellular membrane-bound vesicles which contain powerful digestive enzymes.

Mast cells Large cells found in connective tissues which have a granular appearance. Granules contain chemicals such as heparin, histamine and serotonin.

Mechanical ventilation Artificial means employed to produce respiratory movements in patients who are unable to do this spontaneously.

Medial lemniscus Tract of ascending sensory nerve fibres projecting from the cuneate and gracile fascicles of the medulla to the contralateral ventroposterolateral nucleus of the thalamus.

Medulla oblongata The lower portion of the brainstem — contains the respiratory and cardiovascular control centres.

Megakaryocyte Bone marrow cell which forms platelets.

Melanocyte Skin cell which produces the pigment melanin giving skin coloration.

Menarche Onset of puberty.

Mesenchyme Embryonic form of connective tissue cell from which all adult connective tissues are derived.

Metabolic rate Total body energy expenditure at any particular activity.

Metabolism A term which describes all the chemical reactions that occur in the body.

Metaphysis The middle portion of a bone where growth occurs.

Microglia Brain macrophage cells.

Microvilli Minute folds of the apical plasma membrane of some epithelial cells.

Mitochondria Cellular organelle involved in ATP production. Sometimes referred to as the cell's 'powerhouse'.

Mitral valve Bicuspid valve between the left atrium and the left ventricle.

Monocyte Type of white blood cell involved in phagocytosis of foreign particles and bacteria.

Motoneurone The final common pathway through which activity in the nervous system is transmitted to the muscles and glands of the periphery. These are also sometimes referred to as lower motoneurones and anterior horn cells.

Motor cortex Part of the cerebral cortex lying anterior to the central sulcus in the frontal lobe which is responsible for the final motor output from the brain. It is somatotopically organized.

Motor unit A functional unit consisting of an alpha motoneurone and all the skeletal muscle fibres which it innervates.

Mossy fibre One of the afferent inputs to the cerebellar cortex.

Mucus Viscous fluid secreted by mucous-secreting glands.

Multipolar nerve Neurone with several processes emanating from the cell body, which transmit impulses towards the cell body.

Muscle spindle Sensory receptor located within the bulk of a skeletal muscle and which is sensitive to muscle stretch. Gives rise to type Ia afferent fibres.

Muscular dystrophy Genetically inherited disease that results in muscle degeneration. Affects males only.

Myelin The complex phospholipid sheath produced by Schwann cells that surrounds the axons of certain neurones.

Myocardial infarction Death of heart muscle tissue as a result of impaired blood supply.

Myocardium Heart muscle tissue.

Myofibrils Contractile filaments of a striated muscle.

Myosin Thick contractile protein of muscle cells.

Neuroglia A type of neuronal connective tissue cell.

Neurone A nerve cell.

Neurotransmitter A chemical substance released from the synaptic terminal of a nerve cell which alters the membrane properties of the postsynaptic cell by binding to specific receptor sites on the postsynaptic cell membrane. Examples of neurotransmitters include acetylcholine, noradrenaline, dopamine and gamma-aminobutyric acid (GABA).

Neutrophil Type of white blood cell responsible for defence against infection, by ingesting and killing invading bacteria.

Nociception The sensitivity to noxious stimulation or pain.

Nodes of Ranvier Microscopic gaps in the myelin sheath between Schwann cells.

Noradrenaline Hormone secreted by the adrenal medulla and a neurotransmitter released from sympathetic nerve terminals.

Nucleolus Site of RNA synthesis in the cell's nucleus.

Nucleus (brain) A functional collection of nerve cell bodies within the grey matter of the central nervous system.

Nucleus (cell) The cell organelle that contains the genetic information.

Nystagmus Rhythmic, rapid, involuntary movements of the eye.

OBLA Onset of blood lactate accumulation; a point at either 2 or 4 mmol l^{-1} which is used as a standard reference point during exercise.

Oedema Accumulation of fluid in the extracellular spaces of the body tissues leading to tissue swelling.

Oligodendrocytes Another type of neuronal connective tissue cell.

Organelles Structures within cells that perform specific functions.

Osmosis The movement of water through a semi-permeable membrane to equalize concentrations of solutes on either side of the membrane.

Ossification Laying down and formation of the mineral matrix of bone.

Osteoblasts Cells responsible for the formation of bone.

Osteoclasts Cells which dissolve the mineral matrix of bone releasing calcium.

Osteocyte Adult bone cell which maintains the daily activities of the bone.

Osteomalacia This is a pathological condition in which the mineralization of the bone is incomplete.

Oxyhaemoglobin Haemoglobin bound to oxygen.

Papillary muscles Small projections of muscle tissue on the inner surface of the ventricle walls. They connect to the chordae tendinae and help to prevent eversion of the heart valves during contraction.

Parathyroid glands Endocrine glands that overlie the thyroid gland. They produce parathyroid hormone which regulates calcium levels in the body by promoting calcium release from bones.

Parietal lobe The portion of the cerebral hemispheres which lies behind the central sulcus. Contains the sensory cortex.

Parkinson's disease Degenerative disease of the basal ganglia, affecting the dopaminergic cells of the substantia nigra. Symptoms include resting tremor, slowness of movement and gait abnormalities.

Partial pressure The pressure exerted by a gas in a mixture, calculated as the percentage volume of the gas multiplied by the total pressure exerted by the whole gas mixture. For example, the percentage of oxygen in the atmosphere is 20.9%, while the total atmospheric pressure at sea level is about 760 mmHg. This gives a partial pressure of oxygen (PO_2) of 20.9% of 760 = 158 mmHg.

Peak expiratory flow rate The maximum rate of flow of air out of the lungs during a maximum forced expiration.

Perfusion The flow of blood through the vessels of a tissue.

Periaqueductal grey matter (PAGM) A region of the grey matter which surrounds the cerebral aqueduct in the midbrain. Involved in the modulation of pain transmission.

Perichondrium The connective sheath that covers the outside of cartilage.

Perimysium The connective sheath that separates muscle fibres into bundles.

Periosteum The connective sheath that covers the outside of bones.

Peripheral proteins Proteins of the plasma membrane that lie on one leaflet of the membrane only. They do not span the width of the membrane.

Peroxisomes Membrane-bound cellular vesicles containing specialized enzymes involved with detoxification in certain cells, e.g. liver cells.

Phagocytosis The process where extraneous matter is engulfed by certain cells (phagocytic cells) and destroyed.

Pharynx The throat. A muscular tube extending from the nasal passages, through the oral cavity to connect with the larynx. The pharynx also opens into the oesophagus.

Piezoelectric Minute electrical currents.

Pinocytosis Also known as 'cell drinking'. This is the process where dissolved substances are taken into the cell by the creation of vesicles.

Plasma The fluid component of the blood.

Plasma cells B-lymphocytes that have been activated to produce antibodies for immunity.

Plasmin The plasma enzyme which digests fibrin in order to dissolve blood clots. Plasmin is derived from an inactive precursor – plasminogen.

Platelets Small cell fragments essential for normal blood clotting.

Plyometrics A type of dynamic resistance training whereby it is believed that more motor units are recruited by incorporating the stretch reflex.

Pneumotaxic centre Part of the respiratory centre in the medulla which inhibits the inspiratory area, thus limiting inspiration.

Positive end expiratory pressure (PEEP) Mechanical aid to ventilation produced by application of positive pressure at the end of a normal expiration. This prevents collapse of the alveoli in patients who have a higher than normal elastic recoil of the lung tissue.

Power The rate of performing work.

Precapillary sphincter Smooth muscle ring located at the entrance to the capillary beds which regulates blood flow through the capillaries.

Primary active transport Carrier-mediated transport across the plasma membrane that requires the direct expenditure of ATP.

Proerythroblast A red blood cell precursor.

Proprioception Sensory information from muscles, joints, skin and vestibular apparatus concerning body and limb position.

Propriospinal neurones Spinal cord interneurones which project to different segmental levels of the cord, thereby connecting neurones in different spinal levels.

Pulmonary circulation The blood vessels supplying the lungs.

Pulmonary fibrosis Thickening of the connective tissue of the alveolar walls, causing decreased compliance and an increased diffusion distance for respiratory gases.

Purkinje cells Nerve cells located in the cerebellar cortex which give rise to the only output from the cerebellar cortex to the deep cerebellar nuclei.

Purkinje fibres Conducting fibres found within the ventricles of the heart (see Bundle of His).

Pyramidal cells Cells of the cerebral cortex. The axons of these cells form the main output of the cerebral cortex.

Pyramidal decussation The region in the medulla where the axons of the corticospinal tracts cross the midline.

Renshaw cells Small, inhibitory interneurones which are activated by alpha motoneurones and which have an inhibitory feedback onto the same pool of alpha motoneurones (recurrent inhibition).

Residual volume The volume of air left in the lungs after a maximum expiration.

Respiratory centre Portion of the medulla oblongata and pons responsible for the nervous and chemical control of respiration.

Respiratory quotient (RQ) A ratio defined as the amount of carbon dioxide produced by metabolism divided by the amount of oxygen consumed by metabolism. This can be calculated by measuring carbon dioxide and oxygen concentrations in expired air. The respiratory quotient also gives an indication of the fuel molecules which are being utilized in metabolism. An RQ of 1.0 indicates pure carbohydrate metabolism, since six molecules of carbon dioxide are produced and six molecules of oxygen used up for every molecule of glucose metabolized. A normal resting RQ would have a value of about 0.8, indicating a mixture of carbohydrate and fat metabolism.

Respiratory zone The portion of the lung tissue responsible for respiratory gas exchange.

Reticulin Connective tissue protein.

Rhabdomyolysis A pathological condition most common in race-horses but also in humans where there is an uncoupling of the energy production processes most likely because of an imbalance of ions within the mitochondria.

Ribosome Site of protein synthesis in the cell.

RNA Ribonucleic acid occurring inside cells that is involved in protein synthesis.

Sarcolemma Muscle plasma membrane.

Sarcomeres Repeating contractile units of actin and myosin filaments in striated muscle.

Sarcoplasm Muscle cytoplasm.

Sarcoplasmic reticulum Network of modified endoplasmic reticulum inside muscle cells concerned with the release and storage of calcium.

Schwann cells Connective tissue cells of the nervous system that produce and lay down the myelin sheath.

Sebum Lipid material that is produced by sebaceous glands.

Secondary active transport Carrier-mediated transport across the plasma membrane where substances are moved into the cell down their concentration gradient and where the gradient was generated by a primary active transport mechanism in some other part of the cell.

Simple epithelium A single layer of epithelial cells.

Sino-atrial node The pacemaker region of the heart muscle, located at the entrance of the vena cava to the right atrium.

Sliding filament theory A theory which describes contraction of muscle. The ratchet-like mechanism of actin and myosin ensures shortening of the muscle without shortening of the actin and myosin filaments.

Slow twitch muscle fibre A fibre within skeletal muscle which is slow contracting and has the biochemical attribute to contract for long periods.

Spasticity Increased muscle tone associated with disorders of the motor control systems, characterized by hypertonia and exaggerated reflexes.

Speed endurance Capacity to maintain speed in an environment of endurance factors.

Sphygmomanometer Device used in the measurement of arterial blood pressure, consisting of an inflatable cuff connected to a mercury manometer which measures the pressure inside the cuff. Electronic automated versions of this system are now commercially available.

Spinothalamic tract Sensory pathway of the spinal cord conveying pain and temperature information to the thalamus.

Spirometer Apparatus used to measure and record changes in lung volumes during normal and forced respiratory movements.

Spleen Large organ lying underneath the stomach which is involved in the storage of blood. This organ is also involved in the removal of expended red blood cells from the system. The spleen also has a role to play in immune function.

Spongy bone Type of bone with many large spaces in its structure resembling the structure of an aquatic sponge.

Stage training A type of circuit training whereby each repetition of an exercise is completed before progressing to the next exercise.

Stellate cells Small, star-shaped interneurones of the cerebral cortex.

Strength endurance Capacity to maintain the muscle's contractile force in an environment of endurance factors.

Stroke volume The volume of blood ejected by the ventricles during one heart beat.

Succinic dehydrogenase An enzyme within the tricarboxylic acid (Krebs) cycle which is commonly used as a marker of the aerobic potential of a tissue.

Superior vena cava The large vein which returns blood to the right atrium of the heart from the rest of the systemic circulation.

Surfactant A detergent substance produced by alveolar cells which reduces the alveolar surface tension.

Symporter A membrane carrier protein that can simultaneously transport several substances in the same direction.

Syringomyelia Disease in which cysts form in the central portion of the spinal cord.

Systemic circulation The blood vessels which supply all parts of the body except the lungs.

Systole The period of contraction and ejection during the cardiac cycle.

Tetanus The summative mechanical response of muscle to repeated action potentials at a frequency which is shorter than the twitch time.

Thalamus 'Inner chamber'. The main sensory relay station from the spinal cord to the cerebral cortex. Also involved in relaying motor information between the cortex and the basal ganglia.

Thermoreceptors Specialized sensory receptors for detecting heat and cold.

Thick filaments *see* Myosin

Thin filaments *see* Actin

Thrombocyte Platelet

Thymus gland Organ located in the neck which has a role in lymphocyte maturation and immune function.

Thyroxine Hormone produced by the endocrine thyroid gland.

Tidal volume The volume of air inspired and expired during a normal breath.

Total minute ventilation The total amount of air breathed in and out of the lungs in one minute. Calculated by multiplying tidal volume by the respiratory frequency (number of breaths per minute).

Total peripheral resistance The sum of resistances to flow in all of the peripheral blood vessels. This can be increased or decreased by contraction or relaxation of the smooth muscle in the arteriole walls.

Trabeculae Thin latticework of bone tissue in spongy bone.

Trachea The windpipe. The airway connecting the larynx to the primary bronchi.

Transverse tubules Invaginations of the sarcolemma that project deep into the muscle tissue, which help to transmit muscle action potentials.

Tropomyosin Small protein molecules that are attached to the actin filament which, during rest, block the site for attachment of the myosin heads.

Troponin A further small protein which is anchored to the actin filament and which attaches the tropomyosin.

Triacylglycerol A type of lipid or fat which is stored in tissues. It is composed of glycerol and three fatty acids. Also known as a triglyceride.

Tricarboxylic acid cycle *see* Krebs cycle.

Tunica adventitia The outer coat of the blood vessel wall.

Tunica intima The inner layer of the blood vessel wall.

Tunica media The middle layer of the blood vessel wall.

Twitch The mechanical response of muscle to a single action potential.

Type I muscle fibre A fibre within skeletal muscle which is slow contracting.

Type II muscle fibre A fibre within skeletal muscle which is fast contracting.

Unipolar neurone Type of neurone that has one axon and one dendrite emanating from the same area of the cell body.

Vasoconstriction Decreased diameter of the blood vessels as a result of smooth-muscle contraction in the vessel wall.

Vasodilation Increased diameter of the blood vessels as a result of smooth-muscle relaxation in the vessel wall.

Vein A blood vessel which transports blood back to the heart.

Ventilation:perfusion ratio The ratio of the total amount of ventilation to a lung unit divided by the total amount of blood flow to that lung unit. This ratio may also be applied to portions of the lung or to the whole lung.

Ventral horn The anterior portion of the spinal cord grey matter.

Ventricle One of the lower chambers of the heart.

Ventroposterolateral nucleus One of the thalamic nuclei responsible for relaying sensory information from the spinal cord to the sensory cortex.

Venule Small blood vessel which leads from the capillaries to the venous system.

Vesicle Small membrane-bound sac containing fluid.

Vital capacity The maximum volume of air which can be exhaled following a maximum inspiration.

Volkmann canals A canal through which blood vessels and nerves penetrate the bone from the periosteum.

White adipose tissue A tissue made of adipocytes which are cells that store fat. White adipose tissue mainly acts as a source of energy for metabolism.

White matter The portion of the central nervous system which surrounds the grey matter and which comprises the axons of the neurones which lie within the grey matter. Contains both the ascending and descending tracts of the spinal cord. The myelin sheaths of the axons give the white appearance.

Learning Objectives

By the end of the book the reader should understand:

Chapter 1

1. The structure of the plasma (cell) membrane.
2. The movement of materials across membranes by active and passive processes.
3. The structure and function of cell organelles.
4. The classification and general features of epithelial tissues.
5. The structure and function of exocrine and endocrine glands.
6. The general structure and function of connective tissues.
7. The general structure of bone and its maintenance.
8. The differences in structure between the three main types of muscle tissue.
9. The histological characteristics and functions of the nervous tissue cells.
10. The basic structure and functions of the skin.
11. The basic mechanisms of repair in different tissues.

Chapter 2

1. The pattern of distribution of ions across the nerve cell membrane.
2. The selective ionic permeability of the nerve cell membrane at rest, and the generation of the resting membrane potential.
3. The ionic basis of the action potential.
4. Refractory periods, and the importance of action potential frequency.
5. The principles of action potential propagation.
6. The structure and function of the synapse.
7. Spatial and temporal summation at synapses, and the effects of excitation and inhibition.
8. The basic organization of the brain, brainstem and spinal cord.
9. The structure and function of the autonomic nervous system.

Chapter 3

1. The basic structure and function of spinal reflex circuits.
2. The variety of sensory receptors and their functions.
3. The organization of the motor unit and the regulation of motor output.

4. The organization and functions of reflexes involving group Ia, Ib and II afferents.
5. The functions of interneurones in the spinal cord.
6. The anatomical organization and functions of descending pathways in the spinal cord.
7. The effects of spinal cord lesions on the descending pathways.
8. The anatomical organization and functions of ascending pathways in the spinal cord.
9. The effects of spinal cord lesions on the ascending pathways.
10. The involvement of the motor cortex in the control of movement.
11. The physiological features of spasticity.
12. The basic structure and function of basal ganglia.
13. The motor consequences of basal ganglia dysfunction.
14. The basic structure and function of the cerebellum.
15. The motor consequences of cerebellar dysfunction – cerebellar syndrome.

Chapter 4

1. The peripheral structures and afferent fibres responsible for the detection of noxious stimuli.
2. The central processing of nociceptive information.
3. Physiological mechanisms for pain management, and their application to physiotherapy practice.
4. The concepts of referred pain and phantom limb pain.

Chapter 5

1. The concepts of developmental, functional and adaptive plasticity.
2. The basic mechanisms underlying plastic changes in the nervous system.
3. Restoration of function following plastic changes in the injured nervous system and the role of physiotherapy in supporting this.

Chapter 6

1. The properties of skeletal muscle that allow it to carry out a variety of functions.
2. How skeletal muscle contracts.
3. The ways in which energy is made available to skeletal muscle.
4. The plasticity of skeletal muscle.
5. The process of aging in skeletal muscle.
6. The response of skeletal muscle to injury.
7. The mechanisms for assessing the strength of skeletal muscle.
8. Gender differences in skeletal muscle.
9. The aetiology of muscle soreness.
10. The principles of skeletal muscle regeneration.
11. The causes of fatigue in skeletal muscle.
12. The technology used to understand the intrinsic properties of skeletal muscle.

Chapter 7

1. The general organization of the cardiovascular system.

2. The volumes and composition of the different body fluid compartments.
3. The structure and function of the cellular components of blood.
4. The basis of the ABO blood groups.
5. The basis of blood coagulation and the role of platelets.
6. The general structure and function of the heart.
7. The general physiology of cardiac muscle cells.
8. The origin of the electrocardiogram.
9. The function of the sino-atrial pacemaker and the spread of excitation throughout the heart.
10. Extrinsic and intrinsic regulation of cardiac activity.
11. Starling's law of the heart and its application to cardiac function.
12. The pressure and volume changes in the left heart during the cardiac cycle.
13. The general structure and function of blood vessels.
14. The factors affecting blood pressure, and the measurement and control of blood pressure.
15. The factors governing fluid balance between the circulation and the interstitial spaces.
16. The control of regional blood flow.
17. The acute cardiovascular responses to exercise.
18. The effects of aging on the cardiovascular system.
19. The genesis of atherosclerosis and coronary heart disease.

Chapter 8

1. The general anatomical features of the lungs and respiratory tracts.

2. The general structure of the alveolus.
3. The physical factors that can affect lung function – lung mechanics, lung compliance and airway resistance.
4. The functional importance of the different lung volumes.
5. The general principles of lung function tests using spirometry and the effects of lung pathologies on these tests.
6. The general principles of gas exchange at the alveoli.
7. The gas composition of atmospheric air, alveolar air, arterial and venous blood.
8. The physiological basis of oxygen and carbon dioxide transport in the blood.
9. The role of haemoglobin in gas transport.
10. The chemical and nervous control of respiratory function.
11. The distribution of ventilation and blood flow throughout the lung and the general principles of ventilation–perfusion ratios.
12. The effects of obstructive lung diseases on ventilation–perfusion ratios.
13. The effects of restrictive diseases on respiratory function.
14. The use of oxygen therapy, and its effect on alveolar gas composition.
15. The use of mechanical ventilation techniques.
16. The acute responses of the respiratory system to exercise.
17. The effects of aging on the respiratory system.

Chapter 9

1. The rationale behind the adoption of an exercise programme throughout life.
2. The principles behind the design of an exercise programme for a variety of populations.

3. The nutritional requirements of an individual who is exercising regularly.

4. The principles involved in training for strength, speed and endurance.

5. The effect of chronic exercise on physiological systems.

6. The methods of assessing physiological parameters associated with exercise.

Index